Biostatistics

FOR

DUMMIES

A Wiley Brand

by John C. Pezzullo, PhD

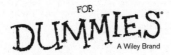

FOR

DUMMIES

A Wiley Brand

Biostatistics For Dummies®

Published by
John Wiley & Sons, Inc.
111 River St.
Hoboken, NJ 07030-5774
www.wiley.com

For general information on our other products and services, please contact our Customer Care Department within the U.S. at 877-762-2974, outside the U.S. at 317-572-3993, or fax 317-572-4002.

For technical support, please visit www.wiley.com/techsupport.

Wiley publishes in a variety of print and electronic formats and by print-on-demand. Some material included with standard print versions of this book may not be included in e-books or in print-on-demand. If this book refers to media such as a CD or DVD that is not included in the version you purchased, you may download this material at http://booksupport.wiley.com. For more information about Wiley products, visit www.wiley.com.

Library of Congress Control Number: 2013936422

ISBN 978-1-118-55398-5 (pbk); ISBN 978-1-118-55395-4 (ebk); ISBN 978-1-118-55396-1 (ebk); ISBN 978-1-118-55399-2 (ebk)

Manufactured in the United States of America

10 9 8 7 6 5 4 3 2

About the Author

John C. Pezzullo, PhD, is an adjunct associate professor at Georgetown University. He has had a half-century of experience supporting researchers in the physical, biological, and social sciences. For more than 25 years, he led a dual life at Rhode Island Hospital as an information technology programmer/analyst (and later director) while also providing statistical and other technical support to biological and clinical researchers at the hospital. He then joined the faculty at Georgetown University as informatics director of the National Institute of Child Health and Human Development's Perinatology Research Branch. He has held faculty appointments in the departments of obstetrics and gynecology, biomathematics and biostatistics, pharmacology, nursing, and internal medicine. He is now semi-retired and living in Florida, but he still teaches biostatistics and clinical trial design to Georgetown students over the Internet. He created the `StatPages.info` website, which provides online statistical calculating capability and other statistics-related resources.

Dedication

To my wife, Betty: Without your steadfast support and encouragement, I would never have been able to complete this book. To Mom and Dad, who made it all possible. And to our kids, our grandkids, and our great-grandkids!

Author's Acknowledgments

My heartfelt thanks to Matt Wagner of Fresh Books, Inc., and to Lindsay Lefevere for the opportunity to write this book; to Tonya Cupp, my special editor, who tutored me in the "Wiley ways" during the first quarter of the chapter-writing phase of the project; to Georgette Beatty, my project editor, who kept me on the path and on target (and mostly on time) throughout the process; to Christy Pingleton, the copy editor, for making sure what I said was intelligible; and to William Miller and Donatello Telesca, the technical reviewers, for making sure that what I said was correct.

Special thanks to Darrell Abernethy for his invaluable suggestions in Chapter 6.

And a special word of appreciation to all my family and friends, who provided so much support and encouragement throughout the whole project.

Publisher's Acknowledgments

We're proud of this book; please send us your comments at http://dummies.custhelp.com. For other comments, please contact our Customer Care Department within the U.S. at 877-762-2974, outside the U.S. at 317-572-3993, or fax 317-572-4002.

Some of the people who helped bring this book to market include the following:

Acquisitions, Editorial, and Vertical Websites

Senior Project Editor: Georgette Beatty

Executive Editor: Lindsay Sandman Lefevere

Copy Editor: Christine Pingleton

Assistant Editor: David Lutton

Editorial Program Coordinator: Joe Niesen

Technical Editors: Dr. William G. Miller, Donatello Telesca

Editorial Manager: Michelle Hacker

Editorial Assistant: Alexa Koschier

Cover Photo: Test tubes © Mike Kemp/ jupiterimages; Graph courtesy of John Pezzullo

Composition Services

Project Coordinator: Sheree Montgomery

Layout and Graphics: Carrie A. Cesavice

Proofreaders: Debbye Butler, John Greenough

Indexer: Ty Koontz

Special Help
Tonya Cupp, Sarah Faulkner, Todd Lothery, Danielle Voirol

Publishing and Editorial for Consumer Dummies

Kathleen Nebenhaus, Vice President and Executive Publisher

David Palmer, Associate Publisher

Kristin Ferguson-Wagstaffe, Product Development Director

Publishing for Technology Dummies

Andy Cummings, Vice President and Publisher

Composition Services

Debbie Stailey, Director of Composition Services

Contents at a Glance

Table of Contents

Introduction

· ·

*B*iostatistics is the practical application of statistical concepts and techniques to topics in biology. Because biology is such a broad field — studying all forms of life from viruses to trees to fleas to mice to people — biostatistics covers a very wide area, including designing biological experiments, safely conducting research on human beings, collecting and verifying data from those studies, summarizing and displaying that data, and analyzing the data to draw meaningful conclusions from it.

No book of reasonable size can hope to span all the subspecialties of biostatistics, including molecular biology, genetics, agricultural studies, animal research (in the lab and in the wild), clinical trials on humans, and epidemiological research. So I've concentrated on the most widely applicable topics and on the topics that are most relevant to research on humans (that is, *clinical* research). I chose these topics on the basis of a survey of graduate-level biostatistics curricula from major universities. I hope it covers most of the topics you're most interested in; but if it doesn't, please tell me what you wish I had included. You can e-mail me at `jcp12345@gmail.com`, and I'll try to respond to your message.

About This Book

I wrote this book as a reference — something you go to when you want information about a particular topic. So you don't have to read it from beginning to end; you can jump directly to the part you're interested in. In fact, I hope you'll be inclined to pick it up from time to time, open it to a page at random, read a page or two, and get a little something useful from it.

This book generally doesn't show you the detailed steps to perform every statistical calculation by hand. That may have been necessary in the mid-1900s, when statistics students spent hours in a "computing lab" (that is, a room that had an adding machine in it) calculating a correlation coefficient, but nowadays computers do all the computing. (See Chapter 4 for advice on choosing statistical software.) When describing statistical tests, my focus is always on the concepts behind the method, how to prepare your data for analysis, and how to interpret the results. I keep mathematical formulas and derivations to a minimum in this book; I include them only when they help explain what's going on. If you really want to see them, you can find them in many biostatistics textbooks, and they're readily available online.

Because good experimental design is crucial for the success of any research, this book gives special attention to the design of clinical trials and, specifically, to calculating the number of subjects you need to study. You find easy-to-apply examples of sample-size calculations in the chapters describing significance tests in Parts III, IV, and V and in Chapter 26.

Conventions Used in This Book

Here are some typographic conventions I use throughout this book:

- When I introduce a new term, I put the term in *italics* and define it. I also use italics occasionally to emphasize important information.

- In bulleted lists, I often place the most important word or phrase of each bulleted item in **boldface** text. The action parts of numbered steps are also boldface.

- I show web links (URLs) as `monotype` text.

- When this book was printed, some web addresses may have needed to break across two lines of text. If that happened, rest assured that I haven't put in any extra characters (like hyphens) to indicate the break. So, when using one of these web addresses, just type in exactly what you see in this book, pretending as though the line break doesn't exist.

- Whenever you see the abbreviation *sd* or *SD,* it always refers to the *standard deviation.*

- Anytime you see the word *significant* in reference to a p value, it means $p \leq 0.05$.

- When you see the lowercase italicized letter *e* in a formula, it refers to the mathematical constant 2.718..., which I describe in Chapter 2. (On the very rare occasions that it stands for something else, I say so.)

- I alternate between using male and female pronouns (instead of saying "he or she," "him or her," and so on) throughout the book. No gender preference is intended.

What You're Not to Read

Although I try to keep technical (that is, mathematical) details to a minimum, I do include them occasionally. The more complicated ones are marked by a Technical Stuff icon. You can skip over these paragraphs, and it won't prevent you from understanding the rest of the material. You can also skip over anything that's in a sidebar (text that resides in a box). Sidebars contain nonessential but interesting stuff, like historical trivia and other "asides."

Foolish Assumptions

I wrote this book to help several kinds of people, and I assume you fall into one of the following categories:

- ✔ Students at the undergraduate or graduate level who are taking a course in biostatistics and want help with the topics they're studying in class

- ✔ People who have had no formal biostatistical training (perhaps no statistical training at all) but find themselves having to deal with data from biological or clinical studies as part of their job

- ✔ Doctors, nurses, and other healthcare professionals who want to carry out clinical research

If you're interested in biostatistics, then you're no dummy. But I bet you sometimes *feel* like a dummy when it comes to biostatistics, or statistics in general, or mathematics. Don't feel bad — I've felt that way many times over the years, and still feel like that whenever I'm propelled into an area of biostatistics I haven't encountered before. (If you haven't taken a basic statistics course yet, you may want to get *Statistics For Dummies* by Deborah J. Rumsey, PhD — published by Wiley — and read parts of that book first.)

The important thing to keep in mind is that you don't have to be a math genius to be a good biological or clinical scientist — one who can intelligently design experiments, execute them well, collect and analyze data properly, and draw valid conclusions. You just have to have a good grasp of the basic concepts and know how to utilize the sophisticated statistical software that has become so widely available.

How This Book Is Organized

I've divided this book into six parts, and each part contains several chapters. The following sections describe what you find in each part.

Part I: Beginning with Biostatistics Basics

This part can be thought of as providing preparation and context for the remainder of this book. Here, I bring you up to speed on math and statistics concepts so that you're comfortable with them throughout this book. Then I provide advice on selecting statistical software. And finally I describe one major setting in which biostatistics is utilized — clinical research.

Part II: Getting Down and Dirty with Data

This part focuses on the raw material that biostatistical analysis works with — *data*. You probably already know the two main types of data: numerical (or quantitative) data, such as ages and heights, and non-numerical data, such as names and genders. Part II gets into the more subtle (but very important) distinctions between different data types.

You discover how to collect data properly, how to summarize it concisely and display it as tables and graphs, and how to describe the quality of the data (its precision and the uncertainties associated with your measured values). And you find out how the precision of your raw data affects the precision of other things you calculate from that data.

Part III: Comparing Groups

This part describes some of the most common statistical analyses you carry out on your data — comparing variables between groups. You discover how to answer questions like these: Does an arthritis medication reduce joint pain more than a placebo? Does a history of diabetes in a parent predict the likelihood of diabetes in the child? And if so, by how much?

You also find out how to show that there's *no meaningful difference* between two groups. Is a generic drug really equivalent to the name brand? Does a new drug *not* interfere with normal heart rhythm? This endeavor entails more than just not proving that there *is* a difference — absence of proof is not proof of absence, and there are special ways to prove that there's no important difference in your data.

Throughout this part, I discuss common statistical techniques for comparing groups such as t tests, ANOVAs, chi-square tests, and the Fisher Exact test.

Part IV: Looking for Relationships with Correlation and Regression

This part takes you through the very broad field of regression analysis — studying the relationships that can exist between variables. You find out how to test for a significant association between two or more variables and how to express that relationship in terms of a formula or equation that predicts the likely value of one variable from the observed values of one or more other variables. You see how useful such an equation can be, both for understanding the underlying science and for doing all kinds of practical things based on that relationship.

After reviewing the simple straight-line and multiple linear regression techniques you probably encountered in a basic stats course, you discover how to handle the more advanced problems that occur in the real world of biological research — *logistic regression* for analyzing yes-or-no kinds of outcomes, like "had a miscarriage"; *Poisson regression* for analyzing the frequency of recurring events, such as the number of hospitalizations for emphysema patients; and *nonlinear regression* when the relationship between the variables can take on a complicated mathematical form.

Part V: Analyzing Survival Data

This part is devoted to the analysis of one very special and important kind of data in biological research — *survival time* (or, more generally, the time to the first occurrence of some particular kind of event). You see what makes this type of data so special and why special methods are needed to deal with it correctly. You see how to calculate survival curves, test for a significant difference in survival between two or more groups of subjects, and apply the powerful and general methods of regression analysis to survival data.

Part VI: The Part of Tens

The final two chapters of this book provide "top-ten lists" of handy information and rules that you'll probably refer to often. Chapter 25 describes ten of the most common statistical distribution functions that you encounter in biostatistical research. Some of these distributions describe how your observed data values are likely to fluctuate, and some are used primarily in conjunction with the common significance tests (t-tests, chi-square tests, and ANOVAs). Chapter 26 contains a set of handy rules of thumb you can use to get quick estimates of the number of subjects you need to study in order to have a good chance of obtaining significant results.

Icons Used in This Book

Icons (the little drawings in the margins of this book) are used to draw your attention to certain kinds of material. Here's what they mean:

This icon signals something that's really worth keeping in mind. If you take away anything from this book, it should be the material marked with this icon.

I use this icon to flag things like derivations and computational formulas that you don't have to know or understand but that may give you a deeper insight into other material. Feel free to skip over any information with this icon.

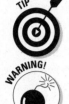

This icon refers to helpful hints, ideas, shortcuts, and rules of thumb that you can use to save time or make a task easier. It also highlights different ways of thinking about some topic or concept.

This icon alerts you to a topic that can be tricky or a concept that people often misunderstand.

Where to Go from Here

You're already off to a good start — you've read this introduction, so you have a good idea of what this book is all about (at least what the major parts of the book are all about). For an even better idea of what's in it, take a look at the Contents at a Glance — this drills down into each part, and shows you what each chapter is all about. Finally, skim through the full-blown table of contents, which drills further down into each chapter, showing you the sections and subsections of that chapter.

If you want to get the big picture of what biostatistics encompasses (at least those parts of biostatistics covered in this book), then read Chapter 1. This is a top-level overview of the basic concepts that make up this entire book. Here are a few other special places you may want to jump into:

- ✔ If you're uncomfortable with mathematical notation, then Chapter 2 is the place to start.
- ✔ If you want a quick refresher on basic statistics (the kind of stuff that would be taught in a Stats 101 course), then read Chapter 3.
- ✔ You can get an introduction to clinical research in Chapters 5 and 6.
- ✔ If you want to know about collecting, summarizing, and graphing data, jump to Part II.
- ✔ If you need to know about working with survival data, you can go right to Part V.
- ✔ If you're puzzled about some particular statistical distribution function, then look at Chapter 25.
- ✔ And if you need to do some quick sample-size estimates, turn to Chapter 26.

Part I
Beginning with Biostatistics Basics

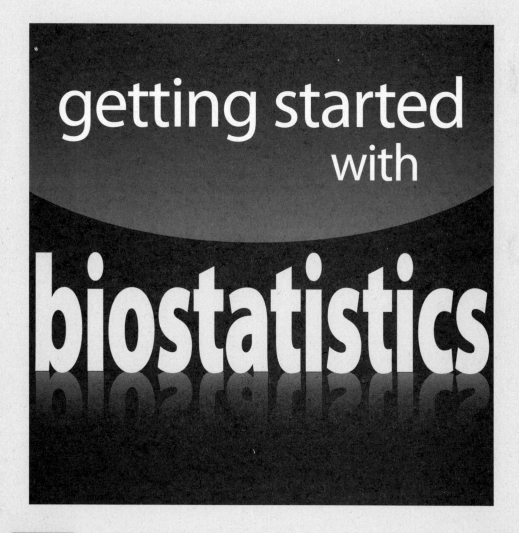

getting started with biostatistics

In this part . . .

✔ Get comfortable with mathematical notation that uses numbers, special constants, variables, and mathematical symbols — a must for all you mathophobes.

✔ Review basic statistical concepts — such as probability, randomness, populations, samples, statistical inference, and more — to get ready for the study of biostatistics.

✔ Choose and acquire statistical software (both commercial and free), and discover other ways to do statistical calculations, such as calculators, mobile devices, and web-based programs.

✔ Understand clinical research — how biostatistics influences the design and execution of clinical trials and how treatments are developed and approved.

Chapter 1

Biostatistics 101

· ·

In This Chapter

▶ Getting up to speed on the prerequisites for biostatistics

▶ Understanding the clinical research environment

▶ Surveying the special procedures used to analyze biological data

▶ Estimating how many subjects you need

▶ Working with distributions

· ·

*B*iostatistics deals with the design and execution of scientific experiments on living creatures, the acquisition and analysis of data from those experiments, and the interpretation and presentation of the results of those analyses.

This book is meant to be a useful and easy-to-understand companion to the more formal textbooks used in graduate-level biostatistics courses. Because most of these courses concentrate on the more clinical areas of biostatistics, this book focuses on that area as well. In this chapter, I introduce you to the fundamentals of biostatistics.

Brushing Up on Math and Stats Basics

Chapters 2 and 3 are designed to bring you up to speed on the basic math and statistical background that's needed to understand biostatistics and to give you some supplementary information (or "context") that you may find generally useful while you're reading the rest of this book.

✔ Many people feel unsure of themselves when it comes to understanding mathematical formulas and equations. Although this book contains fewer formulas than many other statistics books do, I do use them when they help illustrate a concept or describe a calculation that's simple enough to do by hand. But if you're a real mathophobe, you probably dread looking at *any* chapter that has a math expression anywhere in it. That's why

I include Chapter 2 — to show you how to read and understand the basic mathematical notation that I use in this book. I cover everything from basic mathematical operations to functions and beyond.

✔ If you're in a graduate-level biostatistics course, you've probably already taken one or two introductory statistics courses. But that may have been a while ago, and you may not feel too sure of your knowledge of the basic statistical concepts. Or you may have little or no formal statistical training, but now find yourself in a work situation where you interact with clinical researchers, participate in the design of research projects, or work with the results from biological research. If so, then you definitely want to read Chapter 3, which provides an overview of the fundamental concepts and terminology of statistics. There, you get the scoop on topics such as probability, randomness, populations, samples, statistical inference, accuracy, precision, hypothesis testing, nonparametric statistics, and simulation techniques.

Doing Calculations with the Greatest of Ease

This book generally doesn't have step-by-step instructions for performing statistical tests and analyses by hand. That's because in the 21st century you shouldn't be doing those calculations by hand; there are lots of ways to get a computer to do them for you. So this book describes calculations only to illustrate the concepts that are involved in the procedure, or when the calculations are simple enough that it's feasible to do them by hand (or even in your head!).

Unlike some statistics books that assume that you're using a specific software package (like SPSS, SAS, Minitab, and so on), this book makes no such assumption. You may be a student at a school that provides a commercial package at an attractive price or requires that you use a specific product (regardless of the price). Or you may be on your own, with limited financial resources, and the big programs may be out of your reach. Fortunately, you have several options. You can download some excellent free programs from the Internet. And you can also find a lot of web pages that perform specific statistical tests and procedures; collectively they can be thought of as the equivalence of a free online statistical software package. Chapter 4 describes some of these options — commercial products, free programs, web-based calculators, and others.

Concentrating on Clinical Research

This book covers topics that are applicable to all areas of biostatistics, concentrating on methods that are especially relevant to *clinical research* — studies involving people. If you're going to do research on human subjects, you'll want to check out two chapters that deal with clinical trials (and specifically drug development trials). These studies are among the most rigorously designed, closely regulated, expensive, and consequential of all types of scientific research — a mistake here can have disastrous human and financial consequences. So even if you don't expect to ever take part in drug development research, clinical trials (and the statistical issues they entail) are worth a close look.

Two chapters look at clinical research — one from the *inside,* and one from the *outside*.

- ✔ Chapter 5 describes the statistical aspects of clinical trials:

  - **Designing the study:** This aspect includes formulating goals, objectives, and hypotheses; estimating the required sample size; and composing the protocol.

  - **Executing the study:** During this phase, you're dealing with regulatory and subject protection groups, randomization and blinding, and collecting data.

  - **Analyzing the data from the study:** At this point, you're validating data, dealing with missing data and multiplicity, and handling interim analyses.

- ✔ Chapter 6 describes the whole drug development process, from the initial exploration of promising compounds to the final regulatory approval and the subsequent long-term monitoring of the safety of marketed products. It describes the different kinds of clinical trials that are carried out, in a logical progression, at different phases of the development process.

Many researchers have run into problems while analyzing their data because of decisions they made (or failed to make) while designing and executing their study. Many of these early errors arise from not understanding, or appreciating, the different kinds of data that their study can generate. Chapter 7 shows you how to recognize the kinds of data you encounter in biological research (numerical, categorical, and date- and time-oriented data), and how to collect and validate your data. Then in Chapter 8 you see how to summarize each type of data and display it graphically; your choices include bar charts, box-and-whiskers charts, and more.

Drawing Conclusions from Your Data

Most statistical analysis involves *inferring*, or drawing conclusions about the population at large, based on your observations of a small sample drawn from that population. The theory of *statistical inference* is often divided into two broad sub-theories — *estimation* theory and *decision* theory.

Statistical estimation theory

Chapters 9 and 10 deal with *statistical estimation theory*, which addresses the question of how accurately and precisely you can estimate some population parameter (like the mean blood hemoglobin concentration in all adult males, or the true correlation coefficient between body weight and blood pressure in all adult females) from the values you observe in your sample.

 ✔ In Chapter 9, you discover the difference between accuracy and precision (they're not synonymous!), and find out how to calculate the *standard error* (a measure of how precise, or imprecise, your observed value is) for the things you measure or count from your sample.

 ✔ In Chapter 10, you find out how to construct a *confidence interval* (the range that is likely to include the true population parameter) for anything you can measure or count.

But often the thing you measure (or count) isn't what you're really interested in. You may measure height and weight, but really be interested in body mass index, which is calculated from height and weight by a simple formula. If every number you acquire directly has some degree of imprecision, then anything you calculate from those numbers will also be imprecise, to a greater or lesser extent. Chapter 11 explains how random errors propagate through mathematical expressions and shows you how to calculate the standard error (and confidence interval) for anything you calculate from your raw data.

Statistical decision theory

Much of the rest of this book deals with *statistical decision theory* — how to decide whether some effect you've observed in your data (such as the difference in the average value of a variable between two groups or the association between two variables) reflects a real difference or association in the population or is merely the result of random fluctuations in your data or sampling.

Decision theory, as covered in this book, can also be divided into two broad sub-categories — comparing means and proportions between groups (in Part III), and understanding the relationship between two or more variables (in Part IV).

Comparing groups

In Part III, you meet (or get reacquainted with) some of the famous-name tests.

- ✔ In Chapter 12, you see how to compare *average values* between two or more groups by using t tests and ANOVAs, and their counterparts (Wilcoxon, Mann-Whitney, and Kruskal-Wallis tests) that can be used with skewed or other non-normally distributed data.

- ✔ Chapter 13 shows how to compare *proportions* (like cure rates) between two or more groups, using the chi-square and Fisher Exact tests on cross-tabulated data.

- ✔ Chapter 14 focuses on one specific kind of cross-tab — the *fourfold table* (having two rows and two columns). It turns out that you can get a lot of very useful information from a fourfold table, so it's worth a chapter of its own.

- ✔ In Chapter 15, you see how *event rates* (also called *person-time* data) can be estimated and compared between groups.

- ✔ Chapter 16 wraps up Part III with a description of a special kind of analysis that occurs often in biological research — *equivalence* and *non-inferiority* testing, where you try to show that two treatments or products aren't really different from each other or that one isn't any worse than the other.

Looking for relationships between variables

Science is, at its heart, the search for relationships, and regression analysis is the part of statistics that deals with the nature of relationships between different variables:

- ✔ You may want to know whether there's a *significant association* between two variables: Do smokers have a greater risk of developing liver cancer than nonsmokers, or is age associated with diastolic blood pressure?

- ✔ You may want to develop a formula for predicting the value of a variable from the observed values of one or more other variables: Can you predict the duration of a woman's labor if you know how far along the pregnancy is (the gestational age), how many other children she has had in the past (her *parity*), and how much the baby-to-be weighs (from ultrasound measurements)?

✔ You may be fitting a theoretical formula to some data in order to esti-mate one of the parameters appearing in that formula — like determin-ing how fast the kidneys can remove a drug from the body (a terminal elimination rate constant), from measurements of drug concentration in the blood at various times after taking a dose of the drug.

Regression analysis can handle all these tasks, and many more besides. Regression is so important in biological research that this book devotes Part IV to it. But most Stats 101 courses either omit regression analysis entirely or cover only the very simplest type — fitting a *straight line* to a set of points. Even second semester statistics courses may go only as far as *multivariate linear regression,* where you can have more than one predictor variable.

If you know nothing of correlation and regression analysis, read Chapter 17, which provides an introduction to these topics. I cover simple straight-line regression in Chapter 18; I extend that coverage to more than one predictor variable in Chapter 19. These three chapters deal with ordinary linear regres-sion, where you're trying to predict the value of a numerical outcome vari-able (like blood pressure or serum glucose) from one or more other variables (such as age, weight, and gender) by using a formula that's a simple summa-tion of terms, each of which consists of a predictor variable multiplied by a regression coefficient.

But in real-world biological and clinical research, you encounter more com-plicated relationships. Chapter 20 describes *logistic regression,* where the outcome is the occurrence or nonoccurrence of some kind of event, and you want to predict the probability that the event will occur. And you find out about several other kinds of regression in Chapter 21:

✔ *Poisson regression,* where the outcome can be the number of events that occur in an interval of time

✔ *Nonlinear least-squares regression,* where the relationship can be more complicated than a simple summation of terms in a linear model

✔ *LOWESS curve-fitting,* where you may have no explicit formula at all that describes the data

A Matter of Life and Death: Working with Survival Data

Sooner or later, all living things die. And in biological research, it becomes very important to characterize that sooner-or-later part as accurately as possible. But this characterization can get tricky. It's not enough to say that people live an average of 5.3 years after acquiring a certain disease. Does everyone tend to last five or six years, or do half the people die within the first few months, and the other half survive ten years or more? And how do you analyze your data when some subjects may far outlive your clinical study (that is, they're still alive when you have to finish your study and write up the results)? And how do you analyze people who skip town after a few months, so you don't know whether they lived or died after that?

The existence of problems like these led to the development of a special set of techniques specifically designed to deal with survival data. More generally, they also apply to the time of the first occurrence of other (non-death) events as well, like remission or recurrence of cancers, heart attacks, strokes, and first bowel movement after abdominal surgery. These techniques, which span the whole data analysis process, are all collected in Part V.

To discover how to acquire survival data properly (it's not as obvious as you may think), read Chapter 22, where I also show how to summarize and graph survival data, and how to estimate such things as mean and median survival time and percent survival to specified time points. A special statistical test for comparing survival among groups of subjects is covered in Chapter 23. And in Chapter 24, I describe Cox proportional-hazards regression — a special kind of regression analysis for survival data.

Figuring Out How Many Subjects You Need

Of all the statistical challenges a researcher may encounter, none seems to instill as much apprehension and insecurity as calculating the number of subjects needed to provide a sufficiently powered study — one that provides a high probability of yielding a statistically significant result if the hoped-for effect is truly present in the population.

Because sample-size estimation is such an important part of the design of any research project, this book shows you how to make those estimates for the situations you're likely to encounter when doing clinical research. As I describe each statistical test in Parts III, IV, and V, I explain how to estimate the number of subjects needed to provide sufficient power for that test. In addition, Chapter 26 describes ten simple rules for getting a "quick and dirty" estimate of the required sample size.

Getting to Know Statistical Distributions

What statistics book would be complete without a set of tables? Back in the not-so-good old days, when people had to do statistical calculations by hand, they needed tables of the common statistical distributions (Normal, Student t, chi-square, Fisher F, and so on) in order to complete the calculation of the significance test. But now the computer does all this for you, including calculating the exact p value, so these tables aren't nearly as necessary as they once were.

But you should still be familiar with the common statistical distributions that describe how your observations may fluctuate or that may come up in the course of performing a statistical calculation. So Chapter 25 contains a list of the most well-known distribution functions, with explanations of where you can expect to encounter those distributions, what they look like, what some of their more interesting properties are, and how they're related to other distributions. Some of them are accompanied by a small table of critical values, corresponding to significance at the 5 percent level (that is, $p = 0.05$).

Chapter 2

Overcoming Mathophobia: Reading and Understanding Mathematical Expressions

*F*ace it: Most people fear math, and statistics is — to a large extent — mathematical. I want to show you how to read mathematical *expressions* (which are combinations of numbers, letters, math operations, punctuation, and grouping symbols), *equations* (which connect two expressions with an equal sign), and *formulas* (which are equations that tell you how to calculate something), so you can understand what's in a statistics book or article. I also explain how to write formulas, so you can tell a computer how to manipulate your data.

In this chapter, I just use the term *formula* for simplicity to refer to formulas, equations, and expressions.

I show you how to interpret the kinds of mathematical formulas you encounter throughout this book. I don't spend too much time explaining what the more complicated mathematical operations mean; I concentrate on how those operations are indicated in formulas. If you're not sure about the algebra, you can find an excellent treatment of that in *Algebra I For Dummies,* 2nd Edition, and *Algebra II For Dummies;* both titles are written by Mary Jane Sterling and published by Wiley.

Breaking Down the Basics of Mathematical Formulas

For the purposes of this book, you can think of a mathematical formula as a shorthand way to describe how to do a certain calculation. Formulas can have numbers, special constants, and variables, interspersed with various symbols for mathematical operations, punctuation, and typographic effects. They're constructed using rules that have evolved over several centuries and which have been become more or less standardized. The following sections explain two different kinds of formulas (typeset and plain text) that you encounter in this book and describe two of the building blocks (constants and variables) from which formulas are created.

Displaying formulas in different ways

Formulas can be expressed *in print* two ways:

- **A typeset format** utilizes special symbols spread out in a two-dimensional structure, like this:

$$SD = \sqrt{\frac{\sum_{i=1}^{n}(x_i - m)^2}{n-1}}$$

- **A plain text format** strings the formula out as a single, long line, which is helpful if you're limited to the characters on a keyboard:

$$SD = \text{sqrt}(\text{sum}((x[i] - m)^{\wedge}2, i, 1, n)/(n - 1))$$

You must know how to read both types of formula displays — typeset and plain text. The examples in this chapter show both styles.

You may never have to construct a professional-looking typeset formula (unless you're writing a book, like I'm doing right now), but you'll almost certainly have to write plain text formulas as part of organizing, preparing, editing, and analyzing your data.

Checking out the building blocks of formulas

No matter how they're written, formulas are just concise "recipes" that tell you how to calculate something or how something is defined. You just have to know how to read the recipe. To start, look at the building blocks from which formulas are constructed: *constants* (whose values never change) and *variables* (names that stand for quantities that can take on different values at different times).

Constants

Constants can be represented *explicitly* (using the numerals 0–9, with or without a decimal point) or *symbolically* (using a letter in the Greek or Roman alphabet to stand for a value that's especially important in mathematics, physics, or some other discipline). For example:

✔ The Greek letter π (spelled *pi* and pronounced *pie*) almost always represents 3.14159 (plus a zillion more digits), which is the ratio of the circumference of any circle to its diameter.

✔ The strange number 2.71828 (plus a zillion more digits) is called *e* (usually italicized). Later in this chapter, I describe one way *e* is used; you see *e* in statistical formulas throughout this book and in almost every other mathematical and statistical textbook. Whenever you see an italicized *e* in this book, it refers to the number 2.718 unless I explicitly say otherwise.

The official mathematical definition of *e* is the value that the expression $(1+1/n)^n$ approaches as *n* gets larger and larger (approaching infinity). Unlike π, *e* has no simple geometrical interpretation, but one (somewhat far-fetched) example of where *e* pops up is this: Assume you put exactly one dollar in a bank account that's paying 100 percent annual interest, compounded continuously. After exactly one year, your account will have *e* dollars in it. The interest on your original dollar, plus the interest on the interest, would be about $1.72 (to the nearest penny), for a total of $2.72 in your account. Start saving for that summer home!

Mathematicians and scientists use lots of other special Greek and Roman letters as symbols for special numerical constants, but you need only a few of them in your biostatistics work. Pi and *e* are the most common; I define others as they come up.

Variables

The term *variable* has several slightly different meanings in different fields:

✔ **In mathematics and the sciences,** a variable is a symbol (usually a letter of the alphabet) that represents some quantity in a formula. You see variables like x and y in algebra, for example.

✔ **In computer science,** a variable is a name (usually made up of one or more letters (and perhaps also numeric digits) that refers to a place in the computer's memory where one or more numbers (or other kinds of data) can be stored and manipulated. For example, a computer programmer writing a statistical software program may use a variable called *SumXY* to stand for a quantity that's used in the computation of a correlation coefficient.

✔ **In statistics,** a variable is the data element you collect (by counting, measuring, or calculating) and store in a file for analysis. This data doesn't have to be numerical; it can also be categorical or textual. So the variables *Name*, *ID*, *Gender*, *Birthdate*, and *Weight* refer to the data that you acquire on subjects.

Variables names may be written in uppercase or lowercase letters, depending on typographic conventions or preferences, or on the requirements of the software being used.

In typeset format formulas, variables are always italicized; in plain text formulas, they're not.

Focusing on Operations Found in Formulas

A formula tells you how building blocks (numbers, special constants, and variables) are to be combined — that is, what calculations you're supposed to carry out on these quantities. But things can get confusing. One symbol (like the minus sign) can indicate different things, depending on how it's used, and one mathematical operation (like multiplication) can be represented in different ways. The following sections explain the basic mathematical operations you see in formulas throughout this book, show how complicated formulas can be built from combinations of basic operations, and describe two types of equations you'll encounter in statistical books and articles.

Basic mathematical operations

The four basic mathematical operations are addition, subtraction, multiplication, and division (ah, yes — the basics you learned in elementary school). Different symbols indicate these operations, as you discover in the following sections.

Addition and subtraction

Addition and subtraction are always indicated by the + and – symbols, respectively, placed between two numbers or variables. The minus sign has some other tricks up its sleeve, though:

✔ **A minus sign immediately in front of a number** means a negative quantity. For example, –5 could indicate five degrees below 0 or a weight loss of 5 kilograms.

✔ **A minus sign in front of a variable** tells you to reverse the sign of the value of the variable. Therefore, –*x* means that if *x* is positive, you should now make it negative; but if *x* is negative, make it positive. Used this way, the minus sign is referred to as a *unary* operator, because it's acting on only one variable.

Multiplication

Multiplication is indicated in several ways, as shown in Table 2-1.

Table 2-1	Multiplication Options	
What It Is	*Example*	*Where It's Used*
Asterisk	2 * 5	Plain text formulas, but almost never in typeset formulas
Cross	2×5	Typeset formula, between two variables or two constants being multiplied together
Raised dot	$2 \cdot 5$	Typeset formula
Something immediately in front of a parenthesized expression	2(5 + 3) = 16	Typeset formula
Brackets and curly braces	2[6 + (5 + 3)/2] = 20	Typeset formula containing "nested" parentheses
Two or more terms running together	$2\pi r$ (versus $2 \times \pi \times r$)	In typeset formulas only

You can't run terms together to imply multiplication just anytime. For example, you can't replace 5×3 with 53 because 53 is an actual number itself. And you shouldn't replace length × width with *lengthwidth* because people may think you're referring to a single variable named *lengthwidth*. Run terms together to imply multiplication *only* when it's perfectly clear from the context of the formula that the authors are using only single-letter variable names and that they're describing calculations where it makes sense to multiply those variables together.

Division

Like multiplication, division is indicated in several ways:

- ✔ **A slash** (/) in plain text formulas
- ✔ **A division symbol** (÷) in typeset formulas
- ✔ **A long horizontal bar** in typeset formulas:

$$\frac{Distance}{Time}$$

Powers, roots, and logarithms

The next three mathematical operations — working with powers, roots, and logarithms — are all related to the idea of repeated multiplication.

Raising to a power

Raising to a power is a shorthand way to indicate repeated multiplication. You indicate raising to a power by

- ✔ Superscripting in typographic formulas, such as 5^3
- ✔ ** in plain text formulas, such as 5**3
- ✔ ^ in plain text formulas, such as 5^3

All the preceding expressions are read as "five to the third power," or "five cubed," and tell you to multiply three fives together: $5 \times 5 \times 5$, which gives you 125.

These statements about powers are true, too:

- ✔ **A power doesn't have to be a whole number.** You can raise a number to a fractional power. You can't visualize this in terms of repeated multiplications, but your scientific calculator can show you that $2.6^{3.8}$ is equal to approximately 37.748.
- ✔ **A power can be negative.** A negative power indicates the reciprocal of the quantity: x^{-1} really means $1/x$, and, in general, x^{-n} is the same as $1/x^n$.

Remember that constant e (2.718...) described in the earlier section "Numbers and special constants"? Almost every time you see e used in a formula, it's being raised to some power. It's almost as if e were born to be raised to powers. It's so common that raising e to a power (that is, to some exponent) is called *exponentiating,* and another way of representing e^x in plain text is exp(x). And x doesn't have to be a whole number: Using any scientific calculator or spreadsheet, you can show that exp(1.6) equals 4.953 (approximately). You see much more of this in other chapters, for example, Chapters 20 and 25.

Taking a root

Taking a root involves asking the power question backwards: "What base number, when raised to a certain power, gives some specific number?" For example, "What number, when squared, gives 100?" Well, 10×10, or 10^2, gives 100, so the square root of 100 is 10. Similarly, the cube root of 1,000,000 is 100 because $100 \times 100 \times 100$, or 100^3, is a million.

Root-taking is indicated by a *radical sign* ($\sqrt{}$) in a typeset formula, where the entire thing to be square-rooted is located "under the roof" of the radical sign, as shown here: $\sqrt{25}$. You indicate other roots by putting a number in the notch of the radical sign. For example, because 2^8 is 256, the eighth root of 256, or $\sqrt[8]{256}$, is 2. You also can indicate root-taking by using the fact (from algebra) that $\sqrt[n]{x}$ is equal to $x^{1/n}$, or as $x^{\wedge}(1/n)$ in plain text.

Looking at logarithms

In addition to root-taking, another way of asking the power question backwards is "What exponent (or power) must I raise a certain base number to in order to get some specified number?" For root-taking, you specified the power and asked for the base. With logarithms, you specify the base and ask for the power (or exponent).

For example, "What power must I raise 10 to in order to get 1,000?" The answer is 3 because $10^3 = 1,000$. You can say that 3 is the *logarithm* of 1,000 (for the base 10), or, in mathematical terms: $\text{Log}_{10}(1,000) = 3$. Similarly, because $2^8 = 256$, you say that $\text{Log}_2(256) = 8$. And because $e^{1.6} = 4.953$, then $\text{Log}_e(4.953) = 1.6$.

There can be logarithms to any base, but three bases occur frequently enough to have their own nicknames:

- ✔ Base-10 logarithms are called *common logarithms.*
- ✔ Base-*e* logarithms are called *natural logarithms.*
- ✔ Base-2 logarithms are called *binary logarithms.*

The logarithmic function naming is inconsistent among different authors, publishers, and software writers. Sometimes *Log* means natural logarithm, and sometimes it means common logarithm. Often *Ln* is used for natural logarithm, and *Log* is used for common logarithm. Names like *Log10* and *Log2* may also be used to identify the base.

The most common kind of logarithm used in this book is the natural logarithm, so in this book I always use *Log* to indicate natural (base-*e*) logarithms. When I want to refer to common logarithms, I use Log_{10}, and when referring to binary logarithms, I use Log_2.

An *antilogarithm* (usually shortened to *antilog*) is the inverse of a logarithm — if *y* is the log of *x,* then *x* is the antilog of *y.* For example, the base-10 logarithm of 1,000 is 3, so the base-10 antilog of 3 is 1,000.

Calculating an antilog is exactly the same as raising the base to the power of the logarithm. That is, the base-10 antilog of 3 is the same as 10 raised to the power of 3 (which is 10^3, or 1,000). Similarly, the natural antilog of any number is just *e* (2.718) raised to the power of that number: The natural antilog of 5 is e^5, or 148.41, approximately.

Factorials and absolute values

Most mathematical operators are written *between* the two numbers they operate on, or *before* the number if it operates on only one number (like the minus sign used as a unary operator). But factorials and absolute values are two mathematical operators that appear in typeset expressions in peculiar ways.

Factorials

Lots of statistical formulas contain exclamation points. An exclamation point doesn't mean that you should sound excited when you read the formula aloud. An exclamation mark (!) *after* a number is shorthand for calculating that number's *factorial.* To find a number's factorial, you write all the whole numbers from 1 to that number and then multiply them all together. For example, 5! (read as "five factorial") is shorthand for $1 \times 2 \times 3 \times 4 \times 5$, which you can work out on your calculator to get the value 120.

Even though standard keyboards have a ! key, most computer programs and spreadsheets don't let you use ! to indicate factorials; you may have to write 5!, for example, as FACT(5), Factorial(5), or something similar.

Here are a few factorials fun facts:

✔ They grow very fast: You can calculate that 10! is 3,628,800. And 170! is about 7.3×10^{306}, which is close to the largest numbers many computers can deal with.

✔ 0! isn't 0, but is actually 1 (the same as 1!). That may not make any sense, but that's how it is, so burn it into your memory.

✔ The definition of *factorial* can be extended to fractions and even to negative numbers. You don't have to deal with those kinds of factorials in this book.

Absolute values

The *absolute value* is just the value of the number without any minus sign (if it was negative in the first place). Indicate absolute value by placing vertical bars immediately to the left and right of the number. So |5.7| is 5.7, and |–5.7| is also 5.7. Even though most keyboards have the | symbol, the absolute value is usually indicated in plain text formulas as abs(5.7).

Functions

In this book, a *function* is a set of calculations that take one or more numeric values (called *arguments*) and produce a numeric result. A function is indicated in a formula (typeset or plain text) by the name of the function, followed by a set of parentheses that contain the argument or arguments. Here's an example: sqrt(x) indicates the square root of x.

The common functions have been given (more or less) standard names. The preceding sections in this chapter give some: sqrt, exp, log, ln, fact, and abs. The common trigonometric functions are sin, cos, tan, and their inverses: asin, acos, and atan. Statistics makes use of many specialized functions, like FisherF(F, $n1$, $n2$), which calculates the value of the integral of the Fisher F distribution function at a particular value of F, with $n1$ and $n2$ degrees of freedom (see Chapter 25 for some of these probability distribution functions).

When writing formulas using functions, keep in mind that some software is case-sensitive and may require all caps, all lowercase, or first-letter capitalization; other software may not care. Check the documentation of the software you're working with.

Simple and complicated formulas

Simple formulas have one or two numbers and only one mathematical operator (for example, 5 + 3). But most of the formulas you'll encounter are more complicated, with two or more operators.

You need to know the order in which to do calculations, because using different sequences produces different results. Generally, the order in which you evaluate the various operations appearing in a complicated formula is governed by the interplay of several rules, arranged in a hierarchy. Most computer programs try to follow the customary conventions that apply to typeset formulas, but some programs differ; check the software's documentation.

Here's a typical set of operator hierarchy rules. Within each hierarchical level, operations are carried out from left to right:

1. **Evaluate anything within parentheses (or brackets or curly braces or absolute-value bars) first.**

   This includes the parentheses that follow the name of a function.

2. **In a typeset fraction, evaluate the numerator (everything above the horizontal bar) and the denominator (everything below the bar); then divide the numerator by the denominator.**

3. **Evaluate negation, factorials, powers, and roots.**

4. **Evaluate multiplication and division.**

5. **Evaluate addition and subtraction.**

Equations

An *equation* has two expressions with an equal sign between them. Most equations appearing in this book have a single variable name to the left of the equal sign and a formula to the right, like this: $SEM = SD/\sqrt{N}$. This kind of equation defines the variable appearing on the left in terms of the calculations specified on the right. In doing so, it also provides the "cookbook" instructions for calculating (in this case) the *SEM* for any values of *SD* and *N*.

Another type of equation appears in algebra, asserting that the terms on the left side of the equation are equal to the terms on the right. For example, the equation $x + 2 = 3x$ asserts that x is a number that, when added to 2, produces a number that's 3 times as large as the original x. Algebra teaches you how to solve this expression for x, and it turns out that the answer is $x = 1$.

Counting on Collections of Numbers

A variable can refer to one value or to a collection of values, which are generally called *arrays*. Arrays can come with one or more dimensions, which you can think of as rows, columns, and slices.

One-dimensional arrays

A one-dimensional array can be thought of as a simple list of values. For instance, you might record the fasting glucose values (in milligrams per deciliter, mg/dL) of five subjects as 86, 110, 95, 125, and 64, and use the variable name "Gluc" to refer to this collection of five numbers. Gluc is an array of numbers, and each of the five individual glucose values in the collection is an *element* of the Gluc array. The variable name Gluc in a formula refers to the whole collection of numbers (five numbers, in this example).

You can refer to one particular element (that is, to the glucose value of one particular subject) of this array several ways. The number that indicates which element of the array you're referring to is called the *index* of the array.

- ✔ In a typeset formula, indexing is usually indicated by subscripts. For example, $Gluc_3$ refers to the third number in the collection (in this example, 95).

- ✔ In a plain text formula, indexing is usually indicated by brackets, for example, Gluc[3].

The index can be a variable. In that case, Gluc[i] would refer to the ith element of the array. The variable i would, presumably, have some value between 1 and the number of elements in the array (in this example, between 1 and 5).

In some programming languages, the indices start at 0 for the first element, 1 for the second element, and so on, but that can be confusing. In this book, all arrays are indexed starting at 1. But be aware that other books and articles may use an index-0 scheme.

Higher-dimensional arrays

Two-dimensional arrays can be thought of as describing tables of values, with rows and columns (like a block of cells in a spreadsheet), and even higher-dimensional arrays can be thought of as describing a whole collection of tables. Suppose you measure the fasting glucose on five subjects on each of three treatment days. You could think of your 15 measurements being laid out in a 5-x-3 table (five subjects by three days). If you want to represent this entire table with a single variable name like Gluc, you can use *double-indexing*, with the first index specifying the subject (1 through 5) and the second index specifying the day of the measurement (1 through 3). Under that system, Gluc[3,2] indicates the fasting glucose for subject 3 on day 2. And Gluc[i,j] indicates the fasting glucose for the ith subject on the jth day.

Special terms are sometimes used to refer to arrays with one or two dimensions:

- ✔ A one-dimensional array is sometimes called a *vector*. But this can be confusing, because the word *vector* is also used in mathematics, physics, and biology to refer to completely different things.

✔ A two-dimensional array is sometimes called a *matrix* (plural: *matrices*). But this term is usually reserved for two-dimensional arrays of numbers that are going to be manipulated by a special set of mathematical rules called *matrix algebra.* Mathematical descriptions of multiple regression make extensive use of matrix algebra.

Arrays in formulas

If you see an array name in a formula without any subscripts, it usually means you have to evaluate the formula for each element of the array, and the result will be an array with the same number of elements. So, if Gluc refers to the array with the five values 86, 110, 95, 125, and 64, then the expression $2 \times$ Gluc will result in an array with these five values: 172, 220, 190, 250, and 128.

When an array name appears in a formula with subscripts, the meaning depends on the context. It can indicate that the formula is to be evaluated only for some elements of the array, or it can mean that the elements of the array are to be combined in some way before being used (as I describe in the next section).

Sums and products of the elements of an array

This symbol strikes terror into the hearts of so many people who read statistics books and articles: the diabolical Σ (and its less common but even scarier cousin, Π). These symbols are simply two uppercase Greek letters — *sigma* and *pi* — that correspond to the Roman letters S and P, respectively, which stand for *Sum* and *Product.* These symbols are almost always used in front of variables and expressions that represent arrays.

When you see Σ in a formula, just think of it as "add them up." Assuming an array of five numbers (86, 110, 95, 125, and 64) with the name Gluc, you can read the expression $\sum Gluc$ as "the sum of the Gluc array," and simply add all five elements to get $86 + 110 + 95 + 125 + 64$, which equals 480.

Sometimes the Σ notation is in a slightly more complicated form, where the index variable i is displayed under (or to the right of) the sigma and as a subscript of the array name. Read the expression $\sum_i Gluc_i$ as "the sum of the

Gluc array over all values of the index *i*," which produces the same result (480) as the simpler, "naked" sigma. The "subscripted sigma" form is more useful with multidimensional arrays, when you may want to sum over only one of the dimensions. For example, if Ai,j is a two-dimensional array:

10 15 33
25   8   1

then $\sum_i A_{i,j}$ means that you should sum over the *rows* (the *i* subscript) to get the one-dimensional array: 35, 23, and 34. And $\sum_j A_{i,j}$ means to sum across the *columns* (*j*) to get the one-dimensional array: 58, 34.

Finally, you may see the full-blown official mathematical sigma in all its glory, like this:

$$\sum_{i=a}^{b} Gluc_i,$$

which reads "the sum of the Gluc array, over values of the index *i* going from *a* to *b*, inclusive." So if *a* was equal to 1, and *b* was equal to 5, the expression would become:

$$\sum_{i=1}^{5} Gluc_i,$$

which, once again, would say to add up all five elements of the Gluc array (giving you a total of 480 again). But if you wanted to omit the first and last values of the array from the sum, you could have:

$$\sum_{i=2}^{4} Gluc_i,$$

which would say to add up only Gluc2 + Gluc3 + Gluc4, to get 110 + 95 + 125, which would add up to 330.

$$\sum_{i=2}^{4} Gluc_i = Gluc_2 + Gluc_3 + Gluc_4 = 110 + 95 + 125 = 330$$

The pi symbol (Π) works just like Σ, except that you multiply instead of add:

$$\prod_i Gluc = \prod Gluc_i = \prod_{i=1}^{5} Gluc_i = 86 \times 110 \times 95 \times 125 \times 64 = 7{,}189{,}600{,}000$$

Scientific notation: The easy way to work with really big and really small numbers

Statistical analysis sometimes generates very large or very small numbers, but humans are most comfortable working with numbers that are between 1 and 100 (or maybe 1 and 1,000). Numbers much smaller than 1 (like 0.0000000000005) or much larger than 1,000 (like 5,000,000,000,000) make most humans nervous. Working with them (the numbers, not the humans) is difficult and error-prone.

Fortunately, there's *scientific notation* — a nifty way to represent very small or very large numbers. If you see a number like 1.23×10^7 or 1.23E7, or 1.23e+7, it simply means "take the number 1.23, and then slide the decimal point seven spaces to the *right* (adding zeros as needed)." In this case, take 1.23 and think of it as having a lot of extra decimal places with zeros, like 1.2300000000. Then slide the decimal seven places to the right to get 12300000.000 and clean it up to get 12,300,000.

For very small numbers, the number after the e is negative, indicating that you need to slide the decimal point to the *left*. For example, 1.23e−9 is the scientific notation for 0.00000000123.

Note: Don't be misled by the "e" that appears in scientific notation — it doesn't stand for the 2.718 constant. You should read it as "times ten raised to the power of."

Check out *Algebra I For Dummies* by Mary Jane Sterling (published by Wiley) to see other advantages to using scientific notation.

Chapter 3

Getting Statistical: A Short Review of Basic Statistics

This chapter provides a brief overview of some basic concepts that are often taught in a one-semester introductory statistics course. They form a conceptual framework for topics that I cover in more depth throughout this book. Here, you get the scoop on probability, randomness, populations, samples, statistical inference, hypothesis testing, and nonparametric statistics.

Note: I can only summarize the concepts here; they're covered in much more depth in *Statistics For Dummies,* 2nd Edition, and *Statistics II For Dummies,* both written by Deborah J. Rumsey, PhD, and published by Wiley. So you may want to skim through this chapter to get an idea of what topics you're already comfortable with and which ones you need to brush up on.

Taking a Chance on Probability

Defining *probability* without using some word that means the same (or nearly the same) thing can be hard. Probability is the degree of certainty, the chance, or the likelihood that something will happen. Of course, if you then try to define *chance* or *likelihood* or *certainty,* you may wind up using the word *probability* in the definition.

Don't worry; I clear up the basics of probability in the following sections. I explain how to define probability as a number, provide a few simple rules of probability, and compare probability to odds (these two terms are related but not the same thing).

Thinking of probability as a number

Probability describes the relative frequency of the occurrence of an event (like getting heads on a coin flip or drawing the ace of spades from a deck of cards). Probability is a number between 0 and 1, although in casual conversation, you often see probabilities expressed as percentages, often followed by the word *chance* instead of *probability*. For example: If the probability of rain is 0.7, you may hear someone say that there's a 70 percent chance of rain.

Probabilities are numbers between 0 and 1 that can be interpreted this way:

- ✔ **A probability of 0** means that the event definitely won't occur.
- ✔ **A probability of 1** (or 100 percent) means that the event definitely will occur.
- ✔ **A probability between 0 and 1** (like 0.7) means that the event will occur some part of the time (like 70 percent) in the long run.

The probability of one particular thing happening out of N equally likely things that could happen is $1/N$. So with a deck of 52 different cards, the probability of drawing any one specific card (like the ace of spades) is 1/52.

Following a few basic rules

Here are three basic rules, or formulas, of probabilities — I call them the *not rule,* the *and rule,* and the *or rule.* In the formulas that follow, I use *Prob* as an abbreviation for *probability,* expressed as a fraction (between 0 and 1).

Don't use percentage numbers (0 to 100) in probability formulas.

Most of the mathematical underpinning of statistics is based on the careful application of the following basic rules to ever more complicated situations:

- ✔ **The not rule:** The probability of some event X *not* happening is 1 minus the probability of X happening:

    $$\text{Prob}(\text{not } X) = 1 - \text{Prob}(X)$$

    So if the probability of rain tomorrow is 0.7, then the probability of no rain tomorrow is $1 - 0.7$, or 0.3.

- ✔ **The and rule:** For two independent events, X and Y, the probability of event X *and* event Y both happening is equal to the product of the probability of each of the two events:

    $$\text{Prob}(X \text{ and } Y) = \text{Prob}(X) \times \text{Prob}(Y)$$

So, if you flip a fair coin and then draw a card from a deck, what's the probability of getting heads on the coin flip *and* then drawing the ace of spades? The probability of getting heads in a fair coin flip is 1/2, and the probability of drawing the ace of spades from a deck of cards is 1/52, so the probability of having both of these things happen is (1/2)(1/52), or 1/104, or 0.0096 (approximately).

✔ **The or rule:** For two independent events, X and Y, the probability of one or the other or both events happening is given by a more complicated formula, which can be derived from the preceding two rules.

$$\text{Prob}(X \text{ or } Y) = 1 - (1 - \text{Prob}(X)) \times (1 - \text{Prob}(Y))$$

Suppose you roll a pair of dice. What's the probability of at least one of the dice coming up a 4? If the dice aren't loaded, there's a 1/6 chance (a probability of 0.167, approximately) of getting a 4 (or any other specified number) on any die you roll, so the probability of getting a 4 on at least one of the two dice is $1 - (1 - 0.167) \times (1 - 0.167)$, which works out to $1 - 0.833 \times 0.833$, or 0.31, approximately.

The "and" and "or" rules apply only to *independent* events. For example, you can't use these rules to calculate the probability of a person selected at random being obese and hypertensive by using the prevalences (probabilities) of obesity and hypertension in the general population because these two medical conditions tend to be associated — if you have one, you're at greater risk of having the other also.

Comparing odds versus probability

You see the word *odds* used a lot in this book, especially in Chapter 14 (on the fourfold cross-tab table) and Chapter 20 (on logistic regression). Odds and probability are related, but the two words are not synonymous.

Odds equal the probability of something happening divided by the probability of that thing *not* happening. So, knowing that the probability of something not happening is 1 minus the probability of that thing happening (see the preceding section), you have the formula:

Odds = Probability/(1 − Probability)

With a little algebra (which you don't need to worry about), you can solve this formula for probability as a function of odds:

Probability = Odds/(1 + Odds)

Table 3-1 shows how probability and odds are related.

Table 3-1		The Relationship between Probability and Odds
Probability	**Odds**	**Interpretation**
1.0	Infinity	The event will definitely occur.
0.9	9	The event will occur 90% of the time (is nine times as likely to occur as to not occur).
0.75	3	The event will occur 75% of the time (is three times as likely to occur as to not occur).
0.667	2	The event will occur two-thirds of the time (is twice as likely to occur as to not occur).
0.5	1.0	The event will occur about half the time (is equally likely to occur or not occur).
0.333	0.5	The event will occur one-third of the time (is only half as likely to occur as to not occur).
0.25	0.3333	The event will occur 25% of the time (is one-third as likely to occur as to not occur).
0.1	0.1111	The event will occur 10% of the time (is 1/9th as likely to occur as to not occur).
0	0	The event definitely will not occur.

As you can see in Table 3-1, for very low probability, the odds are very close to the probability; but as probability increases, the odds increase faster. By the time probability reaches 0.5, the odds have become 1, and as probability approaches 1, the odds become infinitely large! This definition of odds is consistent with its common-language use. For instance: If the odds of a horse losing a race are 3:1, that means you have three chances of losing and one chance of winning, for a 0.75 probability of losing.

Some Random Thoughts about Randomness

Like probability (which I cover earlier in this chapter), the word *random* is something we use all the time and something we all have some intuitive concept of, but find hard to put into precise language. You can talk about random events and random variables. *Random* is a term that applies to the data you acquire in your experiments. When talking about a sequence of random numbers, *random* means the absence of any pattern in the numbers that can be used to predict what the next number will be.

The important idea is that you can't predict a specific outcome if a random element is involved. But that doesn't mean that you can't make *any* statements about the collection of random numbers. Statisticians can say a lot about how a group of random numbers behave collectively.

The first step in analyzing a set of data is to have a good idea of what the data looks like. This is the job of descriptive statistics — to show you how a set of numbers are spread around and to show you the relationship between two or more sets of data. The basic tool for describing the distribution of values for some variable in a sample of subjects is the *histogram,* or frequency distribution graph (I describe histograms in more detail in Chapter 8). Histograms help you visualize the distributions of two types of variables:

- ✔ **Categorical:** For *categorical variables* (such as gender or race), a histogram is simply a bar chart showing how many observations fall into each category, like the distribution of race in a sample of subjects, as shown in Figure 3-1a.

- ✔ **Continuous:** To make a histogram of a *continuous variable* (such as weight or blood hemoglobin), you divide the range of values into some convenient interval, count how many observations fall within each interval, and then display those counts in a bar chart, as shown in Figure 3-1b (which shows the distribution of hemoglobin for a sample of subjects).

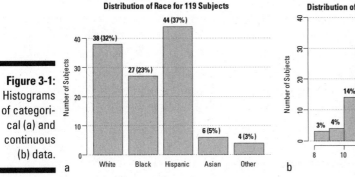
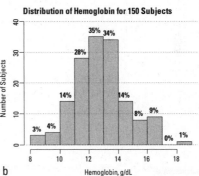

Figure 3-1: Histograms of categorical (a) and continuous (b) data.

Illustration by Wiley, Composition Services Graphics

Picking Samples from Populations

The idea of sampling from a population is one of the most fundamental concepts in statistics — indeed, in all of science. For example, you can't test how a chemotherapy drug will work in *all* people with lung cancer; you can study only a limited sample of lung cancer patients who are available to you and draw conclusions from that sample — conclusions that you hope will be valid for all lung cancer patients.

In the following sections, I explain how samples are only imperfect reflections of the populations they're drawn from, and I describe the basics of probability distributions.

Recognizing that sampling isn't perfect

As used in clinical research, the terms *population* and *sample* can be defined this way:

- ✔ **Population:** All individuals having a precisely defined set of characteristics (for example: human, male, age 18–65, with Stage 3 lung cancer)
- ✔ **Sample:** A subset of a defined population, selected for experimental study

Any sample, no matter how carefully it is selected, is only an imperfect reflection of the population, due to the unavoidable occurrence of random sampling fluctuations. Figure 3-2, which shows IQ scores of a random sample of 100 subjects from the U.S. population, exhibits this characteristic. (IQ scores are standardized so that the average for the whole population is 100, with a standard deviation of 15.)

Figure 3-2:
Distribution of IQ scores in a) the population, and b) a random sample of 100 subjects from that population.

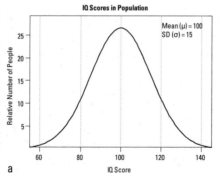
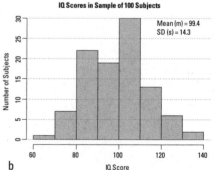

Illustration by Wiley, Composition Services Graphics

The sample is distributed more or less like the population, but clearly it's only an approximation to the true distribution. The mean and standard deviation (I define those terms precisely in Chapter 8) of the sample are close to, but not exactly equal to, the mean and standard deviation of the population, and the histogram doesn't have a perfect bell shape. These characteristics are always true of any random sample.

Histograms are prepared from data you observe in your sample of subjects, and they describe how the values fluctuate in that sample. A histogram of an observed variable, prepared from a random sample of data, is an approximation to what the population distribution of that variable looks like.

Digging into probability distributions

Samples differ from populations because of random fluctuations. Statisticians understand *quantitatively* how random fluctuations behave by developing mathematical equations, called probability distribution functions, that describe how likely it is that random fluctuations will exceed any given magnitude. A probability distribution can be represented in several ways:

- ✔ **As a mathematical equation** that gives the chance that a fluctuation will be of a certain magnitude. Using calculus, this function can be *integrated* — turned into another related function that tells the probability that a fluctuation will be at least as large as a certain magnitude.

- ✔ **As a graph of the distribution,** which looks and works much like a histogram of observed data.

- ✔ **As a table of values** telling how likely it is that random fluctuations will exceed a certain magnitude.

Over the years, hundreds of different probability distributions have been described, but most practical statistical work utilizes only a few of them. You encounter fewer than a dozen probability distributions in this book. In the following sections, I break down two types of distributions: those that describe fluctuations in your data and those that you encounter when performing statistical tests.

Distributions that describe your data

Some distributions describe the random fluctuations you see in your data:

- ✔ **Normal:** The familiar, bell-shaped, *normal* distribution describes (at least approximately) an enormous number of variables you encounter.

- ✔ **Log-normal:** The skewed, *log-normal* distribution describes many laboratory results (enzymes and antibody titers, for example), lengths of hospital stays, and related things like costs, utilization of tests, drugs, and so forth.

- ✔ **Binomial:** The *binomial* distribution describes proportions, such as the fraction of subjects responding to treatment.

- ✔ **Poisson:** The *Poisson* distribution describes the number of occurrences of sporadic random events, such as clicks in a gamma radiation counter or deaths during some period of time.

Chapter 25 describes these and other distribution functions in more detail, and you encounter them throughout this book.

Distributions that come up during statistical testing

Some frequency distributions don't describe fluctuations in observed data, but rather describe fluctuations in numbers that you calculate as part of a statistical test (described in the later section "Honing In on Hypothesis Testing"). These distributions include the Student t, chi-square, and Fisher F distributions (see Chapter 25), which are used to obtain the p values (see the later section "Getting the language down" for a definition of p values) that result from the tests.

Introducing Statistical Inference

Statistical inference is the drawing (that is, *inferring*) of conclusions about a population based on what you see in a sample from that population. In keeping with the idea that statisticians understand how random fluctuations behave, we can say that statistical inference theory is concerned with how we can extract what's real in our data, despite the unavoidable random noise that's always present due to sampling fluctuations or measurement errors. This very broad area of statistical theory is usually subdivided into two topics: statistical *estimation* theory and statistical *decision* theory.

Statistical estimation theory

Statistical estimation theory focuses on the accuracy and precision of things that you estimate, measure, count, or calculate. It gives you ways to indicate how precise your measurements are and to calculate the range that's likely to include the true value. The following sections provide the fundamentals of this theory.

Accuracy and precision

Whenever you estimate or measure anything, your estimated or measured value can differ from the truth in two ways — it can be inaccurate, imprecise, or both.

- ✔ **Accuracy** refers to how close your measurement tends to come to the *true value,* without being systematically biased in one direction or another.

- ✔ **Precision** refers to how close a bunch of replicate measurements come to *each other* — that is, how reproducible they are.

Figure 3-3 shows four shooting targets with a bunch of bullet holes from repeated rifle shots. These targets illustrate the distinction between accuracy and precision — two terms that describe different kinds of errors that can occur when sampling or measuring something (or, in this case, when shooting at a target).

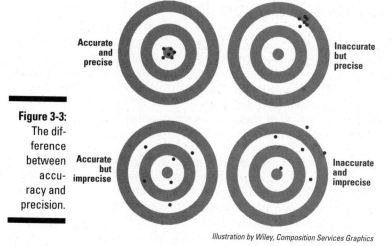

Figure 3-3: The difference between accuracy and precision.

Illustration by Wiley, Composition Services Graphics

You see the following in Figure 3-3:

✔ **The upper-left target** is what most people would hope to achieve — the shots all cluster together (good precision), and they center on the bull's-eye (good accuracy).

✔ **The upper-right target** shows that the shots are all very consistent with each other (good precision), so we know that the shooter was very steady (with no large random perturbations from one shot to the next), and any other random effects must have also been quite small. But the shots were all consistently high and to the right (poor accuracy). Perhaps the gun sight was misaligned or the shooter didn't know how to use it properly. A systematic error occurred somewhere in the aiming and shooting process.

✔ **The lower-left target** indicates that the shooter wasn't very consistent from one shot to another (he had poor precision). Perhaps he was unsteady in holding the rifle; perhaps he breathed differently for each shot; perhaps the bullets were not all properly shaped, and had different aerodynamics; or any number of other random differences may have had an effect from one shot to the next. About the only good thing you can say about this shooter is that at least he tended to be more or less centered around the bull's-eye — the shots don't show any tendency to be consistently high or low, or consistently to the left or right of center. There's no evidence of systematic error (or inaccuracy) in his shooting.

✔ **The lower-right target** shows the worst kind of shooting — the shots are not closely clustered (poor precision) and they seem to show a tendency to be high and to the right (poor accuracy). Both random and systematic errors are prominent in this shooter's shooting.

Sampling distributions and standard errors

The *standard error* (abbreviated SE) is one way to indicate how precise your estimate or measurement of something is. The SE tells you how much the estimate or measured value might vary if you were to repeat the experiment or the measurement many times, using a different random sample from the same population each time and recording the value you obtained each time. This collection of numbers would have a spread of values, forming what is called the *sampling distribution* for that variable. The SE is a measure of the width of the sampling distribution, as described in Chapter 9.

Fortunately, you don't have to repeat the entire experiment a large number of times to calculate the SE. You can usually estimate the SE using data from a single experiment. In Chapter 9, I describe how to calculate the standard errors for means, proportions, event rates, regression coefficients, and other quantities you measure, count, or calculate.

Confidence intervals

Confidence intervals provide another way to indicate the precision of an estimate or measurement of something. A *confidence interval* (CI) around an estimated value is the range in which you have a certain degree of certitude, called the *confidence level* (CL), that the true value for that variable lies. If calculated properly, your quoted confidence interval should encompass the true value a percentage of the time at least equal to the quoted confidence level.

Suppose you treat 100 randomly selected migraine headache sufferers with a new drug, and you find that 80 of them respond to the treatment (according to the response criteria you have established). Your observed response rate is 80 percent, but how precise is this observed rate? You can calculate that the 95 percent confidence interval for this 80 percent response rate goes from 70.8 percent to 87.3 percent. Those two numbers are called the lower and upper 95 percent *confidence limits* around the observed response rate. If you claim that the true response rate (in the population of migraine sufferers that you drew your sample from) lies between 70.8 percent and 87.3 percent, there's a 95 percent chance that that claim is correct.

How did I get those confidence limits? In Chapter 10, I describe how to calculate confidence intervals around means, proportions, event rates, regression coefficients, and other quantities you measure, count, or calculate.

Statistical decision theory

Statistical decision theory is perhaps the largest branch of statistics. It encompasses all the famous (and many not-so-famous) significance tests — Student t tests (see Chapter 12), chi-square tests (see Chapter 13), analysis of variance (ANOVA; see Chapter 12), Pearson correlation tests (see Chapter 17), Wilcoxon and Mann-Whitney tests (see Chapter 12), and on and on.

REMEMBER

In its most basic form, statistical decision theory deals with determining whether or not some real effect is present in your data. I use the word *effect* throughout this book, and it can refer to different things in different circumstances. Examples of effects include the following:

✔ **The average value of something may be different in one group compared to another.** For example, males may have higher hemoglobin values, on average, than females; the effect of gender on hemoglobin can be quantified by the difference in mean hemoglobin between males and females. Or subjects treated with a drug may have a higher recovery rate than subjects given a placebo; the effect size could be expressed as the difference in recovery rate (drug minus placebo) or by the ratio of the odds of recovery for the drug relative to the placebo (the odds ratio).

✔ **The average value of something may be different from zero** (or from some other specified value). For example, the average change in body weight over 12 weeks in a group of subjects undergoing physical therapy may be different from zero.

✔ **Two numerical variables may be associated** (also called *correlated*). For example, if obesity is associated with hypertension, then body mass index may be correlated with systolic blood pressure. This effect is often quantified by the Pearson correlation coefficient.

Homing In on Hypothesis Testing

The theory of statistical hypothesis testing was developed in the early 20th century and has been the mainstay of practical statistics ever since. It was designed to apply the scientific method to situations involving data with random fluctuations (and almost all real-world data has random fluctuations). In the following sections, I list a few terms commonly used in hypothesis testing; explain the steps, results, and possible errors of testing; and describe the relationships between power, sample size, and effect size in testing.

Getting the language down

Here are some of the most common terms used in hypothesis testing:

✔ **Null hypothesis (abbreviated H_0):** The assertion that any apparent effect you see in your data does not reflect any real effect in the population, but is merely the result of random fluctuations.

✔ **Alternate hypothesis (abbreviated H_1 or H_{Alt}):** The assertion that there really is some real effect in your data, over and above whatever is attributable to random fluctuations.

✔ **Significance test:** A calculation designed to determine whether H_0 can reasonably explain what you see in your data.

✔ **Significance:** The conclusion that random fluctuations alone can't account for the size of the effect you observe in your data, so H_0 must be false, and you accept H_{Alt}.

✔ **Statistic:** A number that you obtain or calculate from your data.

✔ **Test statistic:** A number, calculated from your data, usually for the purpose of testing H_0. It's often — but not always — calculated as the ratio of a number that measures the size of the effect (the signal) divided by a number that measures the size of the random fluctuations (the noise).

✔ **p value:** The probability that random fluctuations alone in the absence of any real effect (in the population) can produce an observed effect at least as large as what you observe in your sample. The p value is the probability of random fluctuations making the test statistic at least as large as what you calculate from your data (or, more precisely, at least as far away from H_0 in the direction of H_{Alt}).

✔ **Type I error:** Getting a significant result when, in fact, no effect is present.

✔ **Alpha:** The probability of making a Type I error.

✔ **Type II error:** Failing to get a significant result when, in fact, some effect really is present.

✔ **Beta:** The probability of making a Type II error.

✔ **Power:** The probability of getting a significant result when some effect is really present.

Testing for significance

All the famous statistical significance tests (Student t, chi-square, ANOVA, and so on) work on the same general principle — they evaluate the size of apparent effect you see in your data against the size of the random fluctuations present in your data. I describe individual statistical tests throughout this book — t tests and ANOVAs in Chapter 12, chi-square and Fisher Exact tests in Chapter 13, correlation tests in Chapter 17, and so on. But here I describe the general steps that underlie all the common statistical tests of significance.

1. **Boil your raw data down into a single number, called a *test statistic*.**

   Each test has its own formula, but in general, the test statistic represents the magnitude of the effect you're looking for relative to the magnitude of the random noise in your data. For example, the test statistic for the unpaired Student t test for comparing means between two groups is calculated as a fraction:

$$\text{Student t statistic} = \frac{\text{Mean of Group 1} - \text{Mean of Group 2}}{\text{Standard Error of the Difference}}$$

The numerator is a measure of the effect you're looking for — the difference between the two groups. And the denominator is a measure of the random noise in your data — the spread of values within each group. The larger the observed effect is, relative to the amount of random scatter in your data, the larger the Student t statistic will be.

2. **Determine how likely (or unlikely) it is for random fluctuations to produce a test statistic as large as the one you actually got from your data.**

   The mathematicians have done the hard work; they've developed formulas (really complicated ones) that describe how much the test statistic bounces around if only random fluctuations are present (that is, if H_0 is true).

Understanding the meaning of "p value" as the result of a test

The end result of a statistical significance test is a *p value,* which represents the probability that random fluctuations alone could have generated results that differed from the null hypothesis (H_0), in the direction of the alternate hypothesis (H_{Alt}), by at least as much as what you observed in your data.

If this probability is too small, then H_0 can no longer explain your results, and you're justified in rejecting it and accepting H_{Alt}, which says that some real effect is present. You can say that the effect seen in your data is *statistically significant.*

How small is too small for a p value? This determination is arbitrary; it depends on how much of a risk you're willing to take of being fooled by random fluctuations (that is, of making a Type I error). Over the years, the value of 0.05 has become accepted as a reasonable criterion for declaring significance. If you adopt the criterion that p must be less than or equal to 0.05 to declare significance, then you'll keep the chance of making a Type I error to no more than 5 percent.

Examining Type I and Type II errors

The outcome of a statistical test is a decision to either accept or reject H_0 in favor of H_{Alt}. Because H_0 pertains to the population, it's either true or false for the population you're sampling from. You may never know what that truth is, but an objective truth is out there nonetheless.

The truth can be one of two things, and your conclusion is one of two things, so four different situations are possible; these are often portrayed in a four-fold table, as shown in Figure 3-4 (Chapter 14 has details on these tables).

		The Truth (Based on Entire Population)	
		Nothing Is There (H_0 Is True)	Something Is There (H_0 Is False)
Your Conclusion (Based on Your Sample)	I Don't See Anything (Nonsignificant)	Right!	Wrong (Type II Error)
	I See Something (Significant)	Wrong (Type I Error)	Right!

Figure 3-4: Right and wrong conclusions from a statistical hypothesis test.

Illustration by Wiley, Composition Services Graphics

Here are the four things that can happen when you run a statistical significance test on your data (using an example of testing a drug for efficacy):

✔ You can get a nonsignificant result when there is truly no effect present. This is correct — you don't want to claim that a drug works if it really doesn't. (See the upper-left corner of the outlined box in Figure 3-4.)

✔ You can get a significant result when there truly is some effect present. This is correct — you do want to claim that a drug works when it really does. (See the lower-right corner of the outlined box in Figure 3-4.)

✔ You can get a significant result when there's truly no effect present. This is a Type I error — you've been tricked by random fluctuations that made the drug look effective. (See the lower-left corner of the outlined box in Figure 3-4.) Your company will invest millions of dollars into the further development of a drug that will eventually be shown to be worthless. Statisticians use the Greek letter alpha (α) to represent the probability of making a Type I error.

✔ You can get a nonsignificant result when there truly is an effect present. This is a Type II error (see the upper-right corner of the outlined box in Figure 3-4) — you've failed to see that the drug really works, perhaps because the effect was obscured by the random noise in the data. Further development will be halted, and the miracle drug of the century will be consigned to the scrap heap, along with the Nobel prize you'll never get. Statisticians use the Greek letter beta (β) to represent the probability of making a Type II error.

Limiting your chance of making a Type I error (falsely claiming significance) is very easy. If you don't want to make a Type I error more than 5 percent of the time, don't declare significance unless the p value is less than 0.05. That's called testing at the 0.05 alpha level. If you're willing to make a Type I error 10 percent of the time, use p < 0.10 as your criterion for significance. If you're terrified of Type I errors, use p < 0.000001 as your criterion for significance, and you won't falsely claim significance more than one time in a million.

Why not use a small alpha level (like p < 0.000001) for your significance testing? Because then you'll almost never get significance, even if an effect really is present. Researchers don't like to go through life never making any discoveries. If a drug really is effective, you want to get a significant result when you test it. You need to strike a balance between Type I and Type II errors — between the alpha and beta error rates. If you make alpha too small, beta will become too large, and vice versa. Is there any way to keep both types of errors small? There is, and that's what I describe next.

Grasping the power of a test

The power of a statistical test is the chance that it will come out statistically significant when it should — that is, when the alternative hypothesis is really true. Power is a probability and is very often expressed as a percentage. Beta is the chance of getting a nonsignificant result when the alternative hypothesis is true, so you see that power and beta are related mathematically: Power = 1 – beta.

The power of any statistical test depends on several factors:

- ✔ The alpha level you've established for the test — that is, the chance you're willing to accept of making a Type I error

- ✔ The actual magnitude of the effect in the population, relative to the amount of noise in the data

- ✔ The size of your sample

Power, sample size, effect size relative to noise, and alpha level can't all be varied independently; they're interrelated — connected and constrained by a mathematical relationship involving the four quantities.

This relationship is often very complicated, and sometimes it can't be written down explicitly as a formula, but it does exist. For any particular type of test, you can (at least in theory) determine any one of the four quantities if you know the other three. So there are four different ways to do power calculations, with each way calculating one of the four quantities from arbitrarily specified values of the other three. (I have more to say about this in Chapter 5, where I describe practical issues that arise during the design of research studies.) In the following sections, I describe the relationships between power, sample size, and effect size, and I briefly note how you can perform power calculations.

Power, sample size, and effect size relationships

The alpha level of a statistical test is usually set to 0.05, unless there are special considerations, which I describe in Chapter 5. After you specify the value of alpha, you can display the relationship between the other three variables (power, sample size, and effect size) in several ways. The next three graphs show these relationships for the Student t test; graphs for other statistical tests are generally similar to these:

✔ **Power versus sample size, for various effect sizes:** For all statistical tests, *power always increases as the sample size increases,* if other things (such as alpha level and effect size) are held constant. This relationship is illustrated in Figure 3-5. "Eff" is the effect size — the between-group difference divided by the within-group standard deviation.

Very small samples very seldom produce significant results unless the effect size is very large. Conversely, extremely large samples (many thousands of subjects) are almost always significant unless the effect size is near zero. In epidemiological studies, which often involve hundreds of thousands of subjects, statistical tests tend to produce extremely small (and therefore extremely significant) p values, even when the effect size is so small that it's of no practical importance.

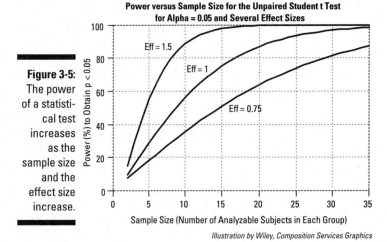

Figure 3-5: The power of a statistical test increases as the sample size and the effect size increase.

Illustration by Wiley, Composition Services Graphics

✔ **Power versus effect size, for various sample sizes:** For all statistical tests, *power always increases as the effect size increases,* if other things (such as alpha level and sample size) are held constant. This relationship is illustrated in Figure 3-6. "N" is the number of subjects in each group.

For very large effect sizes, the power approaches 100 percent. For very small effect sizes, you might think the power of the test would approach zero, but you can see from Figure 3-6 that it doesn't go down all the way to zero; it actually approaches the alpha level of the test. (Keep in mind that the alpha level of the test is the probability of the test producing a significant result when no effect is truly present.)

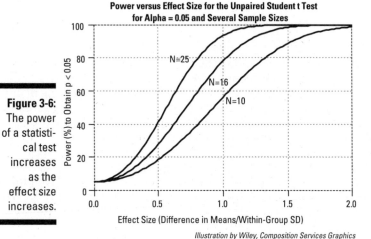

Power versus Effect Size for the Unpaired Student t Test for Alpha = 0.05 and Several Sample Sizes

Figure 3-6: The power of a statistical test increases as the effect size increases.

Illustration by Wiley, Composition Services Graphics

✔ **Sample size versus effect size, for various values of power:** For all statistical tests, *sample size and effect size are inversely related,* if other things (such as alpha level and power) are held constant. Small effects can be detected only with large samples; large effects can often be detected with small samples. This relationship is illustrated in Figure 3-7.

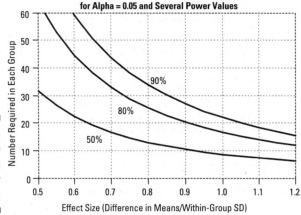

Sample Size versus Effect Size for the Unpaired Student t Test for Alpha = 0.05 and Several Power Values

Figure 3-7: Smaller effects need larger samples.

Illustration by Wiley, Composition Services Graphics

This inverse relationship between sample size and effect size takes on a very simple mathematical form (at least to a good approximation): The required sample size is inversely proportional to the square of the effect size that can be detected. Or, equivalently, the detectable effect size is inversely proportional to the square root of the sample size. So, quadrupling your sample size allows you to detect effect sizes only one-half as large.

How to do power calculations

Power calculations are a crucial part of the design of any research project. You don't want your study to be underpowered (with a high risk of missing real effects) or overpowered (larger, costlier, and more time-consuming than necessary). You need to provide a power/sample-size analysis for any research proposal you submit for funding or any protocol you submit to a review board for approval. You can perform power calculations in several ways:

- ✔ **Computer software:** The larger statistics packages (such as SPSS, SAS, and R) provide a wide range of power calculations — see Chapter 4 for more about these packages. There are also programs specially designed for this purpose (nQuery, StatExact, Power and Precision, PS-Power & Sample Size, and Gpower, for instance).

- ✔ **Web pages:** Many of the more common power calculations can be performed online using web-based calculators. A large collection of these can be found at StatPages.info.

- ✔ **Hand-held devices:** Apps for the more common power calculations are available for most tablets and smartphones.

- ✔ **Printed charts and tables:** You can find charts and tables in textbooks (including this one; see Chapter 12 and this book's Cheat Sheet at www. dummies.com/cheatsheet/biostatistics). These are ideal for quick and dirty calculations.

- ✔ **Rules of thumb:** Some approximate sample-size calculations are simple enough to do on a scrap of paper or even in your head! You find some of these in Chapter 26 and on the Cheat Sheet: Go to www.dummies.com/ cheatsheet/biostatistics.

Going Outside the Norm with Nonparametric Statistics

All statistical tests are derived on the basis of some assumptions about your data, and most of the classical significance tests (such as Student t tests, analysis of variance, and regression tests) assume that your data is distributed according to some classical frequency distribution (most commonly the normal distribution; see Chapter 25). Because the classic distribution functions are all written as mathematical expressions involving parameters (like means and standard deviation), they're called *parametric* distribution functions, and tests that assume your data conforms to a parametric distribution function are called parametric tests. Because the normal distribution is the most common statistical distribution, the term *parametric test* is most often used to mean a test that assumes normally distributed data.

But sometimes your data isn't parametric. For example, you may not want to assume that your data is normally distributed because it may be very noticeably skewed, as shown in Figure 3-8a.

Sometimes, you may be able to perform some kind of transformation of your data to make it more normally distributed. For example, many variables that have a skewed distribution can be turned into normally distributed numbers by taking logarithms, as shown in Figure 3-8b. If, by trial and error, you can find some kind of transformation that normalizes your data, you can run the classical tests on the transformed data. (See Chapter 8.)

Figure 3-8:
Skewed
data (a)
can some-
times be
turned into
normally
distributed
data (b) by
taking loga-
rithms.

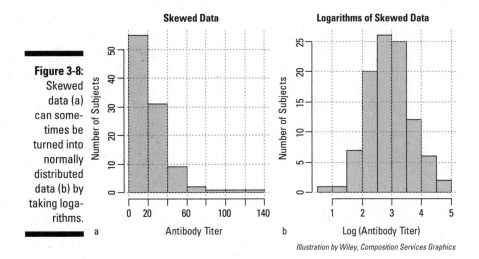

Illustration by Wiley, Composition Services Graphics

But sometimes your data is stubbornly abnormal, and you can't use the parametric tests. Fortunately, statisticians have developed special tests that don't assume normally distributed data; these are (not surprisingly) called nonparametric tests. Most of the common classic parametric tests have nonparametric counterparts. As you may expect, the most widely known and commonly used nonparametric tests are those that correspond to the most widely known and commonly used classical tests. Some of these are shown in Table 3-2.

Table 3-2 Nonparametric Counterparts of Classic Tests	
Classic Parametric Test	*Nonparametric Equivalent*
One-group or paired Student t test (see Chapter 12)	Sign test; Wilcoxon signed-ranks test
Two-group Student t test (see Chapter 12)	Wilcoxon sum-of-ranks test; Mann-Whitney U test
One-way ANOVA (see Chapter 12)	Kruskal-Wallis test
Pearson Correlation test (see Chapter 17)	Spearman Rank Correlation test

Most nonparametric tests involve first sorting your data values, from lowest to highest, and recording the rank of each measurement (the lowest value has a rank of 1, the next highest value a rank of 2, and so on). All subsequent calculations are done with these ranks rather than with the actual data values.

Although nonparametric tests don't assume normality, they do make certain assumptions about your data. For example, many nonparametric tests assume that you don't have any *tied values* in your data set (in other words, no two subjects have exactly the same values). Most parametric tests incorporate adjustments for the presence of ties, but this weakens the test and makes the results nonexact.

Even in descriptive statistics, the common parameters have nonparametric counterparts. Although means and standard deviations can be calculated for any set of numbers, they're most useful for summarizing data when the numbers are normally distributed. When you don't know how the numbers are distributed, medians and quartiles are much more useful as measures of central tendency and dispersion (see Chapter 8 for details).

Chapter 4

Counting on Statistical Software

· ·

· ·

You may be surprised that throughout this book, I tell you *not* to do statistical calculations by hand. With computing power so readily available and with such an abundance of statistical software at your disposal — much of it free — there's just no good reason to put yourself through the misery of mind-numbing calculations and waste your precious time only to (almost certainly) come up with the wrong answer because of some inadvertent error in arithmetic. Just as you would never seriously consider using long division to calculate your car's miles per gallon, you should never consider calculating a correlation coefficient, a t test, or a chi-square test by hand.

In this chapter, I describe some of the many alternatives available to you for performing statistical calculations and analyses. I group them according to the devices on which they run:

- ✔ Personal computers
- ✔ Calculators and mobile devices
- ✔ The web
- ✔ Paper

Desk Job: Personal Computer Software

The first statistical software was developed for the mainframes and minicomputers of the 1960s and 1970s. As personal computers became popular, many of these programs were adapted to run on them. And many more statistical programs were developed from scratch to take advantage of the user-friendly *graphical user interface* (GUI) of Macintosh and Windows computers, including menus, drag-and-drop capability, the point-and-click feature of the mouse, and so forth. More than a hundred of these packages are listed on this web page: `StatPages.info/javasta2.html`.

I describe a few personal computer software products in the following sections. They come in two categories: commercial (the ones you pay for) and free.

Most statistical packages run on Windows; some also run on Mac and Unix or Linux systems. Any Windows package will run on a Mac that has Windows emulation capability (as most of the modern Macs do).

Checking out commercial software

Commercial statistical programs usually provide a wide range of capabilities, personal user support (such as a phone help-line), and some reason to believe (or at least to hope) that the software will be around and supported for many years to come.

Prices vary widely, and the array of pricing options may be bewildering, with single-user and site licenses, nonprofit and academic discounts, one-year and permanent licenses, "basic" and "pro" versions, and so on. Therefore I make only very general statements about relative prices for the commercial packages; check the vendors' websites for details.

Many companies let you download a demo version of their software that's limited in some way — some features may be disabled, the maximum number of cases or variables may be limited, or the software may run for only a certain number of days.

Demo versions are a great way to see whether a software package is easy to use and meets your needs before you shell out the cash for a full version.

In the following sections, I discuss several commercial software programs for you to consider, starting with the biggest, most general, most powerful, and most expensive.

SAS

SAS is one of the most comprehensive statistical packages on the market. It's widely used in all branches of science and is especially pervasive in the pharmaceutical industry. The current versions run on Windows and some Linux systems.

SAS is designed to be run by user-written programs. A GUI module makes the programming task easier, but SAS isn't designed like a typical personal computer program. It doesn't use the familiar "document" paradigm that almost all other personal computer software uses. For example, you don't create a new data file by going to a File menu and selecting New, nor do you open an existing data file by going to File and selecting Open. Most users need SAS training in order to use the program productively.

SAS is large-scale software, designed for large-scale operations. It comes with a wide variety of analyses built in, and its programming language lets you create modules to perform other, less-common kinds of analyses. Its scope has grown beyond just the statistical analysis of data; SAS is now a complete data acquisition, validation, management, analysis, and presentation system.

SAS is also expensive — depending on the optional modules you want to use, it can cost over $1,000 per year. If your organization has a site license, you may be able to use SAS for relatively little or no money for as long as you're affiliated with that organization.

For most readers of this book, SAS is likely to be overkill, but if it's available at your school or organization, it may be worth your time to learn how to use it (especially if you plan to work in pharmaceutical research). See www.sas.com for more details about this program.

SPSS

SPSS is another comprehensive program that can perform all the analyses you're likely to need while remaining quite intuitive and user-friendly. You create and edit data files the same way you'd create and edit word-processing documents and spreadsheets — using the File menu's commands: New, Save, Open, and so forth. SPSS contains a programming language that can automate repetitive tasks and perform calculations and analyses beyond those built into the software. SPSS runs on Windows, Macintosh, and some Linux systems.

SPSS pricing is complicated. Depending on the modules you want to use, it can cost many hundreds of dollars per year. Check out www.spss.com for details on this software.

GraphPad Prism and InStat

Unlike most commercial stats packages, these two programs were designed by and for scientists, not by and for statisticians. GraphPad Prism focuses on the needs of biological and clinical researchers in laboratory settings, and it's quite capable of handling non-laboratory research as well. It offers a powerful combination of parametric and nonparametric tests, extensive regression and curve-fitting (including nonlinear regression), survival analysis, and scientific graphing. It runs on Windows and Mac systems.

GraphPad InStat carries the "scientist, rather than statistician" theme even further, with a user-friendly interface that guides you through the process of selecting the right test based on the structure of your experiment, verifying that your data meets the assumptions of the test, and interpreting all parts of the output in "plain English" with a minimum of statistical jargon. It doesn't have all the capabilities of Prism; its emphasis is on ease of use. If you don't want to have to become a statistician but just want to get your data analyzed properly with minimal fuss, and without a long learning process, check out InStat. It runs on Windows and some Mac systems.

These programs are reasonably priced; academic and student discounts are available, and you can download trial versions to evaluate. They're definitely worth a close look; head to `www.graphpad.com` for details.

Excel and other spreadsheet programs

You can use Excel (and similar spreadsheet programs) to store, summarize, and analyze your raw data and to prepare graphs from your analysis. But using Excel for data storage and analysis has been controversial. Some have argued that Excel is too unstructured to serve as a respectable database (you can put anything into any cell, with no constraints on data types, ranges, and so forth), and you can easily destroy all or parts of your database (by sorting just some columns and not others). Others have said that Excel's built-in mathematical and statistical functions are inaccurate and unreliable. Although some of those criticisms were valid years ago, today's Excel is much improved and is satisfactory for most purposes.

Excel has built-in functions for summarizing data (means, standard deviations, medians, and so on) for the common probability distribution functions and their inverses (normal, Student t, Fisher F, and chi-square) and for performing Student t tests and calculating correlation coefficients and simple linear regression (slope and intercept). If you install the optional Analysis add-in packages provided with Excel, Excel can do more extensive analyses, such as ANOVA and multivariate regression.

Excel runs on both Windows and Macintosh. You can buy it as part of the Microsoft Office suite, and prices vary depending on the version of the suite. For more information, see `office.microsoft.com/en-us/excel`.

Some other packages to consider

Among the many other commercial statistics packages, you may want to look into one or more of these:

- ✔ **Stata:** This package provides a broad range of capabilities through user-written routines. It originally used a command-line interface, but recent versions have implemented a graphical shell. It runs on Windows, Mac, Unix, and Linux systems.

- ✔ **S Plus:** Based on the S programming language (similar to the R language I describe later in this chapter), S Plus provides an extensive graphical user interface. It is highly extensible through user-written routines for almost every imaginable statistical procedure.

- ✔ **Minitab:** With an emphasis on industrial quality control, this package contains many of the capabilities you need for biological research. It runs on Windows systems.

Focusing on free software

Over the years, many dedicated and talented people have developed statistical software packages and made them freely available worldwide. Although some of these programs may not have the scope of coverage or the polish of the commercial packages that I describe earlier in this chapter, they're high-quality programs that can handle most, if not all, of what you probably need to do. The following sections describe several general-purpose statistical packages that perform a wide variety of analyses, an Excel add-in module, and two special-purpose packages that perform power and sample-size calculations.

OpenStat and LazStats

OpenStat, developed by Dr. Bill Miller, is an excellent free program that can perform almost all the statistical analyses described in this book. It has a very friendly user interface, with menus and dialogs that resemble those of SPSS. Dr. Miller provides several excellent manuals and textbooks that support OpenStat, and users can e-mail Dr. Miller directly to get answers to questions or problems they may have. OpenStat runs on Windows systems.

An alternative is LazStats, also from Dr. Miller, which has many of the same capabilities as OpenStat but can run directly (without emulation) on Macintosh and at least some Linux systems.

Fun fact: The "Laz" in "LazStats" doesn't stand for lazy; it stands for the free Lazarus compiler that was used to create the software for Mac and Linux as well as Windows.

Get the scoop on both programs at www.statprograms4U.com.

R

R is a free statistical programming and graphical system that runs on Windows, Macintosh, and Linux systems. It's one of the most powerful computing software packages available, with capabilities surpassing those of many commercial packages. It has built-in support for every kind of statistical analysis described in this book, and many hundreds of add-on packages (also free) extend its capabilities into every area of statistics. You can generate almost every imaginable kind of graph with complete control over every detail (all the technical graphs in this book were made with R).

But R is not easy to use. Its user interface is very rudimentary, and all analyses have to be specified as commands or statements in R's programming language (which is very similar to the S language used by the commercial S-Plus package). It may take you awhile to become proficient in R, but once you do, you'll have almost unlimited capability to carry out any kind of statistical analysis you can think up.

Check out www.r-project.org for more information.

Epi Info

Epi Info, developed by the Centers for Disease Control, was designed to be a fairly complete system to acquire, manage, analyze, and display the results of epidemiological research, although it's useful in all kinds of biostatistical research. It contains modules for creating survey forms, collecting data, and performing a wide range of analyses: t tests, ANOVA, nonparametric statistics, cross tabulations, logistic regression (conditional and unconditional), survival analysis, and analysis of complex survey data. Epi Info runs under Windows. Find the details on this program at wwwn.cdc.gov/epiinfo.

PopTools

PopTools is a free add-in for Excel, written by Greg Hood, an ecologist from Australia. It provides some impressive extensions to Excel — several statistical tests (ANOVA, chi-square, and a few others), a variety of matrix operations, functions to generate random numbers from many different distributions, programs that let you easily perform several kinds of simulations (bootstrapping, Monte-Carlo analysis, and so on), and several handy features for checking the quality of your data. Definitely worth looking at if you're using Excel on a Windows PC (unfortunately, it doesn't work with Mac Excel). Discover more at poptools.org.

PS (Power and Sample Size Calculation) and G*Power

The PS program, from W.D. Dupont and W.D. Plummer of Vanderbilt University, does a few things, and it does them very well. It performs power and sample-size calculations for Student t tests, chi-square tests, several kinds of linear regression, and survival analysis. It has a simple, intuitive user interface and a good help feature, and it provides a verbal description of the analysis (describing the assumptions and interpreting the results) that you can copy and paste into a research proposal or grant application. You can create graphs of power versus sample size or effect size for various scenarios and tweak them until they're of publication quality. For more info, check out biostat.mc.vanderbilt.edu/wiki/Main/PowerSampleSize.

Another excellent power/sample-size program is G*Power. This program handles many more types of statistical analyses than PS, such as multi-factor ANOVAs, ANCOVAs, multiple regression, logistic regression, Poisson regression, and several nonparametric tests. Like PS, it also provides excellent graphics. See www.psycho.uni-duesseldorf.de/abteilungen/aap/gpower3 for details.

G*Power can be more intimidating for the casual user than PS, but because both products are free, you should download and install both of them.

On the Go: Calculators and Mobile Devices

Over the years, as computing has moved from mainframes to minicomputers to personal computers to hand-held devices (calculators, tablets, and smartphones), statistical software has undergone a similar migration. Today you can find statistical software for just about every intelligent (that is, computerized) device there is (with the possible exception of smart toasters).

Scientific and programmable calculators

Many scientific calculators claim to perform statistical calculations, although they may entail no more than calculating the mean and standard deviation of a set of numbers that you key in. Some of the newer scientific calculators also handle correlation and simple linear regression analysis.

Programmable calculators like the TI-83 and HP 35s aren't limited to the calculations that are hard-wired into the device; they let you define your own special-purpose calculations, and therefore can perform almost any computation for which a suitable program has been written.

Mobile devices

Mobile devices (smartphones, tablets, and similar devices) are rapidly becoming the "computer of choice" for many people (according to Mashable. com, 6 billion cellphones were active worldwide in 2011). Indeed, for tasks like e-mail and web browsing, many people find them to be more convenient than desktop or even laptop computers. Perhaps the main reason for their incredible popularity is that they can run an astounding number of custom-written applications, or apps.

Statistics-related apps are available for all the major mobile platforms — Apple iOS, Android, Windows Mobile, and BlackBerry. These range from simple calculators that can do elementary statistical functions (such as means, standard deviations, and some probability functions) to apps that can do fairly sophisticated statistical analyses (such as ANOVAs, multiple regression, and so forth). Prices for these apps range from zero to several hundred dollars. One example is the free StatiCal (short for Statistical Calculator) app for Android systems, which can evaluate the common probability functions and their inverses; calculate confidence intervals; and perform t tests, simple ANOVAs, chi-square tests, and simple correlation and regression analyses.

As of this writing, a tablet or cellphone isn't the ideal platform for maintaining large data files, but it can be very handy for quick calculations on summary data where you need to enter only a few numbers (like chi-square tests on cross-tab tables, or power calculations).

The mobile environment is changing so rapidly that I'm reluctant to recommend specific apps. Go to the "app store" for your particular device (for example, Apple's iTunes App Store or Android's Play Store), and search using terms like *statistics, statistical, anova, correlation,* and so on.

Gone Surfin': Web-Based Software

I define a *web-based* system as one that requires only that your device have a fairly modern web browser (like Microsoft's Internet Explorer, Mozilla Firefox, Opera, Google Chrome, or Apple's Safari) with JavaScript. All modern smartphones and tablets (iPhone, iPad, Android, and Windows) meet this criterion. Properly written web-based software is platform-independent — it doesn't care whether you're running a PC with Windows, a Macintosh, a computer with Linux, an iPhone, an iPad, or an Android phone or tablet. No special software has to be downloaded or installed on your device.

I define a *cloud-based* system as one in which the software and your data files (if any) are stored on servers *in the cloud* (that is, somewhere on the Internet, and you don't care where). Cloud-based systems offer the prospect of letting you access your data, in its most up-to-date form, from any device, anywhere. The ideal web-based/cloud-based system would require only a browser, so it could be accessed from your personal computer, tablet, or smartphone. I'm not aware of any systems currently available that provide all of these capabilities, but they may be coming soon.

Less ambitious than a complete web-based statistics package is a web page that can do one specific statistical calculation or analysis using data that you enter into the page. Many such calculating pages exist, and the website `StatPages.info` lists hundreds of them, organized by type of calculation: descriptive statistics, single-group tests, confidence intervals, two-group comparisons, ANOVAs, cross-tab chi-square tests, correlation and regression analysis, power calculations, and more.

Taken together, all these pages can be thought of as a free, multiplatform, cloud-based statistical software package. But because they've been written by many different people, they don't have a consistent look and feel, they don't exchange data with each other, they don't manage stored data files, and (like anything on the web) individual online calculators tend to come and go over the course of time. But they can be accessed from anywhere at any time; all you need is a device with a browser (a computer, tablet, or smartphone) and an Internet connection.

Besides software, other very useful statistics-related resources are freely available on the web. These include interactive textbooks, tutorials, and other educational materials. Many of these are listed on the `StatPages.info` website.

On Paper: Printed Calculators

I recommend using the options that I list earlier in this chapter for most of your statistical calculations. But there are still a few times when ancient (that is, pre-computer) techniques can be useful. Believe it or not, it's possible to create a printed page that, when used with a ruler or a piece of string, actually becomes a working calculator.

Nomograms, also called *alignment charts,* look something like ordinary graphs, but they're quite different. They usually have three or more straight or curved scales corresponding to three or more variables that are related by some mathematical formula (like height, weight, and body mass index).

The scales are positioned on the paper in such a way that if you lay a ruler (or stretch a string) across them, it will intersect the scales at values that obey the mathematical expression. So if you know the values of any two of the three variables, you can easily find the corresponding value of the third variable.

Nomograms can't be constructed for every possible three-variable expression, but when they can, they're quite useful. Figure 4-1 shows a simple body-mass-index nomogram; several others appear in this book. The dotted line shows that someone who is 5 feet, 9 inches tall and weighs 160 pounds has a BMI of about 24 kilograms per square meter (kg/m^2), near the high end of the normal range.

Body Mass Index Nomogram

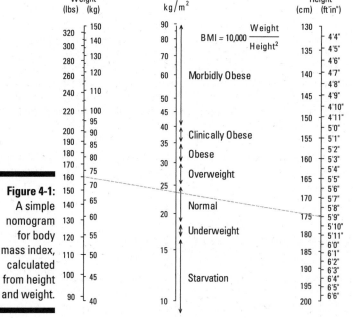

Figure 4-1: A simple nomogram for body mass index, calculated from height and weight.

$$BMI = 10,000 \, \frac{Weight}{Height^2}$$

Illustration by Wiley, Composition Services Graphics

Chapter 5

Conducting Clinical Research

· ·

In This Chapter

▶ Planning and carrying out a clinical research study

▶ Protecting the subjects

▶ Collecting, validating, and analyzing research data

· ·

*T*his chapter and the next one provide a closer look at a special kind of biological research — the clinical trial. This chapter describes some aspects of conducting clinical research; Chapter 6 gives you the "big picture" of pharmaceutical drug trials — an example of a high-profile, high-stakes, highly regulated research endeavor. Although you may never be involved in something as massive as a drug trial, the principles are just as relevant, even if you're only trying to show whether drinking a fruit smoothie every day gives you more energy.

Designing a Clinical Study

Clinical studies should conform to the highest standards of scientific rigor, and that starts with the design of the study. The following sections note some aspects of good experimental design you should keep in mind at the start of any research project.

Identifying aims, objectives, hypotheses, and variables

The *aims* or *goals* of a study are short general statements (often just one statement) of the overall purpose of the trial. For example, the aim of a study may be "to assess the safety and efficacy of drug XYZ in patients with moderate hyperlipidemia."

The *objectives* are much more specific than the aims. Objectives usually refer to the effect of the product on specific safety and efficacy variables, at specific points in time, in specific groups of subjects. An efficacy study may have many individual efficacy objectives, as well as one or two safety objectives; a safety study may or may not have efficacy objectives.

You should identify one or two *primary objectives* — those that are most directly related to the aim of the study and determine whether the product passes or fails in the study. You may then identify up to several dozen *secondary objectives,* which may involve different variables or the same variables at different time points or in different subsets of the study population. You may also list a set of *exploratory objectives*, which are less important, but still interesting. Finally, you list one or more *safety objectives* (if this is an efficacy study) or some efficacy objectives (if this is a safety study).

A typical set of primary, secondary, exploratory, and safety objectives (this example shows one of each type) for an efficacy study might look like this:

- ✔ **Primary efficacy objective:** To compare the effect of drug XYZ, relative to placebo, on changes in serum total cholesterol from baseline to week 12, in patients with moderate hyperlipidemia.

- ✔ **Secondary efficacy objective:** To compare the effect of drug XYZ, relative to placebo, on changes in serum total cholesterol and serum triglycerides from baseline to weeks 4 and 8, in patients with moderate hyperlipidemia.

- ✔ **Exploratory efficacy objective:** To compare the effect of drug XYZ, relative to placebo, on changes in serum lipids from baseline to weeks 4, 8, and 12, in male and female subsets of patients with moderate hyperlipidemia.

- ✔ **Safety objective:** To evaluate the safety of drug XYZ, relative to placebo, in terms of the occurrence of adverse events, changes from baseline in vital signs (blood pressure and heart rate), and safety laboratory results (chemistry, hematology, and so on), in patients with moderate hyperlipidemia.

Hypotheses usually correspond to the objectives but are worded in a way that directly relates to the statistical testing to be performed. So the preceding primary objective may correspond to the following hypothesis: "The mean 12-week reduction in total cholesterol will be greater in the XYZ group than in the placebo group." Alternatively, the hypothesis may be expressed in a more formal mathematical notation and as a null and alternate pair (see Chapters 2 and 3 for details on these terms and the mathematical notation used):

$$H_{Null}: \Delta_{XYZ} - \Delta_{Placebo} = 0$$
$$H_{Alt}: \Delta_{XYZ} - \Delta_{Placebo} > 0$$

where Δ = mean of (TChol$_{Week\ 12}$ – TChol$_{Baseline}$).

Identifying the variables to collect in your study should be straightforward after you've enumerated all the objectives. Generally, you should plan on collecting some or all of the following kinds of data:

- ✔ Basic demographic information (such as date of birth, gender, race, and ethnicity)

- ✔ Information about the subject's participation in the study (for instance, date of enrollment, whether the subject met each inclusion and exclusion criterion, date of each visit, measures of compliance, and final status (complete, withdrew, lost to follow-up, and so on)

- ✔ Basic baseline measurements (height, weight, vital signs, safety laboratory tests, and so forth)

- ✔ Subject and family medical history, including diseases, hospitalizations, smoking and other substance use, and current and past medications

- ✔ Laboratory and other testing (ECGs, X-rays, and so forth) results related to the study's objectives

- ✔ Responses from questionnaires and other subjective assessments

- ✔ Occurrence of adverse events

Some of this information needs to be recorded only once (like birthdate, gender, and family history); other information (such as vital signs, dosing, and test results) may be acquired at scheduled or unscheduled visits, and some may be recorded only at unpredictable times, if at all (like adverse events).

For very simple studies, you may be able to record all your data on a single (albeit large) sheet of ruled paper, with a row for each subject and a column for each variable. But in formal clinical studies, you need to design a *Case Report Form* (CRF). A CRF is often a booklet or binder with one page for the one-time data and a set of identical pages for each kind of recurring data. Many excellent CRF templates can be downloaded from the web, for example from globalhealthtrials.tghn.org/articles/downloadable-templates-and-tools-clinical-research/ (or just enter "CRF templates" in your browser). See the later section "Collecting and validating data" for more information on CRFs.

Deciding who will be in the study

Because you can't examine the entire population of people with the condition you're studying, you must select a representative sample from that population (see Chapter 3 for an introduction to populations and samples). You do this by explicitly defining the conditions that determine whether or not a subject is suitable to be in the study.

✔ **Inclusion criteria** are used during the screening process to identify potential subjects and usually involve subject characteristics that define the population you want to draw conclusions about. A reasonable inclusion criterion for a study of a lipid-lowering treatment would be, "Subject must have a documented diagnosis of hyperlipidemia, defined as Total Cholesterol > 200 mg/dL and LDL > 130 mg/dL at screening."

✔ **Exclusion criteria** are used to identify subjects for whom participation would be unsafe or those whose participation would compromise the scientific integrity of the study (due to preexisting conditions, an inability to understand instructions, and so on). The following usually appears in the list of exclusion criteria: "The subject is, in the judgment of the investigator, unlikely to be able to understand and comply with the treatment regimen prescribed by the protocol."

✔ **Withdrawal criteria** describe situations that could arise during the study that would prevent the subject's further participation for safety or other reasons (such as an intolerable adverse reaction or a serious noncompliance). A typical withdrawal criterion may be "The subject has missed two consecutive scheduled clinic visits."

Choosing the structure of the study

Most clinical trials involving two or more test products have one of the following *structures* (or *designs*), each of which has both pros and cons:

✔ **Parallel:** Each subject receives *one* of the products. Parallel designs are simpler, quicker, and easier for each subject, but you need more subjects. Trials with very long treatment periods usually have to be parallel. The statistical analysis of parallel trials is generally simpler than for crossover trials (see the next bullet).

✔ **Crossover:** Each subject receives *all* the products in sequence during consecutive treatment periods (called *phases*) separated by *washout intervals* (lasting from several days to several weeks). Crossover designs can be more efficient, because each subject serves as his own control, eliminating subject-to-subject variability. But you can use crossover designs only if you're certain that at the end of each washout period the subject will have been restored to the same condition as at the start of the study; this may be impossible for studies of progressive diseases, like cancer or emphysema.

Using randomization

Randomized controlled trials (RCTs) are the gold standard for clinical research. In an RCT, the subjects are randomly allocated into treatment groups (in a parallel trial) or into treatment-sequence groups (in a crossover design). Randomization provides several advantages:

✔ It tends to eliminate *selection bias* — preferentially giving certain treatments to certain subjects (assigning a placebo to the less "likeable" subjects) — and *confounding,* where the treatment groups differ with respect to some characteristic that influences the outcome.

✔ It permits the application of statistical methods to the analysis of the data.

✔ It facilitates blinding. *Blinding* (also called *masking*) refers to concealing the identity of the treatment from subjects and researchers, and can be one of two types:

　• **Single-blinding:** The subjects don't know what treatment they're receiving, but the investigators do.

　• **Double-blinding:** Neither the subjects nor the investigators know which subjects are receiving which treatments.

Blinding eliminates bias resulting from the *placebo effect,* whereby subjects often respond favorably to *any* treatment (even a placebo), especially when the efficacy variables are subjective, such as pain level. Double-blinding also eliminates deliberate and subconscious bias in the investigator's evaluation of a subject's condition.

The simplest kind of randomization involves assigning each newly enrolled subject to a treatment group by the flip of a coin or a similar method. But simple randomization may produce an unbalanced pattern, like the one shown in Figure 5-1 for a small study of 12 subjects and two treatments: Drug (D) and Placebo (P).

Figure 5-1:
Simple randomization.

Subject	1	2	3	4	5	6	7	8	9	10	11	12
Treatment	P	D	P	P	D	P	P	P	D	P	P	P

Illustration by Wiley, Composition Services Graphics

If you were hoping to have six subjects in each group, you won't like having only three subjects receiving the drug and nine receiving the placebo, but unbalanced patterns like this arise quite often from 12 coin flips. (Try it if you don't believe me.)

A better approach is to require six subjects in each group, but to shuffle those six Ds and six Ps around randomly, as shown in Figure 5-2:

Figure 5-2: Random shuffling.

Subject	1	2	3	4	5	6	7	8	9	10	11	12
Treatment	P	D	D	D	D	D	P	P	P	D	P	P

Illustration by Wiley, Composition Services Graphics

This arrangement is better (there are exactly six drug and six placebo subjects), but this particular random shuffle happens to assign more drugs to the earlier subjects and more placebos to the later subjects (again, bad luck of the draw). If these 12 subjects were enrolled over a period of five or six months, seasonal effects might be mistaken for treatment effects (an example of confounding).

To make sure that both treatments are evenly spread across the entire recruitment period, you can use *blocked randomization,* in which you divide your subjects into consecutive blocks and shuffle the assignments within each block. Often the block size is set to twice the number of treatment groups (for instance, a two-group study would use a block size of four), as shown in Figure 5-3.

You can create simple and blocked randomization lists in Excel using the RAND built-in function to shuffle the assignments. You can also use the web page at `graphpad.com/quickcalcs/randomize1.cfm` to generate blocked randomization lists quickly and easily.

Figure 5-3: Blocked randomization.

Subject	1	2	3	4	5	6	7	8	9	10	11	12
Treatment	D	P	D	P	P	P	D	D	P	D	P	D

Illustration by Wiley, Composition Services Graphics

Selecting the analyses to use

You should select the appropriate method for each of your study hypotheses based on the kind of data involved, the structure of the study, and the nature of the hypothesis. The rest of this book describes statistical methods to analyze the kinds of data you're likely to encounter in clinical research. Changes in variables over time and differences between treatments in crossover studies are often analyzed by paired t tests and repeated-measures ANOVAs, and differences between groups of subjects in parallel studies are often analyzed by unpaired t tests and ANOVAs (see Chapter 12 for more on t tests and ANOVAs). Differences in the percentage of subjects responding to treatment or experiencing events are often compared with chi-square or Fisher Exact tests (see Chapters 13 and 14 for the scoop on these tests). The associations between two or more variables are usually analyzed by regression methods (get the lowdown on regression in Part IV). Survival times (and the times to the occurrence of other endpoint events) are analyzed by survival methods (turn to Part V for the specifics of survival analysis).

Defining analytical populations

Analytical populations are precisely defined subsets of the enrolled subjects that are used for different kinds of statistical analysis. Most clinical trials include the following types of analytical populations:

- ✔ **The safety population:** This group usually consists of all subjects who received at least one dose of any study product (even a placebo) and had at least one subsequent safety-related visit or observation. All safety-related tabulations and analyses are done on the safety population.

- ✔ **The intent-to-treat (ITT) population:** This population usually consists of all subjects who received any study product. The ITT population is useful for assessing *effectiveness* — how well the product performs in the real world, where people don't always take the product as recommended (because of laziness, inconvenience, unpleasant side effects, and so on).

- ✔ **The per-protocol (PP) population:** This group is usually defined as all subjects who complied with the rules of the study — those people who took the product as prescribed, made all test visits, and didn't have any serious protocol violations. The PP population is useful for assessing *efficacy* — how well the product works in an ideal world where everyone takes it as prescribed.

Other special populations may be defined for special kinds of analysis. For example, if the study involves taking a special set of blood samples for pharmacokinetic (PK) calculations, the protocol usually defines a PK population consisting of all subjects who provided suitable PK samples.

Determining how many subjects to enroll

You should enroll enough subjects to provide sufficient statistical power (see Chapter 3) when testing the primary objective of the study. The specific way you calculate the required sample size depends on the statistical test that's used for the primary hypothesis. Each chapter of this book that describes hypothesis tests shows how to estimate the required sample size for that test. Also, you can use the formulas, tables, and charts in Chapter 26 and in the Cheat Sheet (at www.dummies.com/cheatsheet/biostatistics) to get quick sample-size estimates.

You must also allow for some of the enrolled subjects dropping out or being unsuitable for analysis. If, for example, you need 64 analyzable subjects for sufficient power and you expect 15 percent attrition from the study (in other words, you expect only 85 percent of the enrolled subjects to have analyzable data), you need to enroll 64/0.85, or 76, subjects in the study.

Putting together the protocol

A *protocol* is a document that lays out exactly what you plan to do in a clinical study. Ideally, every study involving human subjects should have a protocol. The following sections list standard components and administrative information found in a protocol.

Standard elements

A formal drug trial protocol usually contains most of the following components:

- ✔ **Title:** A title conveys as much information about the trial as you can fit into one sentence, including the protocol ID, study name (if it has one), clinical phase, type and structure of trial, type of randomization and blinding, name of the product, treatment regimen, intended effect, and the population being studied (what medical condition, in what group of people). A title can be quite long — this one has all the preceding elements:

  Protocol BCAM521-13-01 (ASPIRE-2) — a Phase-IIa, double-blind, placebo-controlled, randomized, parallel-group study of the safety and efficacy of three different doses of AM521, given intravenously, once per month for six months, for the relief of chronic pain, in adults with knee osteoporosis.

- ✔ **Background information:** This section includes info about the disease (such as its prevalence and impact), known physiology (at the molecular level, if known), treatments currently available (if any), and information about this drug (its mechanism of action, the results of prior testing, and known and potential risks and benefits to subjects).

- ✔ **Rationale:** The rationale for the study states why it makes sense to do this study at this time, including a justification for the choice of doses, how the drug is administered (such as orally or intravenously), and the duration of therapy and follow-up.

- ✔ **Aims, objectives, and hypotheses:** I discuss these items in the earlier section "Aims, objectives, hypotheses, and variables."

- ✔ **Detailed descriptions of all inclusion, exclusion, and withdrawal criteria:** See the earlier section "Deciding who will be in the study" for more about these terms.

- ✔ **Design of study:** The study's design defines its structure (check out the earlier section "Choosing the structure of the study"), the number of treatment groups, and the consecutive stages (screening, washout, treatment, follow-up, and so on). This section often includes a schematic diagram of the structure of the study.

✔ **Product description:** This description details each product that will be administered to the subjects, including the chemical composition (with the results of chemical analysis of the product, if available) and how to store, prepare, and administer the product.

✔ **Blinding and randomization schemes:** These schemes include descriptions of how and when the study will be unblinded (including the emergency unblinding of individual subjects, if necessary); see the earlier section "Using randomization."

✔ **Procedural descriptions:** This section describes every procedure that will be performed at every visit, including administrative procedures (such as enrollment and informed consent) and diagnostic procedures (for example, physical exams and vital signs).

✔ **Safety considerations:** These factors include the known and potential side effects of the product and each test procedure (such as X-rays, MRI scans, and blood draws), including steps taken to minimize the risk to the subjects.

✔ **Handling of adverse events:** This section describes how adverse events will be recorded — description, severity, dates and times of onset and resolution, any medical treatment given for the event, and whether or not the investigator thinks the event was related to the study product. Reporting adverse events has become quite standardized over the years, so this section tends to be very similar for all studies.

✔ **Definition of safety, efficacy, and other analytical populations:** This section includes definitions of safety and efficacy variables and endpoints (variables or changes in variables that serve as indicators of safety or efficacy). See the earlier section "Defining analytical populations."

✔ **Planned enrollment and analyzable sample size:** Justification for these numbers must also be provided.

✔ **Proposed statistical analyses:** Some protocols describe, in detail, every analysis for every objective; others have only a summary and refer to a separate *Statistical Analysis Plan* (SAP) document for details of the proposed analysis. This section should also include descriptions of the treatment of missing data, adjustments for multiple testing to control Type I errors (see Chapter 3), and whether any interim analyses are planned. If a separate SAP is used, it will usually contain a detailed description of all the calculations and analyses that will be carried out on the data, including the descriptive summaries of all data and the testing of all the hypotheses specified in the protocol. The SAP also usually contains mock-ups, or "shells" of all the tables, listings, and figures (referred to as TLFs) that will be generated from the data.

Administrative details

A protocol also has sections with more administrative information:

- ✔ Names of and contact info for the sponsor, medical expert, and primary investigator, plus the physicians, labs, and other major medical or technical groups involved

- ✔ A table of contents, similar to the kind you find in many books (including this one)

- ✔ A synopsis, which is a short (usually around two pages) summary of the main components of the protocol

- ✔ A list of abbreviations and terms appearing in the protocol

- ✔ A description of your policies for data handling, record-keeping, quality control, ethical considerations, access to source documents, and publication of results

- ✔ Financing and insurance agreements

- ✔ Descriptions of all amendments made to the original protocol

Carrying Out a Clinical Study

After you've designed your study and have described it in the protocol document, it's time to set things in motion. The operational details will, of course, vary from one study to another, but a few aspects apply to all clinical studies. In any study involving human subjects, the most important consideration is protecting those subjects from harm, and an elaborate set of safeguards has evolved over the past century. And in any scientific investigation, the accurate collection of data is crucial to the success of the research.

Protecting your subjects

In any research involving human subjects, two issues are of utmost importance:

- ✔ **Safety:** Minimizing the risk of physical harm to the subjects from the product being tested and from the procedures involved in the study

- ✔ **Privacy/confidentiality:** Ensuring that data collected during the study is not made public in a way that identifies a specific subject without the subject's consent

The following sections describe some of the "infrastructure" that helps protect human subjects.

Surveying regulatory agencies

In the United States, several government organizations oversee human subjects' protection:

✔ Commercial pharmaceutical research is governed by the Food and Drug Administration (FDA).

✔ Most academic biological research is sponsored by the National Institutes of Health (NIH) and is governed by the Office for Human Research Protections (OHRP).

Chapter 6 describes the ways investigators interact with these agencies during the course of clinical research.

Other countries have similar agencies. There's also an organization — the International Conference on Harmonization (ICH) — that works to establish a set of consistent standards that can be applied worldwide. The FDA and NIH have adopted many ICH standards (with some modifications).

Working with Institutional Review Boards

For all but the very simplest research involving human subjects, you need the approval of an *IRB* — an Institutional (or Independent) Review Board — before enrolling any subjects into your study. You have to submit an application along with the protocol and an ICF (see the next section) to an IRB with jurisdiction over your research.

Most medical centers and academic institutions — and some pharmaceutical companies — have their own IRBs with jurisdiction over research conducted at their institution. If you're not affiliated with one of these centers or institutions (for example, if you're a physician in private practice), you may need the services of a "free-standing" IRB. The sponsor of the research may suggest (or dictate) an IRB for the project.

Getting informed consent

An important part of protecting human subjects is making sure that they're aware of the risks of a study before agreeing to participate in it. You must prepare an *Informed Consent Form* (ICF) describing, in simple language, the nature of the study, why it is being conducted, what is being tested, what procedures subjects will undergo, and what the risks and benefits are. Subjects must be told that they can refuse to participate and can withdraw at any time for any reason, without fear of retribution or the withholding of regular medical care. The IRB can usually provide ICF templates with examples of their recommended or required wording.

Prior to performing any procedures on a potential subject (including screening tests), you must give the ICF document to the subject and give her time to read it and decide whether she wants to participate. The subject's agreement must be signed and witnessed. The signed ICFs must be retained as part of the official documentation for the project, along with laboratory reports, ECG tracings, and records of all test products administered to the subjects and procedures performed on them. The sponsor, the regulatory agencies, the IRB, and other entities may call for these documents at any time.

Considering data safety monitoring boards and committees

For clinical trials of products that are likely to be of low risk, investigators are usually responsible for being on the lookout for signs of trouble (unexpected adverse events, abnormal laboratory tests, and so forth) during the course of the study. But for studies involving high-risk treatments (like cancer chemotherapy trials), a separate *data safety monitoring board* or *committee* (DSMB or DSMC) may be set up. A DSMB may be required by the sponsor, the investigator, the IRB, or a regulatory agency. A DSMB typically has about six members (usually expert clinicians in the relevant area of research and a statistician) who meet at regular intervals to review the safety data acquired up to that point. The committee is authorized to modify, suspend, or even terminate a study if it has serious concerns about the safety of the subjects.

Getting certified in human subjects protection and good clinical practice

As you've probably surmised from the preceding sections, clinical research is fraught with regulatory requirements (with severe penalties for noncompliance), and you shouldn't try to "wing it" and hope that everything goes well. You should ensure that you, along with any others who may be assisting you, are properly trained in matters relating to human subjects protection. Fortunately, such training is readily available. Most hospitals and medical centers provide yearly training (often as a half-day session), after which you receive a certification in human subjects protection. Most IRBs and funding agencies require proof of certification from all people who are involved in the research. If you don't have access to that training at your institution, you can get certified by taking an online tutorial offered by the NIH (grants.nih. gov/grants/policy/hs/training.htm).

You should also have one or more of the people who will be involved in the research take a course in "good clinical practice" (GCP). GCP certification is also available online (enter "GCP certification" in your favorite browser).

Collecting and validating data

If the case report form (CRF) has been carefully and logically designed, entering each subject's data in the right place on the CRF should be straightforward.

Then you need to get this data into a computer for analysis. You can enter your data directly into the statistics software you plan to use for the majority of the analysis (see Chapter 4 for some software options), or you can enter it into a general database program such as MS Access or a spreadsheet program like Excel. The structure of a computerized database usually reflects the structure of the CRF. If a study is simple enough that a single data sheet can hold all the data, then a single data file (called a *table*) or a single Excel worksheet will suffice. But for most studies, a more complicated database is required, consisting of a set of tables or Excel worksheets (one for each kind of data collection sheet in the CRF). If the design of the database is consistent with the structure of the CRF, entering the data from each CRF sheet into the corresponding data table shouldn't be difficult.

You must retain all the original source documents (lab reports, the examining physician's notes, original questionnaire sheets, and so forth) in case questions about data accuracy arise later.

Before you can analyze your data (see the next section), you must do one more crucially important task — check your data thoroughly for errors! And there *will* be errors — they can arise from transcribing data from the source documents onto the CRF or from entering the data from the CRFs into the computer. Consider some of the following error-checking techniques:

- ✔ Have one person read data from the source documents or CRFs while another looks at the data that's in the computer. Ideally, this is done with all data for all subjects.

- ✔ Have the computer display the smallest and largest values of each variable. Better yet, have the computer display a sorted list of the values for each variable. Typing errors often produce very large or very small values.

- ✔ A more extreme approach, but one that's sometimes done for crucially important studies, is to have two people enter all the data into separate copies of the database; then have the computer automatically compare every single data item between the two databases.

Chapter 7 has more details on describing, entering, and checking different types of data.

Analyzing Your Data

The remainder of this book explains the methods commonly used in biostatistics to summarize, graph, and analyze data. In the following sections, I describe some general situations that come up in all clinical research, regardless of what kind of analysis you use.

Dealing with missing data

Most clinical trials have incomplete data for one or more variables, which can be a real headache when analyzing your data. The statistical aspects of missing data are quite complicated, so you should consult a statistician if you have more than just occasional, isolated missing values. Here I describe some commonly used approaches to coping with missing data:

✔ Exclude a case from an analysis if any of the required variables for that analysis is missing. This approach can reduce the number of analyzable cases, sometimes quite severely (especially in multiple regression, where the whole case must be thrown out, even if only one of the variables in the regression is missing; see Chapter 19 for more information). And if the result is missing for a reason that's related to treatment efficacy, excluding the case can bias your results.

✔ Replace (*impute*) a missing value with the mean (or median) of all the available values for that variable. This approach is quite common, but it introduces several types of bias into your results, so it's not a good technique to use.

✔ If one of a series of sequential measurements on a subject is missing (like the third of a series of weekly glucose values), use the previous value in the series. This technique is called *Last Observation Carried Forward* (LOCF) and is one of the most widely used strategies. LOCF usually produces "conservative" results, making it more difficult to prove efficacy. This approach is popular with regulators, who want to put the burden of proof on the drug.

More complicated methods can also be used, such as estimating the missing value of a variable based on the relationship between that variable and other variables in the data set, or using an analytical method like *mixed-model repeated measures* (MMRM) analysis, which uses all available data and doesn't reject a case just because one variable is missing. But these methods are far beyond the scope of this book, and you shouldn't try them yourself.

Handling multiplicity

Every time you perform a statistical significance test, you run a chance of being fooled by random fluctuations into thinking that some real effect is present in your data when, in fact, none exists. This scenario is called a *Type I error* (see Chapter 3). When you say that you require $p < 0.05$ for significance, you're testing at the 0.05 (or 5 percent) *alpha level* (see Chapter 3) or saying that you want to limit your Type I error rate to 5 percent. But that 5 percent error rate applies to each and every statistical test you run. The more analyses you perform on a data set, the more your overall alpha level increases: Perform two tests and your chance of at least one of them coming out falsely significant is about 10 percent; run 40 tests, and the overall alpha level jumps to 87 percent. This is referred to as the problem of *multiplicity*, or as *Type I error inflation*.

Some statistical methods involving multiple comparisons (like post-hoc tests following an ANOVA for comparing several groups, as described in Chapter 12) incorporate a built-in adjustment to keep the overall alpha at only 5 percent across all comparisons. But when you're testing different hypotheses, like comparing different variables at different time points between different groups, it's up to you to decide what kind of alpha control strategy (if any) you want to implement. You have several choices, including the following:

✔ **Don't control for multiplicity** and accept the likelihood that some of your "significant" findings will be falsely significant. This strategy is often used with hypotheses related to secondary and exploratory objectives; the protocol usually states that no final inferences will be made from these exploratory tests. Any "significant" results will be considered only "signals" of possible real effects and will have to be confirmed in subsequent studies before any final conclusions are drawn.

✔ **Control the alpha level across only the most important hypotheses.** If you have two co-primary objectives, you can control alpha across the tests of those two objectives.

You can control alpha to 5 percent (or to any level you want) across a set of *n* hypothesis tests in several ways; following are some popular ones:

• **The Bonferroni adjustment:** Test each hypothesis at the 0.05/*n* alpha level. So to control overall alpha to 0.05 across two primary endpoints, you need p < 0.025 for significance when testing each one.

• **A hierarchical testing strategy:** Rank your endpoints in descending order of importance. Test the most important one first, and if it gives p < 0.05, conclude that the effect is real. Then test the next most important one, again using p < 0.05 for significance. Continue until you get a nonsignificant result (p > 0.05); then stop testing (or consider all further tests to be only exploratory and don't draw any formal conclusions about them).

• **Controlling the false discovery rate (FDR):** This approach has become popular in recent years to deal with large-scale multiplicity, which arises in areas like genomic testing and digital image analysis that may involve many thousands of tests (such as one per gene or one per pixel) instead of just a few. Instead of trying to avoid even a *single* false conclusion of significance (as the Bonferroni and other classic alpha control methods do), you simply want to control the *proportion* of tests that come out falsely positive, limiting that false discovery rate to some reasonable fraction of all the tests. These positive results can then be tested in a follow-up study.

Incorporating interim analyses

An *interim analysis* is one that's carried out before the conclusion of a clinical trial, using only the data that has been obtained so far. Interim analyses can be blinded or unblinded and can be done for several reasons:

- ✔ An IRB may require an early look at the data to ensure that subjects aren't being exposed to an unacceptable level of risk.

- ✔ You may want to examine data halfway through the trial to see whether the trial can be stopped early for one of the following reasons:

  - The product is *so effective* that going to completion isn't necessary to prove significance.

  - The product is *so ineffective* that continuing the trial is futile.

- ✔ You may want to check some of the assumptions that went into the original design and sample-size calculations of the trial (like within-group variability, recruitment rates, base event rates, and so on) to see whether the total sample size should be adjusted upward or downward.

If the interim analysis could possibly lead to early stopping of the trial for proven efficacy, then the issue of multiplicity comes into play, and special methods must be used to control alpha across the interim and final analyses. These methods often involve some kind of *alpha spending strategy*. The concepts are subtle, and the calculations can be complicated, but here's a very simple example that illustrates the basic concept. Suppose your original plan is to test the efficacy endpoint at the end of the trial at the 5 percent alpha level. If you want to design an interim analysis into this trial, you may use this two-part strategy:

1. **Spend one-fifth of the available 5 percent alpha at the interim analysis.**

   The interim analysis p value must be < 0.01 to stop the trial early and claim efficacy.

2. **Spend the remaining four-fifths of the 5 percent alpha at the end.**

   The end analysis p value must be < 0.04 to claim efficacy.

This strategy preserves the 5 percent overall alpha level while still giving the drug a chance to prove itself at an early point in the trial.

Chapter 6

Looking at Clinical Trials and Drug Development

....

In This Chapter

▶ Understanding preclinical (that is, "before humans") studies

▶ Walking through the phases of clinical studies that test on humans

▶ Checking out other special-purpose clinical trials

....

*M*any of the chapters in this book concentrate on specific statistical techniques and tests, but this chapter gives a bigger picture of one of the main settings where biostatistics is used: clinical research (covered in Chapter 5). As an example, I talk about one particular kind of clinical research: developing a drug and bringing it to market. Many a biostatistician may go his entire career without ever being involved in a clinical drug trial. However, clinical research is worth taking a look at, for several reasons:

✔ It's a broad area of research that covers many types of investigation: laboratory, clinical, epidemiological, and computational experiments.

✔ All the statistical topics, tests, and techniques covered in this book are used at one or more stages of drug development.

✔ It's a high-stakes undertaking, costing hundreds of millions of dollars, and the return on that investment can range from zero dollars to many billions of dollars. So drug developers are highly motivated to do things properly, and that includes using the best statistical techniques throughout the process.

✔ Because of the potential for enormous good — or enormous harm — drug development must be conducted at the highest level of scientific (and statistical) rigor. The process is very closely scrutinized and heavily regulated.

This chapter takes you through the typical steps involved in bringing a promising chemical to market as a prescription drug. In broad strokes, this process usually involves most of the following steps:

1. **Discover a chemical compound or biological agent that shows promise as a treatment for some disease, illness, or other medical or physical condition (which I refer to throughout this chapter as a *target condition*).**

2. **Show that this compound does things at the molecular level (inside the cell) that indicate it may be beneficial in treating the target condition.**

3. **Test the drug in animals.**

   The purpose of this testing is to show that, at least for animals, the drug seems to be fairly safe, and it appears to be effective in treating the target condition (or something similar to it).

4. **Test the drug in humans.**

   This testing entails a set of logical steps to establish the largest dose that a person can tolerate, find the dose (or a couple of doses) that seems to offer the best combination of safety and efficacy, and demonstrate convincingly that the drug works.

5. **Continue to monitor the safety of the drug in an ever-increasing number of users after it's approved and marketed.**

Throughout this chapter, I use the words *effectiveness* and *efficacy* (and their adjective forms *effective* and *efficacious*) to refer to how well a treatment works. These words are not synonymous:

- ✔ **Efficacy** refers to how well a treatment works in an ideal-world situation, where everybody takes it exactly as prescribed.

- ✔ **Effectiveness** refers to how well the treatment works in the real world, where people might refuse to take it as directed (or at all) because of its unpleasantness and/or its side effects. (This is especially relevant in chemotherapy trials, but it comes up in all kinds of clinical testing.)

Both of these aspects of drug performance are important: efficacy perhaps more so in the early stages of drug development, because it addresses the theoretical question of whether the drug can possibly work, and effectiveness more so in the later stages, where the drug's actual real-world performance is of more concern. Common usage doesn't always honor this subtle distinction; the terms "safety and efficacy" and "safe and effective" seem to be more popular than the alternatives "safety and effectiveness" or "safe and efficacious," so I use the more popular forms in this chapter.

Not Ready for Human Consumption: Doing Preclinical Studies

Before any proposed treatment can be tested on humans, there must be at least *some* reason to believe that the treatment might work and that it won't put the subjects at undue risk. So every promising chemical compound or biological agent must undergo a series of tests to assemble this body of evidence before ever being given to a human subject. These "before human" experiments are called *preclinical* studies, and they're carried out in a progressive sequence:

✔ **Theoretical molecular studies *(in silico):*** You can take a chemical structure suggested by molecular biologists, systematically generate thousands of similar molecules (varying a few atoms here and there), and run them through a program that tries to predict how well each variant may interact with a *receptor* (a molecule often in or on the body's cells that plays a role in the development or progression of the target condition). This kind of theoretical investigation is sometimes called an *in silico* study (a term first used in 1989 to describe research conducted by computer simulation of biological molecules, cells, organs, or organisms; it means *in silicon,* referring to semiconductor computer circuits). These techniques are now routinely used to design new *large-molecule drugs* (like naturally occurring or artificially created proteins), for which the computer simulations tend to be quite reliable.

✔ **Chemical studies *(in vitro):*** While computer simulations may suggest promising large molecules, you generally have to evaluate small-molecule drugs in the lab. These studies try to determine the physical, chemical, electrical, and other properties of the molecule. They're called *in vitro* studies, meaning *in glass,* a reference to the tired old stereotype of the chemist in a white lab coat, pouring a colored liquid from one test tube to another. Don't forget your goggles and wild hair.

✔ **Studies on cells and tissues *(ex vivo):*** The next step in evaluating a candidate drug is to see how it actually affects living cells, tissues, and possibly even complete organs. This kind of study is sometimes called *ex vivo,* meaning *out of the living,* because the cells and tissues have been taken out of a living creature. The researchers are looking for changes in these cells and tissues that seem to be related, in some way, to the target condition.

✔ **Animal studies *(in vivo):*** After studies show that a molecule undergoes chemical reactions and interacts the right way with the targeted receptor sites, you can evaluate the drug's effect on complete living organisms to see what the drug actually does *for* them (how effective it is) and what it may do *to* them (how safe it is). These studies are called *in vivo*, meaning *in the living,* because they're conducted on intact living creatures.

In vivo studies tend to be more useful for small-molecule drugs than for large-molecule drugs. Animals and humans may react similarly to small molecules, but the actions of antibodies and proteins tend to be very different between species.

Testing on People during Clinical Trials to Check a Drug's Safety and Efficacy

After a promising candidate drug has been thoroughly tested in the laboratory and on animals, shows the desired effect, and hasn't raised any serious warning flags about dangerous side effects (see the preceding section), then it's time to make the big leap to *clinical trials:* testing on humans. But you can't just give the drug to a bunch of people who have the condition and see whether it helps them. Safety issues become a serious concern when human subjects are involved, and human testing has to be done in a very systematic way to minimize risks.

Clinical drug development is a heavily regulated activity. Every country has an agency that oversees drug development — the U.S. Food and Drug Administration (FDA), Health Canada, the European Medicines Agency (EMEA), the Japanese Ministry of Health and Welfare, and on and on. These agencies have an enormous number of rules, regulations, guidelines, and procedures for every stage of the process. (***Note:*** In this chapter, I use *FDA* to stand not only for the U.S. regulatory agency, but for all such agencies worldwide.)

Before you can test your drug in people, you must show the FDA all the results of the testing you've done in laboratory animals and what you propose to do while testing your drug on humans. The FDA decides whether it's reasonably safe to do the clinical trials. The following sections describe the four phases of a clinical trial.

Phase I: Determining the maximum tolerated dose

An old saying (six centuries old, in fact) is that "dose makes the poison." This adage means that everything is safe in low enough doses (I can fearlessly swallow one microgram of pure potassium cyanide), but anything can be lethal in sufficiently large doses (drinking a gallon of pure water in an hour may well kill me).

So the first step (Phase I) in human drug testing is to determine how much drug you can safely give to a person, which scientists express in more-precisely defined terms:

✔ *Dose-limiting toxicities* (DLTs) are unacceptable side effects that would force the treatment to stop (or continue at a reduced dose). The term *unacceptable* is relative; severe nausea and vomiting would probably be considered unacceptable (and therefore DLTs) for a headache remedy, but not for a chemotherapy drug. For each drug, a group of experts decides what reactions constitute a DLT.

✔ The *maximum tolerated dose* (MTD) is the largest dose that doesn't produce DLTs in a substantial number of subjects (say, more than 5 or 10 percent of them).

The goal of a Phase I trial is to determine the drug's MTD, which will mark the upper end of the range of doses that will be allowed in all subsequent trials of this drug. A typical Phase I trial enrolls subjects into successive groups *(cohorts)* of about eight subjects each. The first cohort gets the drug at one particular dose and its subjects are then watched to see whether they experience any DLTs. If not, then the next cohort is given a larger dose (perhaps 50 percent larger or twice as large). This dose-escalation process continues as long as no DLTs are seen.

As soon as one or more DLTs occur in a cohort, the area around that dose level is explored in more detail in an attempt to nail down the best estimate of the MTD. Depending on how many DLTs are observed at a particular dose level, the protocol may specify testing another cohort at the same dose, at the previous (lower) dose level, or somewhere in between.

Phase I trials are usually done on healthy volunteers because they're mainly about safety. An exception is trials of cancer chemotherapy agents, which have so many unpleasant effects (many of them can actually cause cancer) that it's usually unethical to give them to healthy subjects.

A drug may undergo several Phase I trials. Many drugs are meant to be taken more than once — either as a finite course of treatment (as for chemotherapy) or as an ongoing treatment (as for high blood pressure). The first Phase I trial usually involves a single dosing; others may involve repetitive dosing patterns that reflect how the drug will actually be administered to patients.

The statistical analysis of Phase I data is usually simple, with little more than descriptive summary tables and graphs of event rates at each dose level. Usually, no hypotheses are involved, so no statistical testing is required. Sample sizes for Phase I studies are usually based on prior experience with similar kinds of drugs, not on formal power calculations (see Chapter 3).

The dose level for the first cohort is usually some small fraction of the lowest dose that causes toxicity in animals. You might guess that tolerable drug doses should be proportional to the weight of the animal, so if a 5-kilogram monkey can tolerate 30 milligrams of a drug, a 50-kilogram human should tolerate 300 milligrams. But tolerable doses often don't scale up in such a simple, proportionate way, so researchers often cut the scaled-up dose estimate down by a factor of 10 or more to get a safe starting dose for human trials.

Even with these precautions, the first cohort is always at extra risk, simply because you're sailing in uncharted waters. Besides the possibility of non-proportional scale-up, there's the additional danger of a totally unforeseen serious reaction to the drug. Some drugs (especially antibody drugs) that were perfectly well tolerated in rats, dogs, and monkeys have triggered severe (even fatal) reactions in humans at conservatively scaled-up doses that were thought to be completely safe. So extra precautions are usually put in place for these "first in man" studies.

Besides the primary goal of establishing the MTD for the drug, a Phase I study almost always has some secondary goals as well. After all, if you go to the trouble of getting 50 subjects, giving them the drug, and keeping them under close scrutiny for a day or two afterward, why not take advantage of the opportunity to gather a little more data about how the drug behaves in humans?

With a few extra blood draws, urine collections, and a stool specimen or two, you can get a pretty good idea of the drug's basic *pharmacokinetics:*

- How fast it's absorbed into the bloodstream (if it's taken orally)
- How fast (and by what route) it's eliminated from the body

And, of course, you don't want to pass up the chance to see whether the drug shows any signs of efficacy (no matter how slight).

Phase II: Finding out about the drug's performance

After the Phase I trials, you'll have a good estimate of the MTD for the drug. The next step is to find out about the drug's safety and efficacy at various doses. You may also be looking at several different dosing regimens, including the following options:

- What route (oral or intravenous, for example) to give the drug
- How frequently to give the drug
- For how long (or for what *duration)* to give the drug

Generally, you have several Phase II studies, with each study testing the drug at several different dose levels up to the MTD to find the dose that offers the best tradeoff between safety and efficacy. Phase II trials are called *dose-finding* trials; at the end of Phase II, you should have established the dose (or perhaps two doses) at which you would like to market the drug.

A Phase II trial usually has a parallel, randomized, and blinded design (see Chapter 5 for an explanation of these terms), enrolling a few dozen to several hundred subjects who have the target condition for the drug (such as diabetes, hypertension, or cancer).

You acquire data, before and after drug administration, relating to the safety and efficacy of the drug. The basic idea is to find the dose that gives the highest efficacy with the fewest safety issues. The situation can be viewed in an idealized form in Figure 6-1.

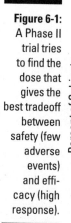

Figure 6-1: A Phase II trial tries to find the dose that gives the best tradeoff between safety (few adverse events) and efficacy (high response).

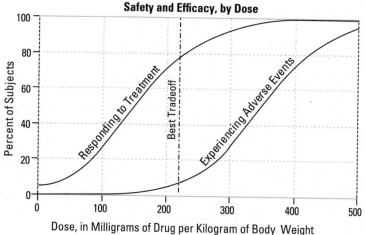

Safety and Efficacy, by Dose

Dose, in Milligrams of Drug per Kilogram of Body Weight

Illustration by Wiley, Composition Services Graphics

Efficacy is usually assessed by several variables (called *efficacy endpoints*) observed during the trial. These depend on the drug being tested and can include:

✔ Changes in measurable quantities directly related to the target condition, such as cholesterol, blood pressure, glucose, and tumor size

✔ Increase in quality-of-life questionnaire scores

✔ Percent of subjects who respond to the treatment (using some acceptable definition of response)

Also, safety has several indicators, including

✔ The percent of subjects experiencing various types of adverse events

✔ Changes in safety lab values, such as hemoglobin

✔ Changes in vital signs, such as heart rate and blood pressure

Usually each safety and efficacy indicator is summarized and graphed by dose level and examined for evidence of some kind of "dose-response" association. (I describe how to test for significant association between variables in Chapter 17.) The graphs may indicate peculiar dose-response behavior; for example, efficacy may increase up to some optimal dose and then decrease for higher doses.

Figure 6-1, in which an overall safety measure and an overall efficacy measure are both shown in the same graph, is useful because it makes the point that (ideally, at least) there should be some range of doses for which the efficacy is relatively high and the rate of side effects is low. In Figure 6-1, that range appears to lie between 150 and 350 milligrams:

- ✔ Below 150 milligrams, the drug is very safe (few adverse events), but less than half as effective as it is at higher doses.

- ✔ Between 150 and 300 milligrams, the drug is quite safe (few adverse events) and seems to be fairly effective (a high response rate).

- ✔ Above 300 milligrams, the drug is very effective, but more than 25 percent of the subjects experience side effects and other safety issues.

The "sweet spot" for this drug is probably somewhere around 220 milligrams, where 80 percent of the subjects respond to treatment and the side-effects rate is in the single digits. The actual choice of best dose may have to be thrashed out between clinicians, businesspeople, bioethicists, and other experts, based on a careful examination of all the safety and efficacy data from all the Phase II studies.

The farther apart the two curves are in Figure 6-1, the wider the range of *good doses* (those with high efficacy and low side effects) is. This range is called the *therapeutic range*. But if the two curves are very close together, there may be *no* dose level that delivers the right mix of efficacy and safety. In that case, it's the end of the road for this drug. The majority of drugs never make it past Phase II.

Between the end of Phase II and the beginning of Phase III, you meet again with the FDA, which reviews all your results up to that point and tells you what it considers an acceptable demonstration of safety and efficacy.

Phase III: Proving that the drug works

If Phase II is successful, it means you've found one or two doses for which the drug appears to be safe and effective. Now you take those doses into the final stage of drug testing: Phase III.

Phase III is kind of like the drug's final exam time. It has to put up or shut up, sink or swim, pass or fail. Up to this point, the drug appears to be safe and effective, and you have reason to hope that it's worth the time and expense to continue development. Now the drug team has to convince the FDA — which demands proof at the highest level of scientific rigor — that the drug, in the dose(s) at which you plan to market it, is safe and effective. Depending on what treatments (if any) currently exist for the target condition, you may have to show that your drug is better than a placebo or that it's at least as good as the current best treatment. (You don't have to show that it's *better* than the current treatments. See Chapter 16.)

The term *as good as* can refer to both safety and efficacy. Your new cholesterol medication may not lower cholesterol as much as the current best treatments, but if it's almost completely free of the (sometimes serious) side effects associated with the current treatments, it may be considered just as good or even better.

Usually you need to design and carry out two *pivotal Phase III studies.* In each of these, the drug must meet the criteria agreed upon when you met with the FDA after Phase II.

The pivotal Phase III studies have to be designed with complete scientific rigor, and that includes absolutely rigorous statistical design. You must

- ✔ Use the most appropriate statistical design (as described in Chapter 5).

- ✔ Use the best statistical methods when analyzing the data.

- ✔ Ensure that the sample size is large enough to provide at least 80 or 90 percent power to show significance when testing the efficacy of the drug (see Chapter 3).

If the FDA decided that the drug must prove its efficacy for two different measures of efficacy *(co-primary endpoints),* the study design has to meet even more stringent requirements.

When Phase III is done, your team submits all the safety and efficacy data to the FDA, which thoroughly reviews it and considers how the benefits compare to the risks. Unless something unexpected comes up, the FDA approves the marketing of the drug.

Phase IV: Keeping an eye on the marketed drug

Being able to market the drug doesn't mean you're out of the woods yet! During a drug's development, you've probably given the drug to hundreds or thousands of subjects, and no serious safety concerns have been raised. But if 1,000 subjects have taken the drug without a single catastrophic adverse event, that only means that the rate of these kinds of events is probably less than 1 in 1,000. When your drug hits the market, tens of millions of people may use it; if the true rate of catastrophic events is, for example, 1 in 2,000, then there will be about 5,000 of those catastrophic events in 10 million users. (Does the term *class action lawsuit* come to mind?)

If the least inkling of possible trouble (or a *signal,* in industry jargon) is detected in all the data from the clinical trials, the FDA is likely to call for ongoing monitoring after the drug goes on the market. This process is referred to as a *risk evaluation mitigation strategy* (REMS), and it may entail preparing guides for patients and healthcare professionals that describe the drug's risks.

The FDA also monitors the drug for signs of trouble. Doctors and other health-care professionals submit information to the FDA on spontaneous adverse events they observe in their patients. This system is called the *FDA Adverse Event Reporting System* (FAERS). FAERS has been criticized for relying on voluntary reporting, so the FDA is developing a system that will use existing automated healthcare data from multiple sources.

If a drug is found to have serious side effects, the official package insert may have to be changed to include a warning to physicians about the problem. This printed warning message is surrounded by a black box for emphasis, and is (not surprisingly) referred to as a black-box warning. Such a warning can doom a drug commercially, unless it is the only drug available for a serious condition. And if really serious problems are uncovered in a marketed drug, the FDA can take more drastic actions, including asking the manufacturer to withdraw the drug from the market or even reversing its original approval of the drug.

Holding Other Kinds of Clinical Trials

The Phase I, II, and III clinical trials previously described are part of the standard clinical testing process for every proposed drug; they're intended to demonstrate that the drug is effective and to create the core of what will become an ever-growing body of experience regarding the safety of the drug. In addition, you'll probably carry out several other special-purpose clinical trials during drug development. A few of the most common ones are described in the following sections.

Pharmacokinetics and pharmacodynamics (PK/PD studies)

The term *pharmacokinetics* (PK) refers to the study of how fast and how completely the drug is absorbed into the body (from the stomach and intestines if it's an oral drug); how the drug becomes distributed through the various body tissues and fluids, called *body compartments* (blood, muscle, fatty tissue, cerebrospinal fluid, and so on); to what extent (if any) the drug is *metabolized* (chemically modified) by enzymes produced in the liver and other organs; and how rapidly the drug is excreted from the body (usually via urine, feces, and other routes).

The term *pharmacodynamics* (PD) refers to the study of the relationship between the concentration of the drug in the body and the biological and physiological effects of the drug on the body or on other organisms (bacteria, parasites, and so forth) on or in the body.

Generations of students have remembered the distinction between PK and PD by the following simple description:

- **Pharmacokinetics** is the study of what the *body* does to the *drug*.
- **Pharmacodynamics** is the study of what the *drug* does to the *body*.

It's common during Phase I and II testing to collect blood samples at several time points before and after dosing and analyze them to determine the plasma levels of the drug at those times. This data is the raw material on which PK and PD studies are based. By graphing drug concentration versus time, you can get some ballpark estimates of the drug's basic PK properties: the maximum concentration the drug attains (C_{Max}), the time at which this maximum occurs (t_{Max}), and the area under the concentration-versus-time curve (AUC). And you may also be able to do some rudimentary PD studies from this data — examining the relationship between plasma drug concentrations and measurable physiological responses.

But at some point, you may want (or need) to do a more formal PK/PD study to get detailed, high-quality data on the concentration of the drug and any of its *metabolites* (molecules produced by the action of your body's enzymes on the original drug molecule) in plasma and other parts of the body over a long enough period of time for almost all the drug to be eliminated from the body. The times at which you draw blood (and other specimens) for drug assays (the so-called *sampling time points*) are carefully chosen — they're closely spaced around the expected t_{Max} for the drug and its metabolites (based on the approximate PK results from the earlier trials) and more spread out across the times when nothing of much interest is going on.

A well-designed PK/PD study yields more precise values of the basic PK parameters (C_{Max}, t_{Max}, and AUC) as well as more sophisticated PK parameters, such as the actual rates of absorption and elimination, information about the extent to which the drug is distributed in various body compartments, and information about the rates of creation and elimination of drug metabolites.

A PK/PD study also acquires many other measurements that indicate the drug's effects on the body, often at the same (or nearly the same) sampling time points as for the PK samples. These PD measurements include:

- **Blood and urine sampling for other chemicals that would be affected by the drug:** For example, if your drug were a form of insulin, you'd want to know glucose concentrations as well as concentrations of other chemicals involved in glucose metabolism.

> ✔ **Vital signs:** Blood pressure, heart rate, and perhaps rate of breathing.
>
> ✔ **Electrocardiographs (ECGs):** Tracings of the heart's electrical activity.
>
> ✔ **Other physiological tests:** Lung function, treadmill, and subjective assessments of mood, fatigue, and so on.

Data from PK/PD studies can be analyzed by methods ranging from the very simple (noting the time when the highest blood concentration of the drug was observed) to the incredibly complex (fitting complicated nonlinear models to the concentrations of drug and metabolites in different compartments over time to estimate reaction rate constants, volumes of distribution, and more). I describe some of these complex methods in Chapter 21.

Bioequivalence studies

You may be making a generic drug to compete with a brand-name drug already on the market whose patent has expired. The generic and brand-name drug are the exact same chemical, so it may not seem reasonable to have to go through the entire drug development process for a generic drug. But because there are differences in the other ingredients that go into the drug (such as fillers and coatings), you have to show that your formula is essentially *bioequivalent* to the name-brand drug. *Bioequivalent* means that your generic product puts the same (or nearly the same) amount of the drug's active ingredient into the blood as the brand-name product.

A *bioequivalence study* is usually a fairly simple pharmacokinetic study, having either a parallel or a crossover design (see Chapter 5 for more on design structure). Each subject is given a dose of the product (either the brand-name or generic drug), and blood samples are drawn at carefully chosen time points and analyzed for drug concentration. From this data, the basic PK parameters (AUC, C_{Max}, and so on) are calculated and compared between the brand-name and generic versions. I describe the statistical design and analysis of bioequivalence studies in Chapter 16.

Thorough QT studies

In the mid-1990s it was recognized that certain drugs interfered with the ability of the heart to "recharge" its muscles between beats, which could lead to a particularly life-threatening form of cardiac arrhythmia called *Torsades de Points* (TdP). Fortunately, warning signs of this arrhythmia show up as a distinctive pattern on an electrocardiogram (ECG) well before it progresses to TdP.

You've seen the typical squiggly pattern of an ECG in movies (usually just before it becomes a flat line). Cardiologists have labeled the various peaks and dips on an ECG tracing with consecutive letters of the alphabet, from P through T, like you see in Figure 6-2.

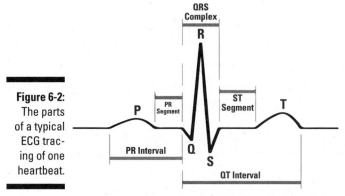

Illustration by Wiley, Composition Services Graphics

That last bump, called the *T-wave,* is the one to look at. It depicts the movement of potassium ions back into the cell (called *repolarization*), getting it ready for the next beat. If repolarization is slowed down, the T-wave will be stretched out. For various reasons, cardiologists measure that stretching out time as the number of milliseconds between the start of the Q wave and the end of the T wave; this is called the *QT interval.*

The QT interval is usually adjusted for heart rate by any of several formulas, resulting in a "corrected" QT interval (*QTc*), which is typically around 400 milliseconds (msec). If a drug prolongs QTc by 50 milliseconds or more, things start to get dicey. Ideally, a drug shouldn't prolong QTc by even 10 milliseconds.

Data from all preclinical and human drug trials are closely examined for the following so-called *signals* that the drug may tend to mess up QTc:

✔ Any *in-silico* or *in-vitro* studies indicate that the drug molecule might mess up ion channels in cell membranes.

✔ Any ECGs (in animals or humans) show signs of QTc prolongation.

✔ Any drugs that are chemically similar to the new drug have produced QT prolongation.

If any such signals are found, the FDA will probably require you to conduct a special *thorough QT trial* (called a *TQT* or *QT/QTc* trial) to determine whether your drug is likely to cause QT prolongation.

A typical TQT may enroll about 100 healthy volunteers and randomize them to receive either the new drug, a placebo, or a drug that's known to prolong QTc by a small amount (this is called a *positive control,* and it's included so that you can make a convincing argument that you'd recognize a QTc prolongation if you saw one). ECGs are taken at frequent intervals after administering the product, clustered especially close together at the times near the expected maximum concentration of the drug and its known metabolites. Each ECG is examined, the QT and heart rate are measured, and the QTc is calculated.

The statistical analysis of a TQT is similar to that of an equivalence trial (which I describe in Chapter 16). You're trying to show that your drug is equivalent to a placebo with respect to QTc prolongation, within some allowable tolerance, which the FDA has decreed to be 10 milliseconds. Follow these steps:

1. **Subtract the QTc of the placebo from the QTc for the drug and for the positive control at the same time point, to get the amount of QTc prolongation at each time point.**

2. **Calculate the 90 percent confidence intervals around the QTc prolongation values, as described in Chapter 10.**

3. **Plot the average differences, along with vertical bars representing the confidence intervals, as shown in Figure 6-3.**

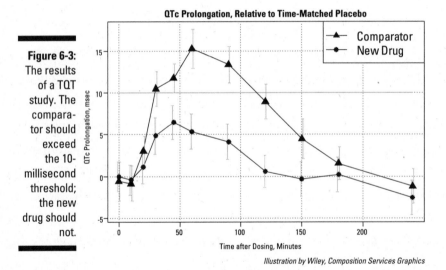

QTc Prolongation, Relative to Time-Matched Placebo

Figure 6-3: The results of a TQT study. The comparator should exceed the 10-millisecond threshold; the new drug should not.

Illustration by Wiley, Composition Services Graphics

To pass the test, the drug's QTc mean prolongation values and their confidence limits must all stay below the 10-millisecond limit. For the positive control drug, the means and their confidence limits should go up; in fact, the confidence limits should lie completely above 0 (that is, there must be a significant increase) at those time points where the control drug is near its peak concentration.

Part II
Getting Down and Dirty with Data

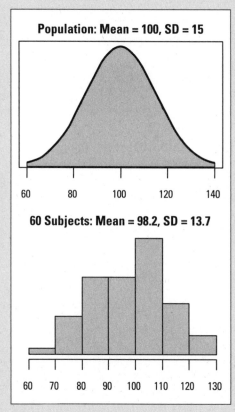

Population: Mean = 100, SD = 15

60 Subjects: Mean = 98.2, SD = 13.7

Illustration by Wiley, Composition Services Graphics

Read about two views of probability — the frequentist view and the Bayesian view — in an article at www.dummies.com/extras/biostatistics.

In this part . . .

- ✔ Collect and validate your data, avoiding common pitfalls upfront that can cause trouble later on.

- ✔ Summarize your data in informative tables and display it in easy-to-understand graphs.

- ✔ Understand the concepts of accuracy and precision. (In a nutshell: *Accuracy* refers to how close a sample statistic tends to come to the corresponding population parameter, and *precision* refers to how close replicate values of a sample statistic are to each other.)

- ✔ Calculate standard errors and confidence intervals for everything you measure, count, or calculate from your data.

Chapter 7

Getting Your Data into the Computer

• •

In This Chapter

▶ Understanding levels of measurement (nominal, ordinal, interval, and ratio)

▶ Defining and entering different kinds of data into your research database

▶ Making sure your data is accurate

▶ Creating a data dictionary to describe the data in your database

• •

*B*efore you can analyze data, you have to collect it and get it into the computer in a form that's suitable for analysis. Chapter 5 describes this process as a series of steps — figuring out what data you need and how it's structured, creating the case report forms (CRFs) and computer files to hold your data, and entering and validating your data.

In this chapter, I describe a crucially important component of that process — storing the data properly in your research data base. Different kinds of data can be represented in the computer in different ways. At the most basic level, there are numbers and categories, and most of us can immediately tell the two apart — you don't have to be a math genius to recognize age as numerical data and gender as categorical info.

So why am I devoting a whole chapter to describing, entering, and checking different types of data? It turns out that the topic of data type is not quite as trivial as it may seem at first — there are some subtleties you should be aware of; otherwise, you may wind up collecting your data the wrong way and finding out too late that you can't run the appropriate analysis on it. Or you may use the wrong statistical technique and get incorrect or misleading results. This chapter explains the different levels of measurements, shows how to define and enter different types of data, suggests ways to check your data for errors, and shows how to formally describe your database so that others are able to work with it if you're not around.

Looking at Levels of Measurement

Around the middle of the 20th century, the idea of levels of measurement caught the attention of biological and social-science researchers, and, in particular, psychologists. One classification scheme, which has become very widely used (at least in statistics textbooks), recognizes four different levels at which variables can be measured: *nominal*, *ordinal*, *interval*, and *ratio*:

- ✓ **Nominal variables** are expressed as mutually exclusive categories, like gender (male or female), race (white, black, Asian, and so forth), and type of bacteria (such as coccus, bacillus, rickettsia, mycoplasma, or spirillum), where the sequence in which you list a variable's different categories is purely arbitrary. For example, listing a choice of races as black, asian, and white is no more or less "natural" than listing them as white, black, and asian.

- ✓ **Ordinal data** has categorical values (or levels) that fall naturally into a logical sequence, like the severity of an adverse event (slight, moderate, or severe), or an agreement scale (strongly disagree, disagree, no opinion, agree, or strongly agree), often called a *Likert scale.* Note that the levels are not necessarily "equally spaced" with respect to the conceptual difference between levels.

- ✓ **Interval data** is a numerical measurement where, unlike ordinal data, the difference (or interval) between two numbers *is* a meaningful measure of the amount of difference in what the variable represents, but the zero point is completely arbitrary and does *not* denote the complete absence of what you're measuring. An example of this concept is the metric Celsius temperature scale. A change from 20 to 25 degrees Celsius represents the same amount of temperature increase as a change from 120 to 125 degrees Celsius. But 0 degrees Celsius is purely arbitrary — it does *not* represent the total absence of temperature; it's simply the temperature at which water freezes (or, if you prefer, ice melts).

- ✓ **Ratio data,** unlike interval data, *does* have a true zero point. The numerical value of a ratio variable is directly proportional to how much there is of what you're measuring, and a value of zero means there's nothing at all. Mass is a ratio measurement, as is the Kelvin temperature scale — it starts at the *absolute zero of temperature* (about 273 degrees below zero on the Celsius scale), where there is no thermal energy at all.

Statisticians tend to beat this topic to death — they love to point out cases that don't fall neatly into one of the four levels and to bring up various counterexamples. But you need to be aware of the concepts and terminology in the preceding list because you'll see them in statistics textbooks and articles, and because teachers love to include them on tests. And, more practically, knowing the level of measurement of a variable can help you choose the most appropriate way to analyze that variable. I make reference to these four levels — nominal, ordinal, interval, and ratio — at various times in this chapter and in the rest of this book.

Classifying and Recording Different Kinds of Data

Although you should be aware of the four levels of measurement described in the preceding section, you also need to be able to classify and deal with data in a more pragmatic way. The following sections describe various common types of data you're likely to encounter in the course of biological or clinical research. I point out some things you need to think through before you start collecting your data.

Few things can mess up a research database, and quite possibly doom a study to eventual failure, more surely than bad decisions (or no decisions) about how to represent the data elements that make up the database. If you collect data the wrong way, it may take an enormous amount of additional effort to go back and get it the right way, if you can retrieve the right data at all.

Dealing with free-text data

It's best to limit *free-text* variables to things like subject comments or write-in fields for *Other* choices in a questionnaire — basically, only those things where you need to record verbatim what someone said or wrote. Don't use free-text fields as a lazy-person's substitute for what should be precisely defined categorical data (which I discuss later in this chapter). Doing any meaningful statistical analysis of free-text fields is generally very difficult, if not impossible.

You should also be aware that most software has field-length limitations for text fields. Current versions of Excel, SPSS, SAS, and so on have very high limits, but other programs (or earlier versions of these programs) may have much lower limits (perhaps 63, 255, or 1,023 characters). Flip to Chapter 4 for an introduction to statistical software.

Assigning subject identification (ID) numbers

Every subject in your study should have a unique *Subject Identifier* (or ID), which is used for recording information, for labeling specimens sent to labs for analysis, and for collecting all a subject's information in the database. In a *single-site study* (one that is carried out at only one geographical location), this ID can usually be a simple number, two to four digits long. It doesn't have to start at 1; it can start at 100 if you want all the ID numbers to be three digits long without leading zeros. In *multi-site studies* (those carried out at several locations, such as different institutions, different clinics, different doctors' offices, and so on), the number often has two parts — a site number and a subject-within-site number, separated by a hyphen, such as 03-104.

Organizing name and address data

A research database usually doesn't need to have the full name or the address of the subject, and sometimes these data elements are prohibited for privacy reasons. But if you do need to store a name (if you anticipate generating mailings like appointment reminders or follow-up letters, for example), use one of the following formats so that you can easily sort subjects into alphabetical order:

- ✔ **A single variable:** Last, First Middle (like Smith, John A)
- ✔ **Two columns:** One for Last, another for First and Middle

You may also want to include separate fields to hold prefixes (Mr., Mrs., Dr., and so on) and suffixes (Jr., III, PhD, and so forth).

Addresses should be stored in separate fields for street, city, state (or province), ZIP code (or comparable postal code), and perhaps country.

Collecting categorical data

Setting up your data collection forms and database tables for categorical data requires more thought than you may expect. Everyone assumes he knows how to record and enter categorical data — you just type what that data is (for example, *Male, White, Diabetes,* or *Headache*), right? Bad assumption! The following sections look at some of the issues you have to deal with.

Carefully coding categories

The first issue is how to "code" the categories (how to represent them in the database). Do you want to enter *Gender* as *Male/Female, M/F, 1* (if male) or *2* (if female), or in some other manner? Most modern statistical software can analyze categorical data with any of these representations, but some older software needs the categories coded as consecutive numbers: *1, 2, 3,* and so on. Some software lets you specify a correspondence between number and text (*1=Male, 2=Female,* for instance); then you can type it in either way, and you can choose to display it in either the numeric or textual form.

Nothing is worse than having to deal with a data set in which *Gender* has been coded as *1* or *2,* with no indication of which is which, when the person who created the file is long gone. So it's probably best to enter the category values as short, meaningful text abbreviations like *M* or *F,* or *Male* or *Female,* which are self-evident and, therefore, self-documenting.

Excel doesn't care what you type in, and this characteristic is one of its biggest drawbacks when it's used as a data repository. You can enter *Gender* as *M* for the first subject, *Male* for the second, *male* for the third, *2* for the fourth, and *m* for the fifth, and Excel couldn't care less. But most statistics programs consider each of these to be a completely different category! Even worse, you may inadvertently type one or more blank spaces before and/or after the text. You may never notice it, but some statistics programs consider *M~* to be different from *~M, ~M~,* and *M~~.* (I use ~ to stand for a blank space.) Therefore, in Excel, it's a good idea to enable AutoComplete for cell values (in the Advanced section of the Options dialog box, located in the File menu). Then when you start typing something in a cell, it suggests something that's already present in that column and begins with the same letter or letters that you typed.

Dealing with more than two levels in a category

When a categorical variable has more than two levels (like the *bacteria type* or *Likert agreement scale* examples I describe in the earlier section "Looking at Levels of Measurement"), things get even more interesting. First, you have to ask yourself, "Is this variable a *Choose only one* or *Choose all that apply* variable?" The coding is completely different for these two kinds of multiple-choice variables.

You handle the *Choose only one* situation just as I describe for *Gender* in the preceding section — you establish a short, meaningful alphabetic code for each alternative. For the *Likert scale* example, you could have a categorical variable called *Attitude,* with five possible values: *SD* (strongly disagree), *D* (disagree), *NO* (no opinion), *A* (agree), and *SA* (strongly agree). And for the *bacteria type* example, if only one kind of bacteria is allowed to be chosen, you can have a categorical variable called *BacType,* with five possible values: *coccus, bacillus, rickettsia, mycoplasma,* and *spirillum.* (Or even better, to reduce the chance of misspellings, you can use short abbreviations such as: *coc, bac, ric, myc,* and *spi.*)

But things are quite different if the variable is *Choose all that apply.* For the *bacteria types* example, if several types of bacteria can be present in the same specimen, you have to set up your database differently. Define separate variables in the database (separate columns in Excel) — one for each possible category value. So you have five variables, perhaps called *BTcoc, BTbac, BTric, BTmyc,* and *BTspi* (the *BT* stands for *bacteria type*). Each variable is a two-value category (perhaps with values *Pres/Abs* — which stand for *present* and *absent* — or *Yes/No,* or *1* or *0*). So, if Subject 101's specimen has coccus, Subject 102's specimen has bacillus and mycoplasma, and Subject 103's specimen has no bacteria at all, the information can be coded as shown in the following table.

Subject	*BTcoc*	*BTbac*	*BTric*	*BTmyc*	*BTspi*
101	Yes	No	No	No	No
102	No	Yes	No	Yes	No
103	No	No	No	No	No

You can handle missing values by leaving the cell blank, but an even better way is to add a category called *Missing* to the regular categories of that variable. If you need several different flavors of *Missing* (like *not collected yet, don't know, other, refused to answer,* or *not applicable*), just add them to the set of permissible levels for that categorical variable. The idea is to make sure that you can always enter something for that variable.

Never try to cram multiple choices into one column — don't enter *coc,bac* into a cell in the *BacType* column. If you do, the resulting column will be almost impossible to analyze statistically, and you'll have to take the time later to painstakingly split your single multi-valued column into separate yes/no columns as I describe earlier. So why not do it right the first time?

Recording numerical data

For numerical data, the main question is how much precision to record. Recording a numerical variable to as many decimals as you have available is usually best. For example, if a scale can measure body weight to the nearest 1/10 of a kilogram, record it in the database to that degree of precision. You can always round off to the nearest kilogram later if you want, but you can never "unround" a number to recover digits you didn't record. Just don't go overboard in this direction — don't record a person's weight as 85.648832 kilograms, even if a digital scale shows it to such ridiculous precision.

Along the same lines, don't group numerical data into intervals when recording it. Don't record *Age* in 10-year intervals (0 to 9, 10 to 19, and so on) if you know the age to the nearest year. You can always have the computer do that kind of grouping later, but you can never recover the age in years if all you record is the decade.

Some programs let you choose between several ways of storing the number in the computer. The program may refer to these different *storage modes* using arcane terms for short, long, or very long *integers* (whole numbers) or *single-precision* (short) or *double-precision* (long) *floating point* (fractional) numbers. Each type has its own limits, which may vary from one program to another or from one kind of computer to another. For example, a short integer might be able to represent only whole numbers within the range from –32,768 to +32,767, whereas a double-precision floating-point number could easily handle a number like $1.23456789012345 \times 10^{250}$. In the old days, the judicious choice of storage modes for your variables could produce smaller files and let the program work with more subjects or more variables. Nowadays, storage is much less of an issue than it used to be, so pinching pennies this way offers little benefit. Go for the most general numeric representation available — usually double-precision floating point, which can represent just about any number you may ever encounter in your research.

Here are a couple things to watch out for with numerical variables in Excel:

✔ Don't put two numbers (such as a blood pressure reading of 135/85 mmHg) into one column of data. Excel won't complain about it, but it will treat it as text because of the embedded "/", rather than as numerical data. Instead, create two separate variables — such as the systolic and diastolic pressures (perhaps called *BPS* for *blood pressure systolic* and *BPD* for *blood pressure diastolic*) — and enter each number into the appropriate variable.

✔ In an obstetrical database, don't enter *6w2d* for a gestational age of 6 weeks and 2 days; even worse, don't enter it as *6.2,* which the computer would interpret as 6.2 weeks. Either enter it as 44 days, or create two variables (perhaps *GAwks* for *gestational age weeks* and *GAdays* for *gestational age days*), to hold the values *6* and *2,* respectively. The computer can easily combine them later into the number of days or the number of weeks (and fractions of a week).

Missing numerical data requires a little more thought than missing categorical data. Some researchers use 99 (or 999, or 9999) to indicate a missing value. If you use that technique, all your analyses will have to ignore those values. Fortunately, many statistics programs let you specify what the missing value indicator is for each variable, and the programs exclude those values from all analyses. But can you *really* be sure you'll *never* have that value pop up as a real value for some very atypical subject? (Some people are 99 years old, and some people can have a blood glucose value of 999 mg/dL). Simply leaving the cell blank may be best; almost all programs treat blank cells as missing data.

Entering date and time data

Now I'm going to tell you something that sounds like I'm contradicting the advice I just gave you (but, of course, I'm not!). Most statistical software can represent dates and times as a single variable (an "instant" on a continuous timeline), so take advantage of that if you can — enter the date and time as one variable (for example, 07/15/2010 08:23), not as a date variable and a time variable. This method is especially useful when dealing with events that take place over a short time interval (like events occurring during labor and delivery).

Most statistical programs store date and time internally as a number, specifying the number of days (and fractions of days) from some arbitrary "zero date." Here are the zero dates for a few common programs:

- ✔ **Excel:** Midnight at the start of December 31, 1899 (this is also the earliest date that Excel can store). So November 21, 2012, at 6:00 p.m., is stored internally as 41,234.75 (the .75 is because 6 p.m. is 3/4 of the way through that day).
- ✔ **SPSS:** October 14, 1582 (the date the Gregorian calendar was adopted to replace the Julian calendar).
- ✔ **SAS:** 01/01/1960 (a totally arbitrary date).

Some programs may store a date and time as a *Julian Date,* whose zero occured at noon, Greenwich mean time, on Jan. 1, 4713 BC. (Nothing happened on that date; it's purely a numerical convenience. See `www.magma.ca/~scarlisl/DRACO/julian_d.html` for an interesting account of this.)

What if you don't know the day of the month? This happens a lot with medical history items; you hear something like "I got the flu in September 2004." Most software insists that a date variable be a complete date and won't accept just a month and a year. In this case, an argument can be made for setting the day to 15 (around mid-month), on the grounds that the error is equally likely to be on either side and therefore tends to cancel out, on average. Similarly, if both the month and day are missing, you can set them to June 30 or July 1 (around mid-year) to achieve the same kind of average error cancellation. If only some records have partial dates, you may want to create another variable to indicate whether the date is complete or partial, so you can tell, if you need to, whether 09/15/2004 really means September 15, 2004, or just September 2004.

Completely missing dates should usually just be left blank; most statistical software treats blank cells as missing data.

Because of the way most statistics programs store dates and times, they can easily calculate intervals between any two points in time by simple subtraction. So it's usually easier and safer to enter dates and times and let the computer calculate the intervals than to calculate them yourself. For example, if you create variables for date of birth (*DOB*) and a visit date (*VisDt*) in Excel, you can often calculate a very accurate *age at the time of the visit* with this formula:

Age = (*VisDt* − *DOB*)/365.25

Similarly, in cancer studies, you can easily and accurately calculate intervals from diagnosis or treatment to remission and recurrence, as well as total survival time, from the dates of the corresponding events.

Checking Your Entered Data for Errors

After you've entered all your data into the computer, there are a few things you can do to check for errors:

- ✔ **Examine the smallest and largest values:** Have the software show you the smallest and largest values for each variable. This check can often catch decimal-point errors (such as a hemoglobin value of 125 g/dL instead of 12.5 g/dL) or transposition errors (for example, a weight of 517 pounds instead of 157 pounds).

- ✔ **Sort the values of variables:** If your program can show you a sorted list of all the values for a variable, that's even better — it often shows misspelled categories as well as numerical outliers.

- ✔ **Search for blanks and commas:** You can have Excel search for blanks in category values that shouldn't have blanks or for commas in numeric variables. Make sure the "Match entire cell contents" option is *deselected* in the Find and Replace dialog box (you may have to click the Options button to see the check box).

- ✔ **Tabulate categorical variables:** You can have your statistics program tabulate each categorical variable (showing you how many times each different category occurred in your data). This check usually finds misspelled categories.

- ✔ **Shrink a spreadsheet's cells:** If you have the PopTools add-in installed in Excel (see Chapter 4), you can use the "Make a map of current sheet" feature, which creates a new worksheet with a miniature view of your data sheet. Each cell in the map sheet is shrunk down to a small square and is color-coded to indicate the type of data in the cell — character, numeric, formula, or blank. With this view, you can often spot typing errors that have turned a numeric variable into text (like a comma instead of a decimal point, or two decimal points).

Chapter 8 describes some other ways you can check for unreasonable data.

Creating a File that Describes Your Data File

Every research database, large or small, simple or complicated, should be accompanied by a *data dictionary* that describes the variables contained in the database. It will be invaluable if the person who created the database is no longer around. A data dictionary is, itself, a data file, containing one record for every variable in the database. For each variable, the dictionary should contain most of the following information (sometimes referred to as *metadata,* which means "data about data"):

- **A short variable name** (usually no more than eight or ten characters) that's used when telling the software what variables you want it to use in an analysis

- **A longer verbal description of the variable** (up to 50 or 100 characters)

- **The type of data** (text, categorical, numerical, date/time, and so on)

  - **If numeric:** Information about how that number is displayed (how many digits are before and after the decimal point)

  - **If date/time:** How it's formatted (for example, 12/25/13 10:50pm or 25Dec2013 22:50)

  - **If categorical:** What the permissible categories are

- **How missing values are represented** in the database (99, 999, "NA," and so on)

Many statistical packages allow (or require) you to specify this information when you're creating the file anyway, so they can generate the data dictionary for you automatically. But Excel lets you enter anything anywhere, without formally defining variables, so you need to create the dictionary yourself (perhaps as another worksheet — which you can call "Data Dictionary" — in the same Excel file that has the data, so that the data dictionary always stays with the data).

Chapter 8

Summarizing and Graphing Your Data

· ·

In This Chapter

▶ Representing categorical data

▶ Characterizing numerical variables

▶ Putting numerical summaries into tables

▶ Displaying numerical variables with bars and graphs

· ·

A large study can involve thousands of subjects, hundreds of different variables, and millions of individual pieces of data. Even a small research project normally generates much more data than you can (or would want to) put into a publication or report. Instead, you need to boil the individual values for each variable down to a few numbers, called *summary statistics,* that give readers an idea of what the whole collection of numbers looks like — that is, how they're *distributed*.

When presenting your results, you may want to arrange these summary statistics into tables that describe how the variables change over time or differ between treatments, or how two or more variables are related to each other. And, because a picture really is worth a thousand words, you probably want to display these distributions, changes, differences, and relationships graphically.

In this chapter, I show you how to summarize and graph two types of data: categorical and numerical. ***Note:*** This chapter doesn't cover *time-to-event* (survival) data. That topic is so important, and the methods for summarizing and charting survival data are so specialized, that I describe them in a chapter all their own — Chapter 22.

Summarizing and Graphing Categorical Data

A categorical variable is summarized in a fairly straightforward way. You just tally the number of subjects in each category and express this number as a count — and perhaps also as a percentage of the total number of subjects in all categories combined. So, for example, a sample of 422 subjects can be summarized by race, as shown in Table 8-1.

Table 8-1	Study Subjects Categorized by Race	
Race	*Count*	*Percent of Total*
White	128	30.3%
Black	141	33.4%
Asian	70	16.6%
Other	83	19.7%
Total	**422**	**100%**

The joint distribution of subjects between two categorical variables (such as Race by Gender), is summarized by a *cross-tabulation* ("cross-tab"), as shown in Table 8-2.

Table 8-2	Cross-Tabulation of Subjects by Two Categorical Variables				
	White	*Black*	*Asian*	*Other*	*Total*
Male	60	60	34	42	196
Female	68	81	36	41	226
Total	128	141	70	83	422

A cross-tab can get very cluttered if you try to include percentages. And there are three different kinds of percentage for each count in a cross-tab. For example, the 60 white males in Table 8-2 comprise 46.9 percent of all white subjects, 30.6 percent of all males, and 14.2 percent of all subjects.

Categorical data is usually displayed graphically as frequency bar charts and as pie charts:

- ✔ **Frequency bar charts:** Displaying the spread of subjects across the different categories of a variable is most easily done by a bar chart (see Figure 8-1a). To create a bar chart manually from a tally of subjects in each category, you draw a graph containing one vertical bar for each category, making the height proportional to the number of subjects in that category. But almost all statistical programs will prepare bar charts for you; you simply select the options you want, such as which categorical variable you want to display and whether you want the vertical axis to show counts or percent of total.

- ✔ **Pie charts:** Pie charts indicate the relative number of subjects in each category by the angle of a circular wedge (a piece of the pie). To create a pie chart manually, you multiply the percent of subjects in each category by 360 (the number of degrees of arc in a full circle), and then divide by 100. You draw a circle with a compass and then split it up into wedges using a protractor (remember those drawing tools from high school?). Much better to have the computer make a pie chart for you — it's no more difficult than having a program make a bar chart.

But comparing the relative magnitude of the different sections of a pie chart is more difficult than comparing bar heights. Can you tell at a glance from Figure 8-1b whether there are more whites or blacks? Or more Asians than "others"? You can make those distinctions immediately from Figure 8-1a. Pie charts are often used to present data to the public (perhaps because the "piece of the pie" metaphor is so intuitive), but they're frowned upon in technical publications.

Many programs let you generate so-called "3D" charts. However, these charts are often drawn with a slanting perspective that renders them almost impossible to interpret, so avoid 3D charts when presenting your data.

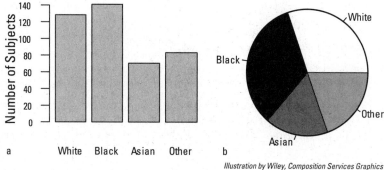

Figure 8-1: A simple bar chart (a) and pie chart (b).

Illustration by Wiley, Composition Services Graphics

Summarizing Numerical Data

Summarizing a numerical variable isn't as simple as summarizing a categorical variable. The summary statistics for a numerical variable should convey, in a concise and meaningful way, how the individual values of that variable are distributed across your sample of subjects, and should give you some idea of the shape of the true distribution of that variable in the population from which you draw your sample. That true distribution can have almost any shape, including the typical shapes shown in Figure 8-2: normal, skewed, pointy-topped, and *bimodal* (two-peaked).

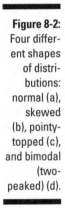

Figure 8-2:
Four different shapes of distributions: normal (a), skewed (b), pointy-topped (c), and bimodal (two-peaked) (d).

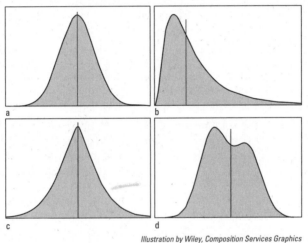

Illustration by Wiley, Composition Services Graphics

How can you convey a general picture of what the true distribution may be using just a few summary numbers? Frequency distributions have some important characteristics, including:

✔ **Center:** Where do the numbers tend to center?

✔ **Dispersion:** How much do the numbers spread out?

✔ **Symmetry:** Is the distribution shaped the same on the left and right sides, or does it have a wider tail on one side than the other?

✔ **Shape:** Is the top of the distribution nicely rounded, or pointier or flatter?

You need to come up with numbers that measure each of these four characteristics; the following sections give you the scoop. (I explain how to graph numerical data later in this chapter.)

Locating the center of your data

Perhaps the most important single thing you want to know about a set of numbers is what value they tend to center around. This characteristic is called, intuitively enough, *central tendency.* Many statistical textbooks describe three measures of central tendency: *mean, median,* and *mode.* These measures don't make a particularly good "top-three" list when it comes to describing experimental data because such a list omits several measures that are quite useful and important, and includes one that's pretty lousy, as I explain in the following sections.

Arithmetic mean

The *arithmetic mean,* also commonly called the *mean,* or the *average,* is the most familiar and most often quoted measure of central tendency. Throughout this book, whenever I use the two-word term *the mean,* I'm referring to the arithmetic mean. (There are several other kinds of means, besides the arithmetic mean, and I describe them later in this chapter.)

The mean of a sample is often denoted by the symbol m or by placing a horizontal bar over the name of the variable, like $\overline{X}$. The mean is obtained by adding up the values and dividing by how many there are. Here's a small sample of numbers — the IQ values of seven subjects, arranged in increasing numerical order: 84, 84, 89, 91, 110, 114, and 116. For the IQ sample:

Arithmetic Mean = (84 + 84 + 89 + 91 + 110 + 114 + 116)/7
= 688/7 = 98.3 (approximately)

You can write the general formula for the arithmetic mean of N number of values contained in the variable X in several ways:

$$\text{Arithmetic Mean} = m = \overline{X} = \frac{\sum_{i=1}^{N} X_i}{N} = \frac{\sum_i X_i}{N} = \frac{\sum X}{N}$$

See Chapter 2 for a refresher on mathematical notation and formulas, including how to interpret the various forms of the summation symbol Σ (the Greek capital sigma). In the rest of this chapter, I use the simplest form (without the i subscripts that refer to specific elements of an array) whenever possible.

Median

Like the mean (see the preceding section), the *median* is a common measure of central tendency (and, in fact, is the only one that really takes the word *central* seriously).

The median of a sample is the middle value in the sorted (ordered) set of numbers. Half the numbers are smaller than the median, and half of them are larger. The median of a *population* frequency distribution function (like the curves shown in Figure 8-2) divides the total area under the curve into two equal parts: half of the *area under the curve* (AUC) lies to the left of the median, and half lies to the right.

The median of the IQ sample from the preceding section (84, 84, 89, 91, 110, 114, and 116) is the fourth of the seven sorted values, which is 91. Three IQs in the sample are smaller than 91, and three are larger than 91. If you have an even number of values, the median is the average of the two middle values.

The median is much less strongly influenced by extreme outliers than the mean. For example, if the largest value in the IQ example had been 150 instead of 116, the mean would have jumped from 98.3 to 103.1, but the median would have remained unchanged at 91. Here's an even more extreme example: If a multibillionaire were to move into a certain state, the *mean* family net worth in that state might rise by hundreds of dollars, but the *median* family net worth would probably rise by only a few cents (if it were to rise at all).

Mode

The *mode* of a sample of numbers is the most frequently occurring value in the sample. The mode is, quite frankly, of very little use for summarizing observed values for continuous numerical variables, for several reasons:

- ✔ If the data were truly continuous (and recorded to many decimal places), there would probably be no exact duplicates, and there would be no mode for the sample.

- ✔ Even when dealing with data that's rounded off to fairly coarse intervals, the mode may not be anywhere near the "center" of the data. In the IQ example, the only value that occurs more than once happens to be the lowest value (84), which is a terrible indicator of central tendency.

- ✔ There could be several different values in your data that occur multiple times, and therefore several modes.

So the mode is not a good summary statistic for sampled data. But it's very useful for characterizing a *population* distribution. It's the place where the peak of the distribution function occurs. Some distribution functions can have two peaks (a *bimodal* distribution), as shown in Figure 8-3d, which often indicates two distinct subpopulations, such as the distribution of a sex hormone in a mixed population of males and females. Some variables can have a distribution with three or even more peaks in certain populations.

Considering some other "means" to measure central tendency

Several other kinds of means are useful measures of central tendency in certain circumstances. They're called *means* because they all involve the same "add them up and divide by how many" process as the arithmetic mean (which I describe earlier in this chapter), but each one adds a slightly different twist to the basic process.

Inner mean

The *inner mean* (also called the *trimmed mean*) of N numbers is calculated by removing the lowest value and the highest value and calculating the arithmetic mean of the remaining $N - 2$ "inner" values. For the IQ example that I use earlier in this chapter (84, 84, 89, 91, 110, 114, and 116), the inner mean equals $(84 + 89 + 91 + 110 + 114)/5 = 488/5 = 97.6$.

An even "inner-er" mean can be calculated by dropping the two (or more) highest and two (or more) lowest values from the data and then calculating the arithmetic mean of the remaining values. In the interest of fairness, you should always chop the same number of values from the low end as from the high end.

Like the median (which I discuss earlier in this chapter), the inner mean is more resistant to outliers than the arithmetic mean. And, if you think about it, if you chop off enough numbers from both ends of the sorted set of values, you'll eventually be left with only the middle one or two values — this "inner-est" mean would actually be the median!

Geometric mean

The *geometric mean* (often abbreviated GM) can be defined by two different-looking formulas that produce exactly the same value. The basic definition has this formula:

$$\text{Geometric Mean} = GM = \sqrt[N]{\Pi X}$$

I describe the product symbol Π (the Greek capital pi) in Chapter 2. This formula is telling you to multiply the values of the N observations together, and then take the Nth root of the product. The IQ example (84, 84, 89, 91, 110, 114, and 116) looks like this:

$$GM = \sqrt[7]{84 \times 84 \times 89 \times 91 \times 110 \times 114 \times 116} = \sqrt[7]{83{,}127{,}648{,}764{,}160} = 93.4$$

This formula can be difficult to evaluate; even computers can run into trouble with the very large product that calculating the GM of a lot of numbers can generate. By using logarithms (which turn multiplications into additions and roots into divisions), you get a "numerically stable" alternative formula:

$$\log(GM) = \frac{\sum \log(X)}{N}, \text{ or } GM = \text{antilog}\left(\frac{\sum \log(X)}{N}\right)$$

This formula may look complicated, but it really just says, "The geometric mean is the *antilog* of the *mean* of the *logs* of the numbers." You take the log of each number, average all those logs the usual way, and then take the anti-log of the average. You can use natural or common logarithms; just be sure to use the same type of antilog. (Flip to Chapter 2 for the basics of logarithms.)

Root-mean-square

The *root-mean-square* (RMS) of a bunch of numbers is defined this way:

$$RMS = \sqrt{\frac{\sum(X^2)}{N}}$$

You square each number, average all those squares the usual way, and then take the square root of the average. For example, the RMS of the two numbers 10 and 20 is $\sqrt{(10^2 + 20^2)/2} = \sqrt{(100+400)/2} = \sqrt{500/2} = \sqrt{250} = 15.81$. The RMS is useful for summarizing the size of random fluctuations, as you see in the later section "Standard deviation, variance, and coefficient of variation."

Describing the spread of your data

After central tendency (see the previous sections), the second most important thing you can say about a set of numbers is how tightly or loosely they tend to cluster around a central value; that is, how narrowly or widely they're *dispersed.* There are several common measures of dispersion, as you find out in the following sections.

Standard deviation, variance, and coefficient of variation

The *standard deviation* (usually abbreviated *SD, sd,* or just *s*) of a bunch of numbers tells you how much the individual numbers tend to differ (in either direction) from the mean (which I discuss earlier in this chapter). It's calculated as follows:

$$SD = sd = s = \sqrt{\frac{\sum_i (d_i)^2}{N-1}}, \text{ where } d_i = X_i - \overline{X}$$

This formula is saying that you calculate the standard deviation of a set of N numbers (X_i) by subtracting the mean from each value to get the *deviation* (d_i) of each value from the mean, squaring each of these deviations, adding up the d_i^2 terms, dividing by $N-1$, and then taking the square root.

This is almost the formula for the root-mean-square deviation of the points from the mean, except that it has $N-1$ in the denominator instead of N. This difference occurs because the sample mean is used as an approximation of the true population mean (which you don't know). If the true mean were available to use, the denominator would be N.

When talking about population distributions, the SD describes the width of the distribution curve. Figure 8-3 shows three normal distributions. They all have a mean of zero, but they have different standard deviations and, there-fore, different widths. Each distribution curve has a total area of exactly 1.0, so the peak height is smaller when the SD is larger.

Figure 8-3: Three dis-tributions with the same mean but different standard deviations.

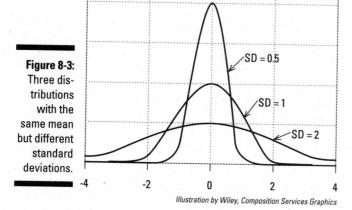

Illustration by Wiley, Composition Services Graphics

For the IQ example that I use earlier in this chapter (84, 84, 89, 91, 110, 114, and 116) where the mean is 98.3, you calculate the SD as follows:

$$SD = \sqrt{\frac{(84-98.3)^2 + (84-98.3)^2 + ... + (116-98.3)^2}{7-1}} = 14.4$$

Standard deviations are very sensitive to extreme values (outliers) in the data. For example, if the highest value in the IQ dataset had been 150 instead of 116, the SD would have gone up from 14.4 to 23.9.

Several other useful measures of dispersion are related to the SD:

- **Variance:** The *variance* is just the square of the SD. For the IQ example, the variance = 14.4^2 = 207.36.

- **Coefficient of variation:** The *coefficient of variation* (CV) is the SD divided by the mean. For the IQ example, CV = 14.4/98.3 = 0.1465, or 14.65 percent.

Range

The *range* of a set of values is the difference between the smallest value (the *minimum* value) and the largest value (the *maximum* value):

Range = maximum value − minimum value

So for the IQ example in the preceding section (84, 84, 89, 91, 110, 114, and 116), the minimum value is 84, the maximum value is 116, and the range is 32 (equal to 116 – 84).

The range is *extremely* sensitive to outliers. If the largest IQ were 150 instead of 116, the range would increase from 32 to 66 (equal to 150 – 84).

Outside of its formal definition in statistics, the term *range* can also refer to two numbers marking the limits of some interval of interest. For example, suppose that a clinical trial protocol (see Chapter 5) specifies that you're to enroll only subjects having glucose values within the range 150 to 250 milligrams per deciliter. You may ask whether a subject with a value of exactly 250 falls "within" that range. This possible ambiguity is usually avoided by using the term *inclusive* or *exclusive* to specify whether a person who is exactly at the limit of a range is considered within it or not. Some ranges can be inclusive at one end and exclusive at the other end.

Centiles

The basic idea of the median (that half of your numbers are less than the median) can be extended to other fractions besides ½.

A *centile* is a value that a certain percentage of the values are less than. For example, ¼ of the values are less than the 25th centile (and ¾ of the values are greater). The median is just the 50th centile. Some centiles have common nicknames:

- ✔ The 25th, 50th, and 75th centiles are called the first, second, and third *quartiles,* respectively.
- ✔ The 20th, 40th, 60th, and 80th centiles are called *quintiles.*
- ✔ The 10th, 20th, 30th, and so on, up to the 90th centile, are called *deciles.*
- ✔ Other Latin-based nicknames include *tertiles, sextiles,* and so forth.

As I explain in the earlier section "Median," if the sorted sequence has no middle value, you have to calculate the median as the average of the two middle numbers. The same situation comes up in calculating centiles, but it's not as simple as just averaging the two closest numbers; there are at least eight different formulas for estimating centiles. Your statistical software may pick one of the formulas (and may not tell you which one it picked), or it may let you choose the formula you prefer. Fortunately, the different formulas usually give nearly the same result.

The *inter-quartile range* (or IQR) is the difference between the 25th and 75th centiles (the first and third quartiles). When summarizing data from strangely shaped distributions, the median and IQR are often used instead of the mean and SD.

Showing the symmetry and shape of the distribution

In the following sections, I discuss two summary statistical measures that are used to describe certain aspects of the symmetry and shape of the distribution of numbers.

Skewness

Skewness refers to whether the distribution has left-right symmetry (as shown in Figures 8-2a and 8-2c) or whether it has a longer tail on one side or the other (as shown in Figures 8-2b and 8-2d). Many different *skewness coefficients* have been proposed over the years; the most common one, often represented by the Greek letter γ (lowercase gamma), is calculated by averaging the cubes (third powers) of the deviations of each point from the mean and scaling by the standard deviation. Its value can be positive, negative, or zero.

A negative skewness coefficient (γ) indicates left-skewed data (long left tail); a zero γ indicates unskewed data; and a positive γ indicates right-skewed data (long right tail), as shown in Figure 8-4.

Figure 8-4: Distributions can be left-skewed (a), symmetric (b), or right-skewed (c).

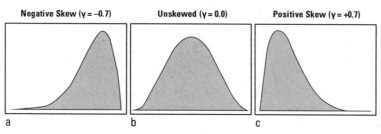

Negative Skew (γ = –0.7)   Unskewed (γ = 0.0)   Positive Skew (γ = +0.7)

a   b   c

Illustration by Wiley, Composition Services Graphics

Of course, the skewness coefficient for any set of real data almost never comes out to exactly zero because of random sampling fluctuations. So how large does γ have to be before you suspect real skewness in your data? A *very rough* rule of thumb for large samples is that if γ is greater than $4/\sqrt{N}$, your data is probably skewed.

Kurtosis

The three distributions shown in Figure 8-5 happen to have the same mean and the same standard deviation, and all three have perfect left-right symmetry (that is, they are *unskewed*). But their shapes are still very different. *Kurtosis* is a way of quantifying these differences in shape.

REMEMBER

If you think of a typical distribution function curve as having a "head" (near the center), "shoulders" (on either side of the head), and "tails" (out at the ends), the term *kurtosis* refers to whether the distribution curve tends to have

- ✔ A pointy head, fat tails, and no shoulders (*leptokurtic*, κ < 3, as shown in Figure 8-5a)

- ✔ Normal appearance (κ = 3; see Figure 8-5b)

- ✔ Broad shoulders, small tails, and not much of a head (*platykurtic*, κ > 3, as shown in Figure 8-5c)

The *Pearson kurtosis index,* often represented by the Greek letter κ (lower-case kappa), is calculated by averaging the fourth powers of the deviations of each point from the mean and scaling by the standard deviation. Its value can range from 1 to infinity and is equal to 3.0 for a normal distribution. The *excess kurtosis* is the amount by which κ exceeds (or falls short of) 3. A *very rough* rule of thumb for large samples is that if κ differs from 3 by more than $8/\sqrt{N}$, your data probably has abnormal kurtosis.

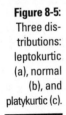
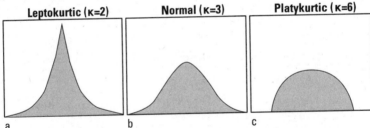

Figure 8-5:
Three distributions: leptokurtic (a), normal (b), and platykurtic (c).

Leptokurtic (κ=2)   Normal (κ=3)   Platykurtic (κ=6)

a   b   c

Illustration by Wiley, Composition Services Graphics

Structuring Numerical Summaries into Descriptive Tables

Now you know how to calculate the basic summary statistics that convey a general idea of how a set of numbers is distributed. So what do you do with those summary numbers? Generally, when presenting your results, you pick a few of the most useful summary statistics and arrange them in a concise way. Many biostatistical reports select N, mean, SD, median, minimum, and maximum, and arrange them something like this:

mean ± SD (N)

median (minimum – maximum)

For the IQ example that I use earlier in this chapter (84, 84, 89, 91, 110, 114, and 116), the preceding arrangement looks like this:

98.3 ± 14.4 (7)

91 (84 – 116)

The real utility of this kind of compact summary is that you can place it in each cell of a table to show changes over time and between groups. For example, systolic blood pressure measurements, before and after treatment with a hypertension drug or a placebo, can be summarized very concisely, as shown in Table 8-3.

Table 8-3	Systolic Blood Pressure Treatment Results	
	Drug	*Placebo*
Before Treatment	138.7 ± 10.3 (40)	141.0 ± 10.8 (40)
	139.5 (117 – 161)	143.5 (111 – 160)
After Treatment	121.1 ± 13.9 (40)	141.0 ± 15.4 (40)
	121.5 (85 – 154)	142.5 (100 – 166)
Change	-17.6 ± 8.0 (40)	-0.1 ± 9.9 (40)
	-17.5 ($-34 - 4$)	1.5 ($-25 - 18$)

This table shows that the drug tended to lower blood pressure by about 18 millimeters of mercury (mmHg), from 139 to 121, whereas the placebo produced no noticeable change in blood pressure (it stayed around 141 mmHg). All that's missing are some p values to indicate the *significance* of the changes over time within each group and of the differences between the groups. I show you how to calculate those in Chapter 12.

Graphing Numerical Data

Displaying information graphically is a central part of interpreting and communicating the results of scientific research. You can easily spot subtle features in a graph of your data that you'd never notice in a table of numbers. Entire books have been written about graphing numerical data, so I can only give a brief summary of some of the more important points here.

Showing the distribution with histograms

Histograms are bar charts that show what fraction of the subjects have values falling within specified intervals. The main purpose of a histogram is to show you how the values of a numerical value are distributed. This distribution is an approximation of the true population frequency distribution for that variable, as shown in Figure 8-6.

The smooth curve in Figure 8-6a shows how IQ values are distributed in an infinitely large population. The height of the curve at any IQ value is proportional to the fraction of the population in the immediate vicinity of that IQ. This curve has the typical "bell" shape of a normal distribution. In the following sections, I explain how histograms are useful when dealing with several types of non-normal distributions.

Figure 8-6:
Population distribution of IQ scores (a) and distribution of a sample from that population (b).

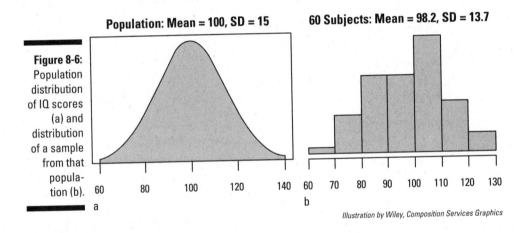

Population: Mean = 100, SD = 15   60 Subjects: Mean = 98.2, SD = 13.7

a   b

Illustration by Wiley, Composition Services Graphics

The histogram in Figure 8-6b indicates how the IQs of 60 subjects randomly sampled from the population might be distributed. Each bar represents an interval of IQ values with a width of ten IQ points, and the height of each bar is proportional to the number of subjects in the sample whose IQ fell within that interval.

Log-normal distributions

Because a sample is only an imperfect representation the population, determining the precise shape of a distribution can be difficult unless your sample size is very large. Nevertheless, a histogram usually helps you spot skewed data, as shown in Figure 8-7a. This kind of shape is typical of a *log-normal* distribution, which occurs very often in biological work (see Chapter 25). It's called *log-normal* because if you take the logarithm of each data value (it doesn't matter what kind of logarithm you take), the resulting logs will have a normal distribution, as shown in Figure 8-7b.

So it's good practice to prepare a histogram for every numerical variable you plan to analyze, to see whether it's noticeably skewed and, if so, whether a logarithmic "transformation" makes the distribution more nearly normal.

Other abnormal distributions

Log-normality isn't the only kind of non-normality that can arise in real-world data. Depending on the underlying process that gives rise to the data, the numbers can be distributed in other ways. For example, event counts often behave according to the Poisson distribution (see Chapter 25) and can be, at least approximately, normalized by taking the square root of each count (instead of the logarithm, as you do for log-normal data). Still other processes can give rise to left-skewed data or to data with two (or more) peaks.

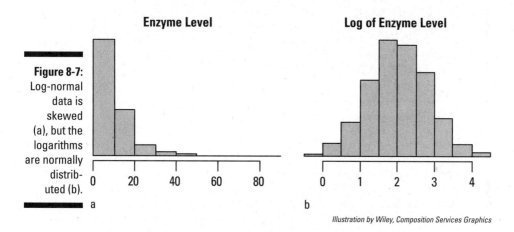

Figure 8-7: Log-normal data is skewed (a), but the logarithms are normally distributed (b).

a   b

Illustration by Wiley, Composition Services Graphics

What if neither the log-normal nor the square-root transformation normalizes your skewed data? One approach is to use the *Box-Cox* transformation, which has this general formula: Transformed $X = (X^A - 1)/A$, where A is an adjustable parameter that you can vary from negative to positive values. Depending on the value of A, this transformation can often make left-skewed or right-skewed data more symmetrical (and more normally distributed). Figure 8-8 shows how the Box-Cox transformation can help normalize skewed data. Some software lets you vary A through a range of positive or negative values using a slider on the screen that you can move with your mouse. As you slide the A value back and forth, you see the histogram change its shape from left-skewed to symmetrical to right-skewed. In Figure 8-8, using $A = 0.12$ normalizes the data quite well.

When A is exactly 0, the Box-Cox formula becomes 0/0, which is indeterminate. But it can be shown that as A approaches 0 (either from the positive or negative side), the Box-Cox formula becomes the same as the logarithm function. So the logarithmic transformation is just a special case of the more general Box-Cox transformation.

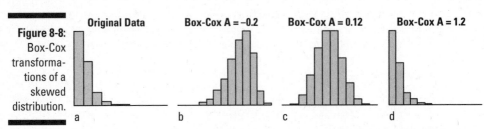

Figure 8-8:
Box-Cox
transforma-
tions of a
skewed
distribution.

Illustration by Wiley, Composition Services Graphics

If you can't find any transformation that makes your data look even approximately normal, then you have to analyze your data using *nonparametric* methods, which don't assume that your data is normally distributed. I describe these methods in Chapter 12.

Summarizing grouped data with bars, boxes, and whiskers

Sometimes you want to show how a variable varies from one group of subjects to another. For example, blood levels of some enzymes vary among the different races. Two types of graphs are commonly used for this purpose: bar charts and box-and-whiskers plots.

Bar charts

One simple way to display and compare the means of several groups of data is with a bar chart, like the one shown in Figure 8-9a, where the bar height for each race equals the mean (or median, or geometric mean) value of the enzyme level for that race. And the bar chart becomes even more informative if you indicate the spread of values for each race by placing lines representing one standard deviation above and below the tops of the bars, as shown in Figure 8-9b. These lines are always referred to as *error bars* (an unfortunate choice of words that can cause confusion when error bars are added to a bar chart).

But even with error bars, a bar chart still doesn't give a very good picture of the *distribution* of enzyme levels within each group. Are the values skewed? Are there outliers? The mean and SD may not be very informative if the values are distributed log-normally or in another unusual way. Ideally, you want to show a histogram for each group of subjects (I discuss histograms earlier in this chapter), but that may take up way too much space. What should you do? Keep reading to find out.

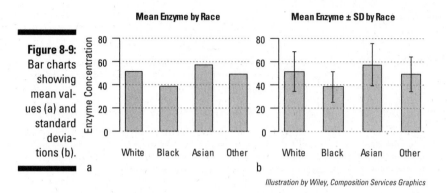

Figure 8-9: Bar charts showing mean values (a) and standard deviations (b).

Illustration by Wiley, Composition Services Graphics

Box-and-whiskers charts

Fortunately, another kind of graph called a *box-and-whiskers plot* (or *B&W*, or just *Box plot*) shows — in very little space — a lot of information about the distribution of numbers in one or more groups of subjects. A simple B&W plot of the same enzyme data illustrated with a bar chart in Figure 8-9 is shown in Figure 8-10a.

The B&W figure for each group usually has the following parts:

- ✔ A box spanning the interquartile range (IQR), extending from the first quartile (25th centile) to the third quartile (75th centile) of the data (see the earlier section "Centiles" for more about this range), and therefore encompassing the middle 50 percent of the data

- ✔ A thick horizontal line, drawn at the median (50th centile), which usually puts it at or near the middle of the box

- ✔ Dashed lines (whiskers) extending out to the farthest data point that's not more than 1.5 times the IQR away from the box

- ✔ Individual points lying outside the whiskers, considered outliers

B&W plots provide a useful summary of the distribution. A median that's not located near the middle of the box indicates a skewed distribution.

Some software draws the different parts of a B&W plot according to different rules (the horizontal line may be at the mean instead of the median; the box may represent the mean ± 1 standard deviation; the whiskers may extend out to the farthest outliers; and so on). Always check the software's documentation and provide the description of the parts whenever you present a B&W plot.

Some software provides various enhancements to the basic B&W plot. Figure 8-10b illustrates two such embellishments you may consider using:

- **Variable width:** The widths of the bars can be scaled to indicate the relative size of each group. You can see that there are considerably fewer Asians and "others" than whites or blacks.

- **Notches:** The box can have notches that indicate the uncertainty in the estimation of the median. If two groups have non-overlapping notches, they probably have significantly different medians. Whites and "others" have similar median enzyme levels, whereas Asians have significantly higher levels and blacks have significantly lower levels.

Figure 8-10:
Box-and-whiskers charts: no-frills (a) and with variable width and notches (b).

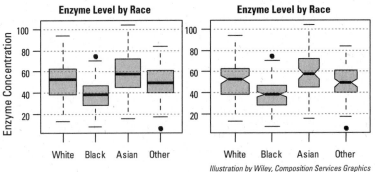

Illustration by Wiley, Composition Services Graphics

Depicting the relationships between numerical variables with other graphs

One of the most important uses for graphs in scientific publications is to show the relationship between two or more numerical variables, such as the associations described in these example questions:

- Is there an association between Hemoglobin A1c (an indicator of diabetes) and Body Mass Index (an indicator of obesity)?

- Is the reduction in blood pressure associated with the administered dose of an antihypertensive drug (in other words, is there a dose-response effect)?

These questions are usually answered with the help of regression analysis, which I describe in Part IV and Chapter 24. In these chapters, I cover the appropriate graphical techniques for showing relationships between variables.

Chapter 9

Aiming for Accuracy and Precision

· ·

In This Chapter

▶ Starting with accuracy and precision fundamentals

▶ Boosting accuracy and precision

▶ Determining standard errors for a variety of statistics

· ·

A very wise scientist once said, "A measurement whose accuracy is completely unknown has no use whatever." Whenever you're reporting a numerical result (and as a researcher, you report numerical results all the time), you must include, along with the numerical value, some indication of how good that value is. A good numeric result is both *accurate* and *precise*. In this chapter, I describe what accuracy and precision are, how you can improve the accuracy and precision of your results, and how you can express quantitatively just how precise your results are.

Beginning with the Basics of Accuracy and Precision

Before you read any further, make sure you've looked at the "Statistical Estimation Theory" section of Chapter 3, which gives an example introducing the concepts of *accuracy* and *precision* and the difference between them. In a nutshell: *Accuracy* refers to how close your numbers come to the *true* values; *precision* refers to how close your numbers come to *each other*. In this section, I define *accuracy* and *precision* more formally in terms of concepts like *sample statistic*, *population parameter*, and *sampling distribution*.

Getting to know sample statistics and population parameters

Scientists conduct experiments on limited *samples* of subjects in order to draw conclusions that (they hope) are valid for a large *population* of people. Suppose you want to conduct an experiment to determine some quantity of interest. For example, you may have a scientific interest in one of these questions:

✔ What is the average fasting blood glucose concentration in adults with diabetes?

✔ What percent of children like chocolate?

✔ How much does blood urea nitrogen (BUN) tend to increase (or decrease) with every additional year after age 60?

To get *exact* answers to questions like these, you'd have to examine every adult diabetic, or every child, or every person over age 60. But you can't examine every person in the population; you have to study a relatively small sample of subjects, in a clinical trial or a survey.

The numeric result that you get from your sample (such as average glucose, the percent of children who like chocolate, or the BUN increase per year) is called a *sample statistic,* and it's your best guess for the value of the corresponding *population parameter,* which is the true value of that average or percent or yearly increase in the entire population. Because of random sampling fluctuations, the sample statistic you get from your study isn't exactly equal to the corresponding population parameter. Statisticians express this unavoidable discrepancy in terms of two concepts: *accuracy* and *precision.* To many people these two terms mean the same thing, but to a statistician they're very different (as you find out in the following section).

Understanding accuracy and precision in terms of the sampling distribution

Imagine a scenario in which an experiment (like a clinical trial or a survey) is carried out over and over again an enormous number of times, each time on a different random sample of subjects. Using the "percent of kids who like chocolate" example, each experiment could consist of interviewing 50 randomly chosen children and reporting what percentage of kids in that sample said that they liked chocolate. Repeating that entire experiment N times (and supposing that N is up in the millions) would require a lot of scientists, take a lot of time, and cost a lot of money, but suppose that you could actually do it. For each repetition of the experiment, you'd get some particular value for the sample statistic you were interested in (the percent of kids in that sample who like chocolate), and you'd write this number down on a (really big) piece of paper.

After conducting your experiment N times, you'd have a huge set of values for the sampling statistic (that is, the percent of kids who like chocolate). You could then calculate the mean of those values by adding them up and dividing by N. And you could calculate the standard deviation by subtracting the mean from each value, squaring each difference, adding up the squares, dividing by $N - 1$, and then taking the square root. And you could construct a histogram of the N percentage values to see how they were spread out, as described in Chapter 8.

Statisticians describe this in a more formal way — they say that all your replicate results are spread out in something called the *sampling distribution* for that sample statistic of your experiment. The idea of a sampling distribution is at the heart of the concepts of accuracy and precision.

- ✔ *Accuracy* refers to how close your observed sample statistic comes to the true population parameter, or more formally, how close the mean of the sampling distribution is to the mean of the population distribution. For example, how close is the mean of all your percentage values to the true percentage of children who like chocolate?

- ✔ *Precision* refers to how close your replicate values of the sample statistic are to each other, or more formally, how wide the sampling distribution is, which can be expressed as the standard deviation of the sampling distribution. For example, what is the standard deviation of your big collection of percentage values?

Thinking of measurement as a kind of sampling

No measuring instrument (ruler, scale, voltmeter, hematology analyzer, and so on) is perfect, so questions of measurement accuracy and precision are just as relevant as questions of sampling accuracy and precision. In fact, statisticians think of measuring as a kind of sampling process. This analogy may seem like quite a stretch, but it lets them analyze measurement errors using the same concepts, terminology, and mathematical techniques that they use to analyze sampling errors.

For example, suppose you happen to weigh exactly 86.73839 kilograms at this very moment. If you were to step onto a bathroom scale (the old kind, with springs and a dial), it certainly wouldn't show exactly that weight. And if you were to step off the scale and then on it again, it might not show exactly the same weight as the first time. A set of repetitive weights would differ from your true weight — and they'd differ from each other — for any of many reasons. For example, maybe you couldn't read the dial that precisely, the scale was miscalibrated, you shifted your weight slightly, or you stood in a slightly different spot on the platform each time.

You can consider your measured weight to be a number randomly drawn from a hypothetical population of possible weights that the scale might produce if the same person were to be weighed repeatedly on it. If you weigh yourself a thousand times, those 1,000 numbers will be spread out into a sampling distribution that describes the accuracy and precision of the process of measuring your weight with that particular bathroom scale.

Expressing errors in terms of accuracy and precision

In the preceding section, I explain the difference between accuracy and precision. In the following sections, I describe what can cause your results to be *inaccurate* and what can cause them to be *imprecise*.

Inaccuracy comes from systematic errors

Inaccuracy results from the effects of *systematic errors* — those that tend to affect all replications the same way — leading to a *biased* result (one that's off in a definite direction). These errors can arise in sampling and in measuring.

Systematic errors in a clinical study can result from causes such as the following:

✔ Enrolling subjects who are not representative of the population that you want to draw conclusions about, either through incorrect inclusion/ exclusion criteria (such as wanting to draw conclusions that apply to males and females but enrolling only males) or through inappropriate advertising (for example, putting a notice in a newspaper, on the web, or on a college cafeteria bulletin board that only part of the target population ever looks at)

✔ Human error (mistakes) such as recording lab results in the wrong units (entering all glucose values as milligrams per deciliter [mg/dL] when the protocol calls for millimoles per liter [mmol/L]) or administering the wrong product to the subject (giving a placebo to a subject who should have gotten the real product)

Systematic errors in a measurement can result from the following types of circumstances:

✔ Physical changes occur in the measuring instrument (for example, wooden rulers might shrink and scale springs might get stiff with age).

✔ The measuring instrument is used improperly (for example, the balance isn't zeroed before weighing).

✔ The measuring instrument is poorly calibrated (or not calibrated at all).

✔ The operator makes mistakes (such as using the wrong reagents in an analyzer).

Systematic errors don't follow any particular statistical distribution — they can be of almost any magnitude in either direction. They're not very amenable to statistical analysis, either. Each kind of systematic error has to be identified, and its source has to be tracked down and corrected.

Imprecision comes from random errors

Imprecision results from the effects of *random fluctuations* — those that tend to be unpredictable — and can affect each replication differently.

Sampling imprecision (as, for example, in a clinical trial) arises from several sources:

- ✔ **Subject-to-subject variability** (for example, different subjects have different weights, different blood pressure, and different tendencies to respond to a treatment)

- ✔ **Within-subject variability** (for example, one person's blood pressure, recorded every 15 minutes, will show random variability from one reading to another because of the combined action of a large number of internal factors, such as stress, and external factors, like activity, noise, and so on)

- ✔ **Random sampling errors** (inherent in the random sampling process itself)

Measurement imprecision arises from the combined effects of a large number of individual, uncontrolled factors, such as

- ✔ **Environmental factors** (like temperature, humidity, mechanical vibrations, voltage fluctuations, and so on)

- ✔ **Physically induced randomness** (such as electrical noise or static, or nuclear decay in assay methods using radioactive isotopes)

- ✔ **Operator variability** (for example, reading a scale from a slightly different angle or estimating digits between scale markings)

Random errors may seem to be more diverse, heterogeneous, indescribable, and, therefore, more unmanageable than systematic errors. But it turns out that random errors are much more amenable to statistical description and analysis than systematic errors, as you see in the next section.

The general magnitude of random sampling and measurement errors is expressed in something called the *standard error* (SE) of the sample statistic or the measured result. The SE is simply the standard deviation of the sampling distribution of the sample statistic or measured value. The smaller the SE is, the higher the precision. (Find out how to calculate the SE for different sample statistics later in this chapter.)

Improving Accuracy and Precision

While perfect accuracy and precision will always be an unattainable ideal, you can take steps to minimize the effects of systematic errors and random fluctuations on your sampled and measured data.

Enhancing sampling accuracy

You improve sampling accuracy by eliminating sources of bias in the selection of subjects for your study. The study's *inclusion* criteria should ideally define the population you want your study's conclusions to apply to. If you want your conclusions to apply to all adult diabetics, for example, your inclusion criteria may state that subjects must be 18 years or older and must have a definitive clinical diagnosis of diabetes mellitus, as confirmed by a glucose tolerance test. The study's *exclusion* criteria should be limited to only those conditions and situations that make it impossible for a subject to safely participate in the study and provide usable data for analysis.

You also want to try to select subjects as broadly and evenly as possible from the total target population. This task may be difficult or even impossible (it's almost impossible to obtain a representative sample from a worldwide population). But the scientific validity of a study depends on having as representative a sample as possible, so you should sample as wide a geographic region as is practically feasible.

Getting more accurate measurements

Measurement accuracy very often becomes a matter of properly calibrating an instrument against known standards. The instrument may be as simple as a ruler or as complicated as a million-dollar analyzer, but the principles are the same. They generally involve the following steps:

1. **Acquire one or more known standards from a reliable source.**

   Known standards are generally prepared and certified by an organization or a company that you have reason to believe has much more accurate instruments than you do, such as the National Institute of Standards and Technology (NIST) or a well-respected company like Hewlett-Packard or Fisher Scientific.

   If you're calibrating a blood glucose analyzer, for example, you need to acquire a set of glucose solutions whose concentrations are known with great accuracy, and can be taken as "true" concentration values (perhaps five vials, with glucose values of 50, 100, 200, 400, and 800 mg/dL).

2. **Run your measuring process or assay, using your instrument, on those standards; record the instrument's results, along with the "true" values.**

   Continuing with the glucose example, you might split each vial into four aliquots (portions), and run these 20 specimens through the analyzer.

3. **Plot your instrument's readings against the true values and fit the best line possible to that data.**

   You'd plot the results of the analysis of the standards as 20 points on a scattergram, with the true value from the standards provider ($Gluc_{True}$) on the X axis, and the instrument's results ($Gluc_{Instr}$) on the Y axis. The best line may not be a straight line, so you may have to do some nonlinear curve-fitting (I describe how to do this in Chapter 21).

4. **Use that fitted line to convert your instrument's readings into the values you report. (You have to do some algebra to rearrange the formula to calculate the X value from the Y value.)**

   Suppose the fitted equation from Step 3 was $Gluc_{Instr} = 1.54 + 0.9573 \times Gluc_{True}$. With a little algebra, this equation can be rearranged to $Gluc_{True} = (Gluc_{Instr} - 1.54)/0.9573$. If you were to run a patient's specimen through that instrument and get a value of 200.0, you'd use the calibration equation to get the corrected value: $(200 - 1.54)/0.9573$, which works out to 207.3, the value you'd report for this specimen.

   If done properly, this process can effectively remove almost all systematic errors from your measurements, resulting in very accurate measurements.

You can find out more about calibration curves from the GraphPad website (www.graphpad.com).

Improving sampling precision

You improve the precision of anything you observe from your sample of subjects by having a larger sample. The *central limit theorem* (or CLT, one of the foundations of probability theory) describes how random fluctuations behave when a bunch of random variables are added (or averaged) together. Among many other things, the CLT describes how the precision of a sample statistic depends on the sample size.

The precision of any sample statistic increases (that is, the SE decreases) in proportion to the square root of the sample size. So, if Trial A has four times as many subjects as Trial B, then the results from Trial A will be twice as precise as (that is, have one-half the SE of) the results from Trial B, because the square root of four is two.

You can also get better precision (and smaller SEs) by setting up your experiment in a way that lessens random variability in the population. For example, if you want to compare a weight-loss product to a placebo, you should try to have the two treatment groups in your trial as equally balanced as possible with respect to every subject characteristic that can conceivably influence weight loss. Identical twins make ideal (though hard-to-find) subjects for clinical trials because they're so closely matched in so many ways. Alternatively, you can make your inclusion criteria more stringent. For example, you can restrict the study groups to just males within a narrow age, height, and weight range and impose other criteria that eliminate other sources of between-subject variability (such as history of smoking, hypertension, nervous disorders, and so on).

But although narrowing the inclusion criteria makes your study sample more homogeneous and eliminates more sources of random fluctuations, it also has some important drawbacks:

✔ It makes finding suitable subjects harder.

✔ Your inferences (conclusions) from this study can now only be applied to the narrower population (corresponding to your more stringent inclusion criteria).

Increasing the precision of your measurements

Here are a few general suggestions for achieving better precision (smaller random errors) in your measurements:

✔ Use the most precise measuring instruments you can afford. For example, a beam balance may yield more precise measurements than a spring scale, and an electronic balance may be even more precise.

✔ Control as many sources of random fluctuations due to external perturbations as you can. Depending on how the measuring device operates, a reading can be influenced by temperature, humidity, mechanical vibrations, electrical power fluctuations, and a host of other environmental factors. Operator technique also contributes to random variability in readings.

✔ When reading an instrument with an analog display, like a dial or linear scale (as opposed to a computerized device with a digital readout), try to *interpolate* (estimate an extra digit) between the divisions and record the number with that extra decimal place. So if you're weighing someone on a scale with a large rotary dial with lines spaced every kilogram, try to estimate the position of the dial pointer to the nearest tenth of a kilogram.

✔ Make replicate readings and average them. This technique is one of the most widely applicable (see the next section for more information).

Calculating Standard Errors for Different Sample Statistics

As I mention in the earlier section "Imprecision comes from random errors," the standard error (SE) is just the standard deviation (SD) of the sampling distribution of the numbers that you get from measuring the same thing over and over again. But you don't necessarily have to carry out this repetitive process in practice. You can usually estimate the SE of a sample statistic obtained from a single experiment by using a formula appropriate for the sample statistic. The following sections describe how to calculate the SE for various kinds of sample statistics.

What if you've calculated something from your raw data by a very complicated set of formulas (like the area under a concentration-versus-time curve)? Ideally, you should be able to quote a standard error for any quantity you calculate from your data, but no SE formula may be available for that particular calculation. In Chapter 11, I explain how SEs propagate through various mathematical formulas, and this information might help you figure out the SE for some calculated quantities. But there is also a very general (and surprisingly simple) method to estimate the SE of centiles, correlation coefficients, AUCs, or anything else you might want to calculate from your data. It involves using your data in a special way (called "resampling") to simulate what might have happened if you had repeated your experiment many times over, each time calculating and recording the quantity you're interested in. The SD of all these simulated values turns out to be a good estimate of the SE of the sample statistic. When this method was first proposed, statisticians were very skeptical and called it the "bootstrap" method, implying that it was like "picking yourself up by your bootstraps" (that is, it was impossible). I describe this method (with an example) in an article at www.dummies.com/extras/biostatistics.

A mean

From the central limit theorem (see the earlier section "Improving sampling precision" for details), the SE of the mean of N numbers (SEM_N) is related to the standard deviation (SD) of the numbers by the formula $SEM_N = SD/\sqrt{N}$. So if you study 25 adult diabetics and find that they have an average fasting blood glucose level of 130 milligrams per deciliter (mg/dL) with an SD of ±40 mg/dL, you can say that your estimate of the mean has a precision (SE) of $40/\sqrt{25}$, which is equal to ±40/5, or ±8 mg/dL.

Making three or four replicates of each measurement and then reporting the average of those replicates is typical practice in laboratory research (though less common in clinical studies). Applied to measurements, the central limit theorem tells you that the SEM_N is more precise than any one individual measurement (SE_1) by a factor of the square root of N: $SEM_N = SE_1/\sqrt{N}$.

The mean of four measurements has an SE that's one-half the SE of a single measurement; that is, it's twice as precise. So averaging three or four independent measurements often provides an easy and relatively inexpensive way to improve precision. But because of the square-root relationship, it becomes a matter of diminishing returns — to get 1 extra digit of precision (a tenfold reduction in SE), you have to average 100 independent replicates. Also, averaging doesn't improve accuracy; systematic errors affecting all the replicates are not reduced by averaging.

A proportion

If you were to survey 100 typical children and find that 70 of them like chocolate, you'd estimate that 70 percent of children like chocolate. How precise is that estimated 70-percent figure?

Based on the properties of the binomial distribution (see Chapters 3 and 25), which generally describes observed proportions of this type, the standard error (SE) of an observed proportion (p), based on a sample size of N, is given by this approximate formula:

$$SE = \sqrt{p(1-p)/N}$$

For small values of N, this formula underestimates SE, but for $N = 10$ or more, the approximation is very good.

Plugging in the numbers, the SE of the observed 70 percent (0.7 proportion) in 100 children is

$$SE = \sqrt{0.7(1-0.7)/100} = 0.046$$

So you report the percentage of children who like chocolate as 70 percent $\pm$ 4.6 percent, being sure to state that the $\pm$ number is the standard error of the percentage.

Event counts and rates

Closely related to the binomial case in the preceding section (where you have some number of events observed out of some number of opportunities for the event to occur) is the case of the observed number of sporadic events over some interval of time or space.

For example, suppose that there were 36 fatal highway accidents in your county in the last three months. If that's the only safety data you have to go on, then your best estimate of the monthly fatal accident rate is simply that observed count divided by the length of time during which they were observed: 36/3, or 12.0 fatal accidents per month. How precise is that estimate?

Based on the properties of the Poisson distribution (see Chapters 3 and 25), which generally describes the sporadic occurrences of independent events, the standard error (*SE*) of an event rate (*R*), based on the occurrence of *N* events in *T* units of time, is given by this approximate formula:

$$SE = \sqrt{N}/T$$

For small values of *N*, this formula underestimates the SE, but for an *N* of ten or more, the approximation is very good.

Plugging in the numbers, the SE for an observed count of 36 fatalities (*N*) in 3 months (*T*) is

$$\sqrt{36}/3 = 6/3 = 2.0$$

So you would report that the estimated rate is 12.0 ± 2.0 fatal accidents per month, being sure to state that the $\pm$ number is the SE of the monthly rate.

Another common example is an isotope-based lab assay, which counts individual nuclear disintegrations. These instruments can be programmed to count for a certain amount of time or to count until a certain number of disintegrations have been observed. Either way, the disintegration rate is the number of counts divided by the amount of time. If you set the instrument to count for one second and you get about 100 clicks, that number is good to ± 10 clicks, or about 10 percent relative precision. But if you count for one minute and get about 6,000 clicks, that number is good to ± 77 clicks, or about 1.3 percent relative precision. So there's a clear tradeoff between speed and precision — the longer you count, the more precise the event rate (and in this case, the assay result).

A regression coefficient

Suppose you're interested in whether or not blood urea nitrogen (BUN), a measure of kidney performance, tends to naturally increase after age 60 in generally healthy adults. You enroll a bunch of generally healthy adults age 60 and above, record their ages, and measure their BUN. Next, you create a scatter plot of BUN versus age, and then you fit a straight line to the data points, using *regression analysis* (see Chapter 18 for details). The regression analysis gives you two *regression coefficients:* the slope and the intercept of the fitted straight line. The slope of this line has units of (mg/dL)/year, and tells you how much, on average, a healthy person's BUN goes up with every additional year of age after age 60. Suppose the answer you get is a 1.4 mg/dL glucose increase per year. How precise is that estimate of yearly increase?

This is one time you don't need any formula. Any good regression program (like the ones I describe in Chapter 3 and in the regression-related chapters later in this book) should provide the SE for every parameter (regression coefficient) it fits to your data, so it should give you the SE for the slope of the fitted straight line. Be thankful the program does this, because you wouldn't want to attempt the SE calculations yourself — they're really complicated!

Estimating the sample size needed to achieve the precision you want

All the SE formulas shown in this chapter contain a $\sqrt{N}$ term. (Precision is almost always proportional to the square root of N.) This fact leads to a simple way to estimate the sample size required for any desired SE — just use some algebra to solve the SE formula for N.

For example, if you're designing a study to estimate the success rate of some treatment, and you want your estimate to have an SE of ±5 percentage points, how many subjects do you have to treat? The formula for the SE of a proportion, as you find out earlier in this chapter, is $SE = \sqrt{p(1-p)/N}$. Using some high-school algebra, you can solve this equation for N to get $N = p(1-p)/(SE^2)$.

You can substitute 0.05 for SE (keep in mind that numbers have to go into the formulas as proportions, not as percentages). You also need a guess for the expected proportion of successes. Suppose you expect your treatment to have an 80 percent success rate; you enter 0.8 for p (remember: proportions, not percentages). You have $N = 0.8(1-0.8)/(0.05^2)$, which works out to about 64 subjects. Similarly, you can calculate that if you want ±1 percent precision, you need 1,600 subjects (it's hard to estimate proportions very precisely!).

The same idea can be applied to other sample statistics, even those for which no explicit SE formula is available. For example, Chapter 18 describes a way to estimate how many observations you need in order to estimate a regression coefficient with a certain precision.

Chapter 10

Having Confidence in Your Results

. . . .

In This Chapter

▶ Investigating the basics of confidence intervals

▶ Determining confidence intervals for a number of statistics

▶ Linking significance testing to confidence intervals

. . . .

*I*n Chapter 9, I show you how to express the precision of a numeric result using the standard error (SE) and how to calculate the SE (or have a computer calculate it for you) for the most common kinds of numerical results you get from biological studies — means, proportions, event rates, and regression coefficients. But the SE is only one way of specifying how precise your results are. In this chapter, I describe another commonly used indicator of precision — the *confidence interval* (CI).

I assume that you're familiar with the concepts of populations, samples, and statistical estimation theory (see Chapter 3 if you're not) and that you know what standard errors are (see Chapter 9 if you don't). Always keep in mind that when you conduct any kind of research study, such as a clinical trial, you're studying a small *sample* of subjects (like 50 adult volunteers with diabetes) that you've randomly selected as representing a large, hypothetical *population* (all adults with diabetes). And any numeric quantity (called a *sample statistic*) that you observe in this sample is just an imperfect estimate of the corresponding *population parameter* — the true value of that quantity in the population.

Feeling Confident about Confidence Interval Basics

Before jumping into the main part of this chapter (how to calculate confidence intervals around the sample statistics you get from your experiments), it's important to be comfortable with the basic concepts and terminology related to confidence intervals. This is an area where nuances of meaning can be tricky, and the right-sounding words can be used the wrong way.

Defining confidence intervals

Informally, a *confidence interval* indicates a range of values that's likely to encompass the truth. More formally, the CI around your sample statistic is calculated in such a way that it has a specified chance of surrounding (or "containing") the value of the corresponding population parameter.

Unlike the SE, which is usually written as a ± number immediately following your measured value (for example, a blood glucose measurement of 120 ± 3 mg/dL), the CI is usually written as a pair of numbers separated by a dash, like this: 114–126. The two numbers that make up the lower and upper ends of the confidence interval are called the lower and upper *confidence limits* (CLs). Sometimes you see the abbreviations written with a subscript L or U, like this: CL_L or CL_U, indicating the lower and upper confidence limits, respectively.

Although SEs and CIs are both used as indicators of the precision of a numerical quantity, they differ in their focus (sample or population):

- ✔ A standard error indicates how much your observed sample statistic may fluctuate if the same experiment is repeated a large number of times, so the SE focuses on the *sample*.
- ✔ A confidence interval indicates the range that's likely to contain the true population parameter, so the CI focuses on the *population*.

One important property of confidence intervals (and standard errors) is that they vary inversely with the square root of the sample size. For example, if you were to quadruple your sample size, it would cut the SE and the width of the CI in half. This "square root law" is one of the most widely applicable rules in all of statistics.

Looking at confidence levels

The probability that the confidence interval encompasses the true value is called the *confidence level* of the CI. You can calculate a CI for any confidence level you like, but the most commonly seen value is 95 percent. Whenever you report a confidence interval, you must state the confidence level, like this: 95% CI = 114–126.

In general, higher confidence levels correspond to wider confidence intervals, and lower confidence level intervals are narrower. For example, the range 118–122 may have a 50 percent chance of containing the true population parameter within it; 115–125 may have a 90 percent chance of containing the truth, and 112–128 may have a 99 percent chance.

Betting on the truth

You can think of confidence intervals in terms of the following imaginary scenario. Say you conduct an experiment on a random sample from some population, and you obtain a value for some sample statistic. You calculate a 95 percent CI around this value, and then you assert that your CI contains the true population value. If the true value were ever to become known, your assertion would be revealed as either true or false. In the long run, if you were to carry out many such experiments, calculating the 95 percent confidence interval each time, your assertions would prove to be true at least 95 percent of the time.

If you're the devious type, you may be thinking, "I know how to guarantee that I'll be right just about *all* the time, and I don't have to do any calculations at all. I'll just always quote an absurdly wide confidence interval." For example, you could quote a confidence interval for mean blood glucose that goes from 0 to 1 billion mg/dL. Both of those extremes are physically impossible, of course, so the true value has to lie somewhere within that ridiculously large interval. Clearly, that's not what you want a CI to be. A good CI must be as narrow as possible while still guaranteeing that it encompasses the true value at least a specified fraction (the confidence level) of the time.

The confidence level is sometimes abbreviated CL, just like the confidence limit, which can be confusing. Fortunately, the distinction is usually clear from the context in which CL appears; when it's not clear, I spell out what CL stands for.

Taking sides with confidence intervals

Properly calculated 95 percent confidence intervals contain the true value 95 percent of the time and fail to contain the true value the other 5 percent of the time. Usually, 95 percent confidence limits are calculated to be balanced so that the 5 percent failures are split evenly — the true value is less than the lower confidence limit 2.5 percent of the time and greater than the upper confidence limit 2.5 percent of the time. This is called a two-sided, *balanced* CI.

But the confidence limits don't have to be balanced. Sometimes the consequences of overestimating a value may be more severe than underestimating it, or vice versa. You can calculate an *unbalanced,* two-sided, 95 percent confidence limit that splits the 5 percent exceptions so that the true value is smaller than the lower confidence limit 4 percent of the time, and larger than the upper confidence limit 1 percent of the time. Unbalanced confidence limits extend farther out from the estimated value on the side with the smaller percentage.

In some situations, like noninferiority studies (described in Chapter 16), you may want *all* the failures to be on one side; that is, you want a *one-sided* confidence limit. Actually, the other side goes out an infinite distance. For example, you can have an observed value of 120 with a one-sided confidence interval that goes from minus infinity to +125 or from 115 to plus infinity.

Calculating Confidence Intervals

Just as the SE formulas in Chapter 9 depend on what kind of sample statistic you're dealing with (whether you're measuring or counting something or getting it from a regression program or from some other calculation), confidence intervals (CIs) are calculated in different ways depending on how you obtain the sample statistic. In the following sections, I describe methods for the most common situations, using the same examples I use in Chapter 9 for calculating standard errors.

You can use a "bootstrap" simulation method to calculate the SE of any quantity you can calculate from your data; you can use the same technique to generate CIs around those calculated quantities. You use your data in a special way (called "resampling") to simulate what might have happened if you had repeated your experiment many times over, each time calculating and recording the quantity you're interested in. The CI is simply the interval that encloses 95 percent of all these simulated values. I describe this method (with an example) in an online article at www.dummies.com/extras/biostatistics.

Before you begin: Formulas for confidence limits in large samples

Most of the approximate methods I describe in the following sections are based on the assumption that your observed value has a sampling distribution that's (at least approximately) normally distributed. Fortunately, there are good theoretical and practical reasons to believe that almost every sample statistic you're likely to encounter in practical work will have a nearly normal sampling distribution, for large enough samples.

For any normally distributed sample statistic, the lower and upper confidence limits can be calculated very simply from the observed value (V) and standard error (SE) of the statistic:

$$CL_L = V - k \times SE$$
$$CL_U = V + k \times SE$$

Confidence limits computed this way are often referred to as *normal-based, asymptotic,* or *central-limit-theorem* (CLT) confidence limits. (The CLT, which I introduce in Chapter 9, provides good reason to believe that almost any sample statistic you're likely to encounter will be nearly normally distributed for large samples.) The value of k in the formulas depends on the desired confidence level and can be obtained from a table of critical values for the normal distribution or from a web page such as `StatPages.info/pdfs.html`. Table 10-1 lists the k values for some commonly used confidence levels.

Table 10-1   Multipliers for Normal-Based Confidence Intervals

Confidence Level	Tail Probability	k Value
50%	0.50	0.67
80%	0.20	1.28
90%	0.10	1.64
95%	0.05	1.96
98%	0.02	2.33
99%	0.01	2.58

For the most commonly used confidence level, 95 percent, k is 1.96, or approximately 2. This leads to the very simple approximation that 95 percent confidence limits are about two standard errors above and below the observed value.

The distance of each confidence limit from the measured value, $k \times SE$, is called the *margin of error* (ME). Because MEs are almost always calculated at the 95 percent confidence level, they're usually about twice as large as the corresponding SEs. MEs are most commonly used to express the precision of the results of a survey, such as "These poll results have a margin of error of ±5 percent." This usage can lead to some confusion because the SE is also usually expressed as a ± number. For this reason, it's probably best to use the CI instead of the ME to express precision when reporting clinical research results. In any event, be sure to state which one you're using when you report your results.

The confidence interval around a mean

Suppose you study 25 adult diabetics ($N = 25$) and find that they have an average fasting blood glucose level of 130 mg/dL with a standard deviation (SD) of ±40 mg/dL. What is the 95 percent confidence interval around that 130 mg/dL estimated mean?

To calculate the confidence limits around a mean using the formulas in the preceding section, you first calculate the standard error of the mean (the SEM), which (from Chapter 9) is $SEM = SD/\sqrt{N}$, where SD is the standard deviation of the N individual values. So for the glucose example, the SE of the mean is $SEM = 40/\sqrt{25}$, which is equal to 40/5, or 8 mg/dL.

Using $k = 1.95$ for a 95 percent confidence level (from Table 10-1), the lower and upper confidence limits around the mean are

$$CL_L = 130 - 1.96 \times 8 = 114.3$$
$$CL_U = 130 + 1.96 \times 8 = 145.7$$

You report your result this way: mean glucose = 130 mg/dL, 95%CI = 114–146 mg/dL. (Don't report numbers to more decimal places than their precision warrants. In this example, the digits after the decimal point are practically meaningless, so the numbers are rounded off.)

A more accurate version of the formulas in the preceding section uses k values derived from a table of critical values of the Student t distribution. You need to know the number of degrees of freedom, which, for a mean value, is always equal to $N - 1$. Using a Student t table (see Chapter 25) or a web page like `StatPages.info/pdfs.html`, you can find that the Student-based k value for a 95 percent confidence level and 24 degrees of freedom is equal to 2.06, a little bit larger than the normal-based k value. Using this k value instead of 1.96, you can calculate the 95 percent confidence limits as 113.52 and 146.48, which happen to round off to the same whole numbers as the normal-based confidence limits. Generally you don't have to use the more-complicated Student-based k values unless N is quite small (say, less than 10).

What if your original numbers (the ones being averaged) aren't normally distributed? You shouldn't just blindly apply the normal-based CI formulas for non-normally distributed data. If you know that your data is log-normally distributed (a very common type of non-normality), you can do the following:

1. **Take the logarithm of every individual subject's value.**

2. **Find the mean, SD, and SEM of these logarithms.**

3. **Use the normal-based formulas to get the confidence limits (CLs) around the mean of the logarithms.**

4. **Calculate the antilogarithm of the mean of the logs.**

    The result is the geometric mean of the original values. (See Chapter 8.)

5. **Calculate the antilogarithm of the lower and upper CLs.**

    These are the lower and upper CLs around the geometric mean.

If you don't know what distribution your values have, you can use the boot-strapping approach described later in this chapter.

The confidence interval around a proportion

If you were to survey 100 typical children and find that 70 of them like chocolate, you'd estimate that 70 percent of children like chocolate. What is the 95 percent CI around that 70 percent estimate?

There are many approximate formulas for confidence intervals around an observed proportion (also called *binomial* confidence intervals). The simplest method is based on approximating the binomial distribution by a normal distribution (see Chapter 25). It should be used only when N (the denominator of the proportion) is large (at least 50), and the proportion is not too close to 0 or 1 (say, between 0.2 and 0.8). You first calculate the SE of the proportion as described in Chapter 9, $SE = \sqrt{p(1-p)/N}$, and then you use the normal-based formulas in the earlier section "Before you begin: Formulas for confidence limits in large samples."

Using the numbers from the preceding example, you have $p = 0.7$ and $N = 100$, so the SE for the proportion is $\sqrt{0.7(1-0.7)/100}$, or 0.046. From Table 10-1, k is 1.96 for 95 percent confidence limits. So $CL_L = 0.7 - 1.96 \times 0.046$ and $CL_U = 0.7 + 1.96 \times 0.046$, which works out to a 95 percent CI of 0.61 to 0.79. To express these fractions as percentages, you report your result this way: "The percentage of children in the sample who liked chocolate was 70 percent, 95%CI = 61–79%."

Many other approximate formulas for CIs around observed proportions exist, most of which are more reliable when N is small. There are also several exact methods, the first and most famous of which is called the *Clopper-Pearson method,* named after the authors of a classic 1934 article. The Clopper-Pearson calculations are too complicated to attempt by hand, but fortunately, many statistical packages can do them for you.

You can also go to the "Binomial Confidence Intervals" section of the online web calculator at `StatPages.info/confint.html`. Enter the numerator (70) and denominator (100) of the fraction, and press the Compute button. The page calculates the observed proportion (0.7) and the exact confidence limits (0.600 and 0.788), which you can convert to percentages and express as 95%CI = 60–79%. For this example, the normal-based approximate CI (61–79%) is very close to the exact CI, mainly because the sample size was quite large. For small samples, you should report exact confidence limits.

The confidence interval around an event count or rate

Suppose that there were 36 fatal highway accidents in your county in the last three months. If that's the only safety data you have to go on, then your best estimate of the monthly fatal accident rate is simply the observed count (N), divided by the length of time (T) during which the N counts were observed: 36/3, or 12.0 fatal accidents per month. What is the 95 percent CI around that estimate?

There are many approximate formulas for the CIs around an observed event count or rate (also called a *Poisson* CI). The simplest method is based on approximating the Poisson distribution by a normal distribution (see Chapter 25). It should be used only when N is large (at least 50). You first calculate the SE of the event rate as described in Chapter 9, $SE = \sqrt{N}/T$; then you use the normal-based formulas in the earlier section "Before you begin: Formulas for confidence limits in large samples."

Using the numbers from the fatal-accident example, $N = 36$ and $T=3$, so the SE for the even rate is $\sqrt{25}/3$, or 1.67. According to Table 10-1, k is 1.96 for 95 percent CLs. So $CL_L = 12.0 - 1.96 \times 1.67$ and $CL_U = 12.0 + 1.96 \times 1.67$, which works out to 95 percent confidence limits of 8.73 and 15.27. You report your result this way: "The fatal accident rate was 12.0, 95%CI = 8.7–15.3 fatal accidents per month."

To calculate the CI around the event count itself, you estimate the SE of the count N as $SE = \sqrt{N}$, then calculate the CI around the observed count using the formulas in the earlier section "Before you begin: Formulas for confidence limits in large samples." So the SE of the 36 observed fatal accidents in a three-month period is simply $\sqrt{36}$, which equals 6.0. So $CL_L = 36.0 - 1.96 \times 6.0$ and $CL_H = 36.0 + 1.96 \times 6.0$, which works out to a 95 percent CI of 24.2 to 47.8 accidents in a three-month period.

Many other approximate formulas for CIs around observed event counts and rates are available, most of which are more reliable when N is small. There are also several exact methods. They're too complicated to attempt by hand, involving evaluating the Poisson distribution repeatedly to find values for the true mean event count that are consistent with (that is, not significantly different from) the count you actually observed. Fortunately, many statistical packages can do these calculations for you.

 You can also go to the "Poisson Confidence Intervals" section of the online web calculator at StatPages.info/confint.html. Enter the observed count (36) and press the Compute button. The page calculates the exact 95 percent CI (25.2–49.8). For this example, the normal-based CI (24.2–47.8) is only a rough approximation to the exact CI, mainly because the event count was only 36 accidents. For small samples, you should report exact confidence limits.

The confidence interval around a regression coefficient

Suppose you're interested in whether or not blood urea nitrogen (BUN), a measure of kidney performance, tends to increase after age 60 in healthy adults. You can enroll a bunch of generally healthy adults age 60 and above, record their ages, and measure their BUN. Then you can create a scatter plot of BUN versus age and fit a straight line to the data points (see Chapter 18). The slope of this line would have units of (mg/dL)/year and would tell you how much, on average, a healthy person's BUN goes up with every additional year of age after age 60. Suppose the answer you get is that glucose increases 1.4 mg/dL per year. What is the 95 percent CI around that estimate of yearly increase?

This is one time you don't need any formulas. Any good regression program (like the ones described in Chapter 4) can provide the SE for every parameter it fits to your data. (Chapter 18 describes where to find the SE for the slope of a straight line.) The regression program may also provide the confidence limits for any confidence level you specify, but if it doesn't, you can easily calculate the confidence limits using the formulas in the earlier section "Before you begin: Formulas for confidence limits in large samples."

Relating Confidence Intervals and Significance Testing

You can use confidence intervals (CIs) as an alternative to some of the usual significance tests (see Chapter 3 for an introduction to the concepts and terminology of significance testing and Chapters 12–15 for descriptions of specific significance tests). To assess significance using CIs, you first define a number that measures the amount of effect you're testing for. This effect size can be the difference between two means or two proportions, the ratio of two means, an odds ratio, a relative risk ratio, or a hazard ratio, among others. The complete absence of any effect corresponds to a difference of 0, or a ratio of 1, so I call these the "no-effect" values.

The following are always true:

- If the 95 percent CI around the observed effect size *includes the no-effect value* (0 for differences, 1 for ratios), then the effect is *not* statistically significant (that is, a significance test for that effect will produce p > 0.05).

- If the 95 percent CI around the observed effect size *does not include the no-effect value*, then the effect *is* significant (that is, a significance test for that effect will produce p ≤ 0.05).

The same kind of correspondence is true for other confidence levels and significance levels: 90 percent confidence levels correspond to the p = 0.10 significance level, 99 percent confidence levels correspond to the p = 0.01 significance level, and so on.

So you have two different, but related, ways to prove that some effect is present — you can use significance tests, and you can use confidence intervals. Which one is better? The two methods are consistent with each other, but many people prefer the CI approach to the p-value approach. Why?

- ✔ The p value is the result of the complex interplay between the observed effect size, the sample size, and the size of random fluctuations, all boiled down into a single number that doesn't tell you whether the effect was large or small, clinically important or negligible.

- ✔ The CI around the mean effect clearly shows you the observed effect size, along with an indicator of how uncertain your knowledge of that effect size is. It tells you not only whether the effect is statistically significant, but also can give you an intuitive sense of whether the effect is clinically important.

    The CI approach lends itself to a very simple and natural way of comparing two products for equivalence or noninferiority, as I explain in Chapter 16.

Chapter 11

Fuzzy In Equals Fuzzy Out: Pushing Imprecision through a Formula

*I*n Chapters 9 and 10, I describe how you can estimate the precision of anything you can measure (like height and weight) or count (such as hospital admissions, adverse events, and responses to treatment). In this chapter, I show you how to estimate the precision of things you calculate from the things you measure or count (for example, you can calculate body mass index from height and weight measurements). I explain the concept of *error propagation,* and I describe some simple rules you can use for simple expressions, such as those involving only addition, subtraction, multiplication, and division. Then I show you how to deal with simple or complicated expressions without having to do any calculations at all, using readily available software to do all the hard work for you.

Knowing how to make these calculations is important because often you can't directly measure the thing you're really interested in; you have to calculate it from one or more other things that you *can* measure. You have to be able to determine the precision of these calculated numbers as well, because any number whose accuracy or precision is completely unknown is completely worthless.

Note: For the purposes of this chapter, it doesn't matter whether you choose to express precision as a standard error (SE) or as a *margin of error* (the distance from the number to the ends of a confidence interval, as I describe in Chapter 10). I refer to SE throughout this chapter, but the techniques I describe work for margin of error as well.

Understanding the Concept of Error Propagation

A less extreme form of the old saying "garbage in equals garbage out" is "fuzzy in equals fuzzy out." Random fluctuations in one or more measured variables produce random fluctuations in anything you calculate from those variables. This process is called the *propagation of errors*. You need to know how measurement errors propagate through a calculation that you perform on a measured quantity.

Here's a simple way to estimate the SE of a variable (Y) that's calculated from almost any mathematical expression that involves a single variable (X). Starting with the observed X value (which I call Xo), and its standard error (SE), just do the following 3-step calculation:

1. **Evaluate the expression, substituting the value of $Xo - SE$ for X in the formula. Call the result Y_1.**

2. **Evaluate the expression, substituting the value of $Xo + SE$ for X in the formula. Call the result Y_2.**

3. **The SE of Y is simply $(Y_2 - Y_1)/2$.**

Here's an example that shows how (and why) this process works.

Suppose you measure the diameter (d) of a coin as 2.3 centimeters, using a caliper or ruler that you know (from past experience) has an SE of ±0.2 centimeters. Now say that you want to calculate the area (A) of the coin from the measured diameter. If you know that the area of a circle is given by the formula $A = (\pi/4) d^2$, you can immediately calculate the area of the coin as $(\pi/4)2.3^2$, which you can work out on your calculator to get 4.15475628 square centimeters. Of course, you'd never report the area to that many digits because you didn't measure the diameter very precisely. So just how precise is your calculated area? In other words, how does that ±0.2-centimeter SE of d propagate through the formula $A = (\pi/4)d^2$ to give the SE of A?

One way to answer this question would be to consider an *interval of uncertainty* around the observed diameter (*d*) that goes from one SE below *d* to one SE above *d*. *Interval of uncertainty* isn't an official statistical term, but it has a great abbreviation (IOU), so I use it in this section. The IOU, as I've just defined it, is always two SEs wide. In the coin example, the diameter's IOU extends from 2.3 – 0.2 to 2.3 + 0.2, or from 2.1 to 2.5 centimeters.

Now figure out the areas corresponding to the diameters at the lower and upper ends of the IOU. Using 2.1 for *d* in the area formula gives *A* = 3.46, and using 2.5 for *d* gives *A* = 4.91. So the IOU for the area of the coin goes from 3.46 to 4.91 square centimeters. The width of this IOU is 4.91 – 3.46, or 1.45 square centimeters, which represents two SEs for the area. So the SE of the area is 1.45/2, or 0.725 square centimeter.

These calculations are illustrated in Figure 11-1. The curved line represents the formula $A = (\pi/4) \times d^2$. The dark arrows show how the measured diameter (2.3 centimeters), when plugged into the formula, produces a calculated area of about 4.15 square centimeters. The lighter colored gray arrows represent the lower and upper ends of the IOU and show how the IOU for the diameter produces an IOU for the area.

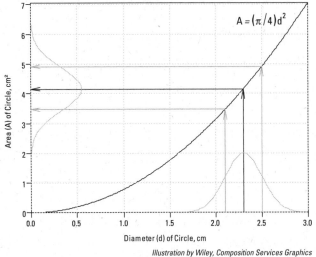

Figure 11-1:
How uncertainty in diameter becomes uncertainty in area.

Relationship between Diameter and Area of a Circle

$A = (\pi/4)d^2$

Area (A) of Circle, cm²

Diameter (d) of Circle, cm

Illustration by Wiley, Composition Services Graphics

The SE of the area depends on the SE of the diameter and the slope of the curve. In fact, the SE of the area is equal to the SE of the diameter multiplied by the slope of the curve. I express this relationship as a formula later in this chapter.

Unfortunately, the simple procedure illustrated in this example can't be generalized to handle functions of two or more variables, such as calculating a person's body mass index from height and weight. Mathematicians have derived a very general formula for calculating (approximately) how SEs in one or more variables propagate through any expression involving those variables, but it's very complicated, and to use it you have to be really good at calculus or you'll almost certainly make mistakes along the way.

Fortunately, there are much better alternatives, all of which I cover in the rest of this chapter:

- You can use some simple error-propagation formulas for simple expressions.
- Even easier, you can go to a web page that does the error-propagation calculations for functions of one or two variables.
- You can use a very general simulation approach that can easily analyze how errors propagate through even the most complicated expressions, involving any number of variables.

Using Simple Error Propagation Formulas for Simple Expressions

Even though some general error-propagation formulas are very complicated (as I note in the preceding section), the rules for propagating SEs through some simple mathematical expressions are much easier to work with. Here are some of the most common simple rules.

All the rules that involve two or more variables assume that those variables have been measured independently; they shouldn't be applied when the two variables have been calculated from the same raw data.

Adding or subtracting a constant doesn't change the SE

Adding (or subtracting) an exactly known numerical constant (that has no SE at all) doesn't affect the SE of a number. So if $x = 38 \pm 2$, then $x + 100 = 138 \pm 2$. Likewise, if $x = 38 \pm 2$, then $x - 15 = 23 \pm 2$.

Multiplying (or dividing) by a constant multiplies (or divides) the SE by the same amount

Multiplying a number by an exactly known constant multiplies the SE by that same constant. This situation arises when converting units of measure. For example, to convert a length from meters to centimeters, you multiply by exactly 100, so a length of an exercise track that's measured as 150 ± 1 meters can also be expressed as $15,000 \pm 100$ centimeters.

For sums and differences: Add the squares of SEs together

When adding or subtracting two independently measured numbers, you square each SE, then add the squares, and then take the square root of the sum, like this:

$$SE(x+y) = \sqrt{SE(x)^2 + SE(y)^2}$$

$$SE(x-y) = \sqrt{SE(x)^2 + SE(y)^2}$$

For example, if each of two measurements has an SE of ± 1, and those numbers are added together (or subtracted), the resulting sum (or difference) has an SE of $\sqrt{1^2 + 1^2}$, which is $\sqrt{2}$ or about ± 1.4.

A useful rule to remember is that the SE of the sum or difference of two equally precise numbers is about 40 percent larger than the SE of one of the numbers.

When two numbers of different precision are combined (added or subtracted), the precision of the result is determined mainly by the less precise number (the one with the larger SE). If one number has an SE of ± 1 and another has an SE of ± 5, the SE of the sum or difference of these two numbers is $\sqrt{1^2 + 5^2}$, which is $\sqrt{26}$, which is 5.1, or only slightly larger than the larger of the two individual SEs.

For averages: The square root law takes over

The SE of the average of N equally precise numbers is equal to the SE of the individual numbers divided by the square root of N.

For example, if your lab analyzer can determine a blood glucose value with an SE of ±5 milligrams per deciliter (mg/dL), then if you split up a blood sample into four specimens, run them through the analyzer, and average the four results, the average will have an SE of $5/\sqrt{4}$, or ±2.5 mg/dL. The average of four numbers is twice as precise as (has one-half the SE of) each individual number.

For products and ratios: Squares of relative SEs are added together

The rule for products and ratios is similar to the rule for adding or subtracting two numbers that I describe earlier in this chapter, except that you have to work with the *relative* SE instead of the SE itself. The *relative SE* of x is the SE of x divided by the value of x. So, a measured weight of 50 kilograms with an SE of 2 kilograms has a relative SE of 2/50, which is 0.04 or 4 percent. When multiplying or dividing two numbers, square the relative standard errors, add the squares together, and then take the square root of the sum. This gives you the relative SE of the product (or ratio). The formulas are

$$SE(xy) = xy\sqrt{\left(\frac{SE(x)}{x}\right)^2 + \left(\frac{SE(y)}{y}\right)^2}$$

$$SE\left(\frac{x}{y}\right) = \left(\frac{x}{y}\right)\sqrt{\left(\frac{SE(x)}{x}\right)^2 + \left(\frac{SE(y)}{y}\right)^2}$$

This formula may look complicated, but it's actually very easy to use if you work with percent errors (relative precision). Then it works just like the "add the squares" rule for addition and subtraction. So if one number is known to have a relative precision of ± 2 percent, and another number has a relative precision of ± 3 percent, the product or ratio of these two numbers has a relative precision (in percentage) of $\sqrt{2^2 + 3^2}$, which is $\sqrt{13}$ or ±3.6 percent.

Note that multiplying a number by an exactly known constant doesn't change the relative SE. For example, doubling a number represented by x would double its SE, but the relative error (SE/x) would remain the same because both the numerator and the denominator would be doubled.

For powers and roots: Multiply the relative SE by the power

For powers and roots, you have to work with relative SEs. When x is raised to any power k, the relative SE of x is multiplied by k; and when taking the kth root of a number, the SE is divided by k. So squaring a number doubles its relative SE, and taking the square root of a number cuts the relative SE in half.

For example, because the area of a circle is proportional to the square of its diameter, if you know the diameter with a relative precision of ±5 percent, you know the area with a relative precision of ±10 percent.

Take another look at the example from the beginning of this chapter. The diameter of the coin is 2.3 ± 0.2 centimeters, for a relative precision of $0.2/2.3 = 0.087$, or an 8.7 percent relative SE. And the area of the circle is calculated as 4.155 ± 0.725 square centimeters for a relative precision of $0.725/4.155 = 0.1745$, or a 17.45 percent relative SE, which is almost exactly twice the relative SE of the diameter. Notice that the constant ($\pi/4$) is completely ignored because relative errors aren't affected by multiplying or dividing by a known constant.

If k is negative (such as x^{-2}, which is $1/x^2$), you ignore the minus sign and use the absolute value of k. So the relative SE of $1/x^2$ is twice the relative SE of x. A special case of this rule is the simple reciprocal: The relative SE of $1/x$ is equal to the relative SE of x. In other words, if x is precise to ±1 percent, then $1/x$ is also precise to ±1 percent.

For example, under certain assumptions, the *half-life* ($t_{1/2}$) of a drug in the body is related to the *terminal elimination rate constant* (k_e) for the drug by the formula: $t_{1/2} = 0.693/k_e$. A pharmacokinetic regression analysis (see Chapter 21) might produce the result that $k_e = 0.1633 \pm 0.01644$ (k_e has units of "per hour"). You can calculate that $t_{1/2} = 0.693/0.1633 = 4.244$ hours. How precise is this half-life value? First you calculate the relative SE of the k_e value as $SE(k_e)/k_e$, which is $0.01644/0.1633 = 0.1007$, or about 10 percent. Because k_e has a relative precision of ± 10 percent, $t_{1/2}$ also has a relative precision of ± 10 percent, because $t_{1/2}$ is proportional to the reciprocal of k_e (you can ignore the 0.693 entirely, because relative errors are not affected by multiplying or dividing by a known constant). If the $t_{1/2}$ value of 4.244 hours has a relative precision of 10 percent, then the SE of $t_{1/2}$ must be 0.4244 hours, and you report the half-life as 4.24 ± 0.42 hours.

Handling More Complicated Expressions

Sometimes you have an expression that can't be handled by the simple rules described earlier in this chapter. The expression may be a very complicated expression and may involve logarithms, exponentials, or trigonometric functions. In these situations, you still have some options, as you find out in the following sections.

Using the simple rules consecutively

A complicated expression can often be broken down into a sequence of simple operations, which can then be analyzed by the rules described earlier in this chapter. For example, you can calculate the SE of the result of $xy + z$ from the SEs of x, y, and z by first using the product rule to get the SE of xy. Then you can use the addition rule with the SE of xy and the SE of z to get the SE of $xy + z$. But you have to be very careful going back and forth between SEs and relative SEs because you're likely to make a mistake somewhere in the calculations. It's much easier (and safer) to have the computer do all the calculations for you. Keep reading!

Checking out an online calculator

The web page at `statpages.info/erpropgt.html` calculates how precision propagates through almost any expression involving one or two variables. It even handles the case of two variables with correlated fluctuations. You simply enter the following items:

✔ The expression, using a fairly standard algebraic syntax (JavaScript)

✔ The values of the variable or variables

✔ The corresponding SEs

The web page then evaluates the general error-propagation formulas and shows you the value of the resulting number, along with its SE. Figure 11-2 shows how the web page handles the simple coin-area example I use in the earlier section "Understanding the Concept of Error Propagation."

Figure 11-2:
Using the web page to calculate error propagation through an expression with one variable.

> **For a single variable: z=f(x)**
>
> 1. Enter the measured value of the variable (x) and its standard error of estimate:
> x = [2.3]   +/- [0.2]
>
> 2. Enter the expression involving x: For example: 1/(10-x)
> z = [(Pi/4)*x*x]
>
> 3. Click on this button: [Propagate]
>
> The value of the resulting expression, z, and its standard error:
> z = [4.154756284] +/- [0.722566310]

Screenshot courtesy of John C. Pezzullo, PhD

The expression must refer to the variable (diameter) as *x*, and the squaring of *x* must be indicated as *x* * *x*, because JavaScript doesn't allow x^2. The web page knows what the value of pi is. It calculates an area of 4.15 square centimeters and an SE of 0.72 square centimeter, in good agreement with the calculations I describe earlier.

The web page can also analyze error propagation through expressions involving two measured values. Suppose you want to calculate body mass index (BMI, in kilograms per square meter) from a measured value of height (in centimeters) and weight (in kilograms), using the formula: BMI = 10,000weight/height^2. Suppose the measured height is 175 ± 1 centimeter, and the weight is 77 ± 1 kilograms (where the ± numbers are the SEs). The BMI is easily calculated as 10,000 × 77/175^2, or 25.143 kg/m^2. But what's the SE of that BMI? Figure 11-3 shows how the web page performs that calculation.

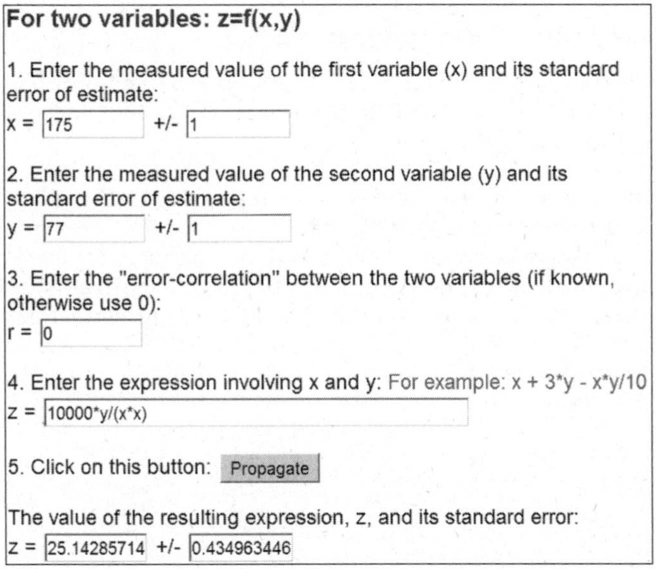
For two variables: z=f(x,y)
1. Enter the measured value of the first variable (x) and its standard error of estimate:
x = 175 +/- 1
2. Enter the measured value of the second variable (y) and its standard error of estimate:
y = 77 +/- 1
3. Enter the "error-correlation" between the two variables (if known, otherwise use 0):
r = 0
4. Enter the expression involving x and y: For example: x + 3*y - x*y/10
z = 10000*y/(x*x)
5. Click on this button: Propagate
The value of the resulting expression, z, and its standard error:
z = 25.14285714 +/- 0.434963446

Figure 11-3: Using the web page to calculate error propagation through an expression with two variables.

Screenshot courtesy of John C. Pezzullo, PhD

The page requires that height and weight be called *x* and *y*, respectively. I entered the square of the height as (*x* * *x*), because JavaScript doesn't allow x^2. I entered 0 for the error-correlation term because height and weight are two independent measurements (using different instruments). The resulting BMI produced by the web page was 25.1 ± 0.4 kilograms per square meter.

Simulating error propagation — easy, accurate, and versatile

Finally, I briefly describe what is probably the most general error-propagation technique (also called *Monte-Carlo analysis*). You can use this technique to solve many difficult statistical problems. Calculating how SEs propagate through a formula for *y* as a function of *x* works like this:

1. **Generate a random number from a normal distribution whose mean equals the value of *x* and whose standard deviation is the SE of *x*.**

2. **Plug the *x* value into the formula and save the resulting *y* value.**

3. **Repeat this step a large number of times.**

   The resulting set of *y* values will be your simulated sampling distribution for *y*.

4. **Calculate the SD of the *y* values.**

   The SD of the simulated *y* values is your estimate of the SE of *y*. (Remember, the SE of a number is the SD of the sampling distribution for that number.)

You can perform these calculations very easily using the free program Statistics 101 (see Chapter 4). With very little extra effort, this software can give you the confidence interval and even a histogram of the simulated areas. And simulation can easily and accurately handle non-normally distributed measurement errors. For the coin-area example, the program (only four lines long) generates the output shown in Figure 11-4. The SE of the coin area from this simulation is about 0.72, in good agreement with the value obtained by the other methods I describe earlier in this chapter.

Figure 11-4:
Using
Statistics
101 to simu-
late error
propagation.

```
1' Generate 100,000 Random diameters with mean=2.3, sd=0.2
2  normal 100000 2.3 0.2 d
3' For each one, calculate the area of the circle
4  let A = 3.1416*(d/2)^2
5' Calculate the SD of the simulated areas; this is the SE
6  stdev A SEofA
7' Print out the SE of the Area
8  PRINT TABLE "Standard Error of the Area" SEofA
```

```
Standard Error of the Area
SEofA
0.72341
```

Screenshot courtesy of John C. Pezzullo, PhD

Part III
Comparing Groups

Observed Counts		Outcome		
		Lived	Died	Total
Treatment	Drug:	33	27	60
	Placebo:	10	30	40
	Total:	43	57	100

Expected Counts if the Null Hypothesis Is True		Outcome		
		Lived	Died	Total
Treatment	Drug:	25.8	34.2	60
	Placebo:	17.2	22.8	40
	Total:	43	57	100

Illustration by Wiley, Composition Services Graphics

Discover the uses and steps of the simulation approach in a free article at www.dummies.com/extras/biostatistics.

In this part . . .

- ✔ Compare averages between two or more groups, using t tests, ANOVAs, and nonparametric tests.

- ✔ Compare proportions between two or more groups, using the chi-square and Fisher Exact tests.

- ✔ Analyze fourfold tables (also known as 2x2 cross-tabs) to get relative risks, odds ratios, and loads of other useful measures of association.

- ✔ Compare event rates, also known as person-time data.

- ✔ Test for equivalence between two products (like generic and brand-name drugs) and for noninferiority with respect to an established treatment (when you can't compare to a placebo).

Chapter 12

Comparing Average Values between Groups

Comparing average values between groups of numbers is part of the analysis of almost every biological experiment, and over the years statisticians have developed dozens of tests for this purpose. These tests include several different flavors of the Student t test, analyses of variance (ANOVA) and covariance (ANCOVA), and a dizzying collection of tests with such exotic-sounding names as Welch, Wilcoxon, Mann-Whitney, Kruskal-Wallis, Friedman, Tukey-Kramer, Dunnett, and Newman-Keuls, to name just a few. The number of possibilities is enough to make your head spin, and it leaves many researchers with the uneasy feeling that they may be using an inappropriate statistical test on their data.

In this chapter, I guide you through the menagerie of statistical tests for comparing groups of numbers, explaining why so many tests are out there, which ones are right for which situations, how to run them on a computer, and how to interpret the output. I focus on those tests that are usually provided by modern statistical programs (like those in Chapter 4).

Knowing That Different Situations Need Different Tests

You may wonder why there are so many tests for such a simple task as comparing averages. Well, "comparing averages" doesn't refer to a single task; it's a broad term that can apply to a lot of situations that differ from each other on the basis of:

- ✔ Whether you're looking at changes over time within one group of subjects or differences between groups of subjects (or both)

- ✔ How many time points or groups of subjects you're comparing

- ✔ Whether or not the numeric variable you're comparing is nearly normally distributed

- ✔ Whether or not the numbers have the same *spread* (standard deviation) in all the groups you're comparing

- ✔ Whether you want to compensate for the possible effects of some other variable on the variable you're comparing

These different conditions can occur in any and all combinations, so there are lots of possible situations. In the following sections, I look at the kinds of comparisons you may frequently encounter when analyzing biological data and tell you which tests are appropriate for each kind.

Comparing the mean of a group of numbers to a hypothesized value

Comparison of an observed mean to a particular value arises in studies where, for some reason, you can't have a control group (such as a group taking a placebo or an untreated group), so you have to compare your results to a *historical control,* such as information from the literature. It also comes up when you're dealing with data like test scores that have been scaled to have some specific mean in the general population (such as 100 for IQ scores).

This data is usually analyzed by the *one-group Student t test* that I describe in the later section "Surveying Student t tests." For non-normal data, the *Wilcoxon Signed-Ranks (WSR) test* can be used instead.

Comparing two groups of numbers

Perhaps the most common situation is one in which you're comparing two groups of numbers. You may want to compare some proposed biomarker of a medical condition between a group of subjects known to have that condition and a group known to not have it. Or you may want to compare some measure of drug efficacy between subjects treated with the drug and subjects treated with a placebo. Or maybe you want to compare the blood level of some enzyme between a sample of males and females.

Such comparisons are generally handled by the famous *unpaired* or *"independent sample" Student t test* (usually just called *the t test*) that I describe in the later section "Surveying Student t tests." But the t test is based on two assumptions about the distribution of data in the two groups:

✔ **The numbers are normally distributed** (called the *normality assumption*). For non-normal data you can use the nonparametric *Mann-Whitney (M-W) test,* which your software may refer to as the *Wilcoxon Sum-of-Ranks (WSOR) test.* The WSOR was developed first but was restricted to equal-size groups; the M-W test generalized the WSOR test to work for equal or unequal group sizes.

✔ **The standard deviation (SD) is the same for both groups** (called the *equal-variance* assumption because the variance is simply the square of the SD; thus, if the two SDs are the same, the two variances will also be the same). Chapter 8 provides more information about standard deviations. If the two groups have noticeably different variances (if, for example, the SD of one group is more than 1.5 times as large as the SD of the other), then the t test may not give reliable results, especially with unequal size groups. Instead, you can use a special modification to the Student t test, called the *Welch test* (also called the *Welch t test,* or the *unequal-variance t test;* see the later section "Surveying Student t tests" for details).

Comparing three or more groups of numbers

Comparing three or more groups of numbers is an obvious extension of the two-group comparison in the preceding section. For example, you may compare some efficacy endpoint, like response to treatment, among three treatment groups (for example, drug A, drug B, and placebo). This kind of comparison is handled by the *analysis of variance* (ANOVA) that I describe later in this chapter. When there is one grouping variable, like treatment, you have a *one-way ANOVA.* If the grouping variable has three levels (like drug A, drug B, and placebo in the earlier example), it's called a *one-way, three-level ANOVA.*

The null hypothesis of the one-way ANOVA is that all the groups have the same mean; the alternative hypothesis is that at least one group is different from at least one other group. The ANOVA produces a single p value, and if that p is less than your chosen criterion (such as $p < 0.05$), you can conclude that something's different somewhere (see Chapter 3 for more info on hypothesis testing and p values). But the ANOVA doesn't tell you which groups are different from which others. For that, you need to follow a significant ANOVA with one or more so-called *post-hoc* tests (described later in this chapter), which look for differences between each pair of groups.

You can also use the ANOVA to compare just two groups; this *one-way, two-level ANOVA* produces exactly the same p value as the classic unpaired equal-variance Student t test.

Analyzing data grouped on several different variables

The ANOVA is a very general method; it can accommodate several grouping variables at once, such as comparing treatment response among different treatment groups, genders, and medical conditions. An ANOVA involving three different grouping variables is called a *three-way ANOVA*.

In ANOVA terminology, the term *way* refers to how many grouping variables are involved, and the term *level* refers to the number of different groups within any one grouping variable.

Like the t test, the ANOVA also assumes normally distributed numbers with equal standard deviations in all the groups. If your data is non-normal, you can use the *Kruskal-Wallis test* instead of the one-way ANOVA, and if the groups have very dissimilar standard deviations, you can use the *Welch unequal-variance ANOVA*. You can use a *Friedman test* instead of a two-way ANOVA if only one of the two categorical variables is of interest, and the other is just a "nuisance" variable whose effect you want to mathematically compensate for (see the next section).

Adjusting for a "nuisance variable" when comparing numbers

Sometimes you know that the variable you're comparing (like reduction in blood pressure) is influenced not only by which group the subject belongs to (for example, antihypertension drug or placebo), but also by one or more other variables, such as age, medical condition, smoking status, and so forth. These variables may not be evenly distributed across the groups you're comparing (even in a randomized trial).

You can mathematically compensate for the effects of these "nuisance" variables, more properly called *confounders* (variables that can affect the outcome and may not be evenly balanced between groups), by using an *analysis of covariance* (ANCOVA). An ANCOVA is like an ANOVA in that it compares the mean value of an outcome variable between two or more groups. But an ANCOVA also lets you specify one or more *covariates* (as they're called in ANCOVA lingo) that you think may influence the outcome. The ANCOVA tells you whether the mean of the outcome variable is different between groups after compensating (that is, mathematically cancelling out) any influence of the covariates on the outcome.

Comparing sets of matched numbers

All the t tests, ANOVAs, ANCOVAs, and their nonparametric counterparts previously described deal with comparisons between two or more groups of independent samples of data, such as different groups of subjects, where there's no logical connection between a specific subject in one group and a specific subject in another group. But you often want to compare sets of data where precisely this kind of pairing exists. Matched-pair data comes up in several situations (illustrated here for two sets of data, but applicable to any number of sets):

- ✔ The values come from the same subject, but at two or more different times, such as before and after some kind of treatment, intervention, or event.

- ✔ The values come from a crossover clinical trial (see Chapter 6 for more about this structure), in which the same subject receives two or more treatments at two or more consecutive phases of the trial.

- ✔ The values come from two or more different individuals who have been paired, or matched, in some way. They may be twins or they may be matched on the basis of having similar characteristics (such as age, gender, and so on).

Comparing matched pairs

Paired comparisons are usually handled by the *paired student t test* that I describe later in this chapter. If your data isn't normally distributed, you can use the nonparametric *Wilcoxon Signed-Ranks test* instead.

The paired Student t test and the one-group Student t test are really the same test. When running a paired t test, you first calculate the difference between each pair of numbers (for example, subtract the pretreatment value from the post-treatment value), and then test those differences against the hypothesized value 0 using a one-group test.

Comparing three or more matched numbers

When you have three or more matched numbers, you can use *repeated-measures analysis of variance* (RM-ANOVA). The RM-ANOVA can also be used when you have only two groups; then it gives *exactly* the same p value as the classic paired Student t test.

If the data is non-normally distributed, you can use the nonparametric *Friedman test*. (Be careful — there are several different Friedman tests, and this isn't the same one that's used in place of a two-way ANOVA!)

Another problem to be aware of with RM-ANOVA and more than two levels is the issue of *sphericity* — an extension of the idea of equal variance to three or more sets of paired values. Sphericity refers to whether the paired differences have the same variance for all possible pairs of levels. Sphericity is assessed by the *Mauchly test,* and if the data is significantly nonspherical, special adjustments are applied to the RM-ANOVA by the software.

Comparing within-group changes between groups

Comparing within-group changes between groups is a special situation, but one that comes up very frequently in analyzing data from clinical trials. Suppose you're testing several arthritis drugs against a placebo, and your efficacy variable is the subject's reported pain level on a 0-to-10 scale. You want to know whether the drugs produce a greater improvement in pain level than the placebo. So you record each subject's pain level before starting the treatment (known as the *baseline* or *pretreatment*) and again at the end of the treatment period *(post-treatment).*

One obvious way to analyze this data would be to subtract each subject's pretreatment pain level from the post-treatment level to get the amount of change resulting from the treatment, and then compare the changes between the groups with a one-way ANOVA (or unpaired t test if there are only two groups). Although this approach is statistically valid, clinical trial data usually isn't analyzed this way; instead, almost every clinical trial nowadays uses an ANCOVA to compare changes between groups.

In an ANCOVA, the outcome (called the *dependent variable*) being compared between groups is not the change from pre- to post-treatment, but rather the post-treatment value itself. The pretreatment value is entered into the ANCOVA as the covariate. In effect, the ANCOVA subtracts a multiple of the pretreatment value from the post-treatment value before comparing the differences. That is, instead of defining the change as (Post – Pre), the ANCOVA calculates the change as (Post – $f \times$ Pre), where f is a number that the ANCOVA figures out. The f multiplier can be greater or less than 1; if it happens to come out exactly equal to 1, then the ANCOVA is simply comparing the pre-to-post change, just like the ANOVA.

Statisticians prefer the ANCOVA approach because it's usually slightly more efficient than the simple comparison of changes, and also because it can compensate (at least partially) for several other complications that often afflict clinical trial data.

An ANCOVA can be considered a form of multiple linear regression (see Chapter 19), and, in fact, all the classical methods I describe earlier (paired and unpaired t tests, ANOVAs, and ANCOVAs) can be formulated as multiple regression problems. Some statistical packages bundle some or all of these analyses into a single analysis called the general linear model.

Trying the Tests Used for Comparing Averages

After you see what tests are used when, you can take a closer look at the different kinds of tests — the basic concepts behind them, how to run them, and how to interpret the output. The following sections cover a variety of Student t tests, the ANOVA, and nonparametric tests.

I don't clutter this chapter with pages of mathematical formulas for the following tests, because you'll probably never have to do one of these tests by hand. If you really want to see the formulas, you can find them in most statistics textbooks and on the Internet. Just enter the name of the test in your search engine's browser.

Surveying Student t tests

In this section, I present the basic idea of a Student t test, show the computational steps common to the different kinds of t tests (one-group, paired, unpaired equal- or unequal-variance), and explain the computational differences between the different types. Then I describe how to run the t tests using typical statistical software and show how to interpret the output produced by one software package (OpenStat).

Understanding the basic idea of a t test

All the Student t tests for comparing sets of numbers are trying to answer the same question, "*Is the observed difference larger than what you would expect from random fluctuations alone?*" The t tests all answer this question in the same general way, which you can think of in terms of the following steps:

1. **Calculate the difference (D) between the groups or the time points.**

2. **Calculate the precision of the difference (the magnitude of the random fluctuations in that difference), in the form of a standard error (*SE*, described in Chapter 9) of that difference.**

3. **Calculate a test statistic (*t*), which expresses the size of the difference relative to the size of its standard error.**

   That is: $t = D/SE$.

4. **Calculate the degrees of freedom (*df*) of the *t* statistic.**

   Degrees of freedom is a tricky concept; as a practical matter, when dealing with t tests, it's the total number of observations minus the number of means you calculated from those observations.

5. **Calculate the p value (how likely it is that random fluctuations alone could produce a t value at least as large as the value you just calculated) using the Student t distribution.**

The Student t statistic is always calculated as D/SE; each kind of t test (one-group, paired, unpaired, Welch) calculates *D*, *SE,* and *df* in a way that makes sense for that kind of comparison, as summarized in Table 12-1.

Table 12-1   How t Tests Calculate Difference, Standard Error, and Degrees of Freedom

	One-Group	*Paired*	*Unpaired t* *Equal Variance*	*Welch t* *Unequal Variance*
D	Difference between mean of observations and a hypothesized value (*h*)	Mean of paired differences	Difference between means of the two groups	Difference between means of the two groups
SE	SE of the observations	SE of paired differences	SE of difference, based on a pooled estimate of SD within each group	SE of difference, from SE of each mean, by propagation of errors
df	Number of observations − 1	Number of pairs − 1	Total number of observations − 2	"Effective" df, based on the size and SD of the two groups

Running a t test

Almost all modern statistical software packages can perform all four kinds of t tests (see Chapter 4 for more about these packages). Preparing your data for a t test is quite easy:

✔ **For the one-group t test,** you need only one column of data, containing the variable whose mean you want to compare to the hypothesized value (H). The program usually asks you to specify a value for H and assumes 0 if you don't specify it.

✔ **For the paired t test,** you need two columns of data representing the pair of numbers (before and after, or the two matched subjects). For example, if you're comparing the before and after values for 20 subjects, or values for 20 sets of twins, the program will want to see a data file with 20 rows and two columns.

✔ **For the unpaired test (Student t or Welch),** most programs want you to have all the measured values in one variable, in one column, with a separate row for every observation (regardless of which group it came from). So if you were comparing test scores between a group of 30 subjects and a group of 40 subjects, you'd have a file with 70 rows and 2 columns. One column would have the test scores, and the other would have a numerical or text value indicating which group each subject belonged to.

Interpreting the output from a t test

Figure 12-1 shows the output of an unpaired t test from the OpenStat program (which you can find at www.statprograms4u.com/OpenStatMain.htm). Other programs usually provide the same kind of output, although it may be arranged and formatted differently.

```
COMPARISON OF TWO MEANS

Variable        Mean    Variance  Std.Dev.  S.E.Mean  N
Group 1         4.46     7.51      2.74      0.97    8
Group 2         5.55     9.81      3.13      0.90    12
Assuming equal variances, t =    -0.798 with probability = 0.4353 and  18
           degrees of freedom
Difference =     -1.09 and Standard Error of difference =     1.36
Confidence interval = (   -3.95,    1.78)
Assuming unequal variances, t =    -0.821 with probability = 0.4236 and
         16.52 degrees of freedom
Difference =     -1.09 and Standard Error of difference =     1.33
Confidence interval = (   -3.89,    1.72)
F test for equal variances =    1.306, Probability = 0.3730

NOTE: t-tests are two-tailed tests.
```

Figure 12-1: OpenStat output from an unpaired Student t test.

Illustration by Wiley, Composition Graphics Services

The first few lines provide the usual summary statistics (the mean, variance, standard deviation, standard error of the mean, and count of the number of observations) for each group. The program gives the output for both kinds of unpaired t tests (you don't even have to ask):

✔ **The classic Student t test** (which assumes equal variances)

✔ **The Welch test** (which works for unequal variances)

For each test, the output shows the value of the t statistic, the p value (which it calls *probability*), and the degrees of freedom (df), which, for the Welch test, might not be a whole number. The program also shows the difference between the means of the two groups, the standard error of that difference, and the 95 percent confidence interval around the difference of the means (see Chapter 10 for details on confidence intervals). The program leaves it up to you to use the results from the appropriate test (Student t or Welch t) and ignore the other test's results.

But how do you know which set is appropriate? The program very helpfully performs what's called an *F test for equal variances* between the two groups. Look at the p value from this F test:

- ✔ If p > 0.05, use the "Assuming equal variances" results.
- ✔ If p ≤ 0.05, use the "Assuming unequal variances" results.

In this example, the *F test* gives a p value of 0.373, which (being greater than 0.05) says that the two variances are not significantly different. So you can use the classic equal variances t test, which gives a p value of 0.4353. This p value (being greater than 0.05) says that the means of the two groups are not significantly different. In this case, the unequal variances (Welch) t test also gives a nonsignificant p value of 0.4236 (the two t tests often produce similar p values when the variances are nearly equal).

Assessing the ANOVA

In this section, I present the basic concepts underlying the analysis of variance (ANOVA) for comparing three or more groups of numbers and describe some of the more popular post-hoc tests. Then I show how to run an ANOVA using the OpenStat software package and how to interpret the output.

Understanding the basic idea of an ANOVA

When comparing two groups (A and B), you test the difference (A – B) between the two groups with a Student t test. So when comparing three groups (A, B, and C) it's natural to think of testing each of the three possible two-group comparisons (A – B, A – C, and B – C) with a t test. But running an exhaustive set of two-group t tests can be risky, because as the number of groups goes up, the number of two-group comparisons goes up even more. The general rule is that *N* groups can be paired up in $N(N-1)/2$ different ways, so in a study with six groups, you'd have $6 \times 5/2$, or 15 two-group comparisons.

In Chapter 6, I explain that when you do a lot of significance tests, you run an increased chance of making a *Type I error* — falsely concluding significance. This type of error is also called an *inflated alpha*. So if you want to know whether a bunch of groups all have consistent means or whether one or more of them are different from one or more others, you need a *single* test producing a *single* p value that answers that question.

The one-way ANOVA is exactly that kind of test. It doesn't look at the differences between pairs of group means; instead, it looks at how the entire collection of group means is spread out and compares that to how much you might expect those means to spread out if all the groups were sampled from the same population (that is, if there were no true difference between the groups). The result of this calculation (I'll spare you the details) is expressed in a test statistic called the *F ratio* (designated simply as *F*), the ratio of how much variability there is *between* the groups relative to how much there is *within* the groups. If the null hypothesis is true (in other words, if no true difference exists between the groups), then the F ratio should be close to 1, and its sampling fluctuations should follow the *Fisher F distribution* (see Chapter 25), which is actually a family of distribution functions characterized by two numbers:

- **The numerator degrees of freedom:** This number is often designated as df_N or df_1, which is one less than the number of groups.

- **The denominator degrees of freedom:** This number is designated as df_D or df_2, which is the total number of observations minus the number of groups.

The p value can be calculated from the values of *F*, df_1, and df_2, and the software will perform this calculation for you. If the p value from the ANOVA is significant (less than 0.05 or your chosen alpha level), then you can conclude that the groups are not all the same (because the means varied from each other by too large an amount).

Picking through post-hoc tests

But now you're back to your original question: *Which groups are different from which others?* Over the years, statisticians have developed a lot of tests for comparing means between several groups. These are called *post-hoc tests* (*post hoc* is Latin for "after this," meaning "after this ANOVA," and post-hoc tests are typically done after an ANOVA comes out significant). Most statistical packages that do ANOVAs offer one or more post-hoc tests as optional output. The packages (and many elementary statistics textbooks) may state, or at least imply, that these post-hoc tests guard against increased Type I error rates (an inflated alpha), but the truth isn't that simple. Controlling alpha to 0.05 across a lot of hypothesis tests is not a trivial task — a lot of subtle issues arise, which statisticians are still grappling with today. I could devote the rest of this book to that topic alone, but instead, I just describe some of the tests that most statistical programs offer as optional output from an ANOVA and make a few comments to help you choose which one to use.

- **The Bonferroni test** analyzes each pair of groups with a t test, but controls the overall alpha to 0.05 by requiring the p value for any comparison to be less than 0.05 divided by the total number of comparisons: $N(N-1)/2$, where N is the number of groups.

  Note: The Bonferroni test really shouldn't be used as a post-hoc test following an ANOVA; it's more appropriate when testing completely different hypotheses, not a set of interrelated ones. But many statistical packages offer it as a post-hoc test.

✔ **Fisher's LSD (least significant difference) test** analyzes all pairs of groups, but it doesn't properly control the overall alpha level across all comparisons. (As great a statistician as R. A. Fisher was, he blew it on this one.) Don't use LSD!

✔ **Tukey's HSD ("honestly" significant difference) test** analyzes all pairs of groups, but it correctly controls alpha across all the comparisons. It's a good, safe, "workhorse" post-hoc test, but it's limited to equal-size groups (called *balanced* groups).

✔ **The Tukey-Kramer test** is a generalization of the original Tukey HSD test to handle different-size *(unbalanced)* groups.

✔ **Scheffe's test** compares all pairs of groups and also lets you bundle certain groups together, if doing so makes physical sense. For example, if you have three treatment groups, A = Drug A, B = Drug B, and C = Placebo, you may want to determine whether the drug (regardless of which drug) is different from the placebo; that is, you may want to test A and B as one group against C. Scheffe's test is the most conservative and safest test to use if you absolutely hate Type I errors, but it's less powerful than the other tests, so you'll miss real differences more often.

✔ **Dunnett's test** is used when one of the groups is special — a *reference* group (typically placebo) against which you want to test each of the other groups. Because it doesn't have to compare as many pairs of groups as the other post-hoc tests, the Dunnett test is more powerful at detecting differences between the reference group and the others.

For a more detailed treatment of post-hoc tests, go to the excellent GraphPad website: www.graphpad.com and search within that site for *post hoc*.

Running an ANOVA

Running a one-way ANOVA is no more difficult than running an unpaired Student t test (see the earlier section "Running a t test"). You create two columns of data — one containing the numerical values being compared and another identifying the group the subject belongs to (just as with the t test, but now the group variable can have more than two levels). Then you specify what optional outputs you want to see (descriptive summaries for each group, tests for equal variance, graphs of group means, post-hoc tests [if any] you'd like to have, and so on).

Interpreting the output of an ANOVA

Figure 12-2 shows the output from an ANOVA run on a data set of pain scores of 40 subjects in three treatment groups (a placebo and two drugs), using OpenStat statistical software. Other programs usually provide the same kind of output, although it may be arranged and formatted differently.

The output begins with what's called a *variance table,* most of which you don't have to pay much attention to. You can spot the two degrees-of-freedom numbers: 2 between groups (# of groups – 1) and 37 within groups

(# of observations − # of groups). The test statistic for the ANOVA is the Fisher F ratio (6.61 in this table). The most important number in the table is the p value (the probability that random fluctuations would produce at least as large an F value as what your data produced), which is designated as "PROB.>F" in the table. The value 0.00 (which the program rounded off from a more accurate value of 0.0035) means that you can reject the null hypothesis (all group means are equal) and conclude that there's a difference somewhere among the groups.

```
ONE WAY ANALYSIS OF VARIANCE RESULTS
Dependent variable is: Score, Independent variable is: Group
SOURCE    D.F.     SS       MS        F        PROB.>F    OMEGA SQR.
BETWEEN    2      22.33    11.17     6.61      0.00       0.22
WITHIN    37      62.50     1.69
TOTAL     39      84.83


MEANS & VARIABILITY OF DEPENDENT VARIABLE FOR LEVELS OF THE INDEPENDENT VARIABLE
GROUP    MEAN     VARIANCE  STD.DEV.  N
  1      6.39      1.22      1.10    14
  2      5.08      2.10      1.45    13
  3      4.65      1.79      1.34    13
TOTAL    5.40      2.18      1.47    40


TESTS FOR HOMOGENEITY OF VARIANCE
Hartley Fmax test statistic =       1.72 with deg.s freem: 3 and    13.
Cochran C statistic =       0.41 with deg.s freem: 3 and    13.
Bartlett Chi-square =       0.91 with   2 D.F. Prob. > Chi-Square =  0.635


                    Scheffe contrasts among pairs of means.
                         alpha selected = 0.05
Group vs Group  Difference  Scheffe   Critical  Significant?
                            Statistic  Value
   1        2       1.31      2.61     2.550     YES
   1        3       1.74      3.47     2.550     YES
   2        3       0.43      0.85     2.550     NO


              Tukey-Kramer Test for (Differences Between Means
                         alpha selected = 0.05
Groups    Difference  Statistic      Probability  Significant?
 1 -  2     1.308     q =  3.696       0.0337       YES
 1 -  3     1.739     q =  4.913       0.0037       YES
 2 -  3     0.431     q =  1.195       0.6778       NO


              Bonferroni Test for (Differences Between Means
                    Overall alpha selected = 0.05
Comparisons made at alpha / no. comparisons = 0.017
Groups    Difference  Statistic  Prob > Value  Significant?
 1 -  2     1.308       2.651      0.014         YES
 1 -  3     1.739       3.695      0.001         YES
 2 -  3     0.431       0.788      0.438         NO
```

Figure 12-2: OpenStat output for one-way analysis of variance.

Illustration by Wiley, Composition Graphics Services

The ANOVA table is followed by a simple summary table of the mean, variance, standard deviation, and count of the observations in each group. Looking at the MEAN column, you see that Groups 2 and 3 have fairly similar averages (5.08 and 4.65, respectively), while Group 1 is noticeably higher (6.39). So Group 1 seems to be different from the others — but could this apparent difference be merely the result of random fluctuations? The rest of the output answers that question.

The summary table is followed by a test for *homogeneity of variances* (whether all groups have nearly the same standard deviations). OpenStat performs several variance tests (software packages often give you more than you want or need); the important one here is the Bartlett test. The last number in this row is the p value of 0.635, indicating that the variances (and therefore the standard deviations) do not differ significantly among the three groups, so you can use the ordinary ANOVA with confidence.

Finally, there are several post-hoc tests, comparing Group 1 to Group 2, Group 1 to Group 3, and Group 2 to Group 3. I had asked the program to perform the Scheffe, Tukey-Kramer, and Bonferroni tests from among the several that it offered. OpenStat is nice enough to interpret the tests for you and tell you, at the end of each row of output, whether the difference between the means for that pair of groups is significant or not.

In this example, all three post-hoc tests reached the same conclusions. That doesn't always happen, but it's very comforting when it does. All three tests agree that Groups 1 and 2 are different; Groups 1 and 3 are different, and Groups 2 and 3 are not significantly different. So Group 1, with its suspiciously high mean of 6.39, really is different from Groups 2 and 3, with their lower means. (By the way, in this example, Group 1 was the placebo.)

Running Student t tests and ANOVAs from summary data

You don't have to have the individual observations to perform a t test or one-way ANOVA; these tests need only the summary statistics (counts, means, and standard deviations or standard errors) of the numbers in each group (or of the paired differences, for the paired t test). This fact can be very useful when you want to perform these tests on published results, where only the summary statistics are available. Here are two online calculators you can use:

- ✔ StatPages.info/anova1sm.html lets you run an unpaired t test or a one-way ANOVA from summary data (count, mean, and standard deviation or standard error) for two or more (up to eight) groups. The program will produce an ANOVA table with the p value. (Keep in mind that an ANOVA with only two groups is identical to an unpaired Student t test.)

> ✔ `graphpad.com/quickcalcs/ttest1.cfm` lets you run paired and unpaired (equal or unequal variance) t tests from summary data or from individual observations (up to 50 rows).

The site `Statpages.info` lists many other web pages that perform various kinds of t tests and ANOVAs.

Running nonparametric tests

Running a nonparametric test (like the Wilcoxon, Mann-Whitney, Kruskal-Wallis, or Friedman test) is generally no more difficult than running the corresponding parametric t test or ANOVA. The data is set up in exactly the same way — one column for a one-group test, a pair of columns for a paired test; two columns (one numeric and one categorical) for unpaired tests, and so on. And you specify the variables to the program using commands or dialog boxes that are usually structured in the same way.

The nonparametric tests generally don't compare group means or test for a nonzero mean difference; rather, they compare group medians or test for a median difference of zero. So the output of a nonparametric test will look slightly different from the output of the corresponding parametric test — you'll probably see medians instead of means, and centiles instead of standard deviations. And you won't see any t or F values, but you should be able to find the p value indicating whether the groups have significantly different medians (or whether the median difference is significantly different from zero).

Estimating the Sample Size You Need for Comparing Averages

As you find out in the following sections, there are several ways to estimate the sample size you need in order to have a good chance of getting a significant result on a t test or an ANOVA. (Check out Chapter 3 for a refresher on the concepts of power and sample size.)

Simple formulas

Chapter 26 provides a set of simple formulas that let you estimate how many subjects you need for several kinds of t tests and ANOVAs. As with all sample-size calculations, you need to specify the *effect size of importance* (the smallest between-group difference that's worth knowing about), and you need an estimate of the amount of *random variability* in your data (the within-group standard deviation).

Software and web pages

Many modern statistics programs (SPSS, SAS, R, and so on; see Chapter 4) provide power and sample-size calculations for most of the standard statistical tests. The PS program performs these calculations for paired and unpaired t tests, and the free G-Power program handles all the t tests and many kinds of ANOVAs and ANCOVAs.

The website `StatPages.info` lists several dozen web pages that perform power and sample-size calculations for t tests and ANOVAs.

A sample-size nomogram

In Chapter 3, I explain that for any statistical test, four quantities (called statistical study design parameters) — power, alpha level, sample size, and effect size — are interrelated; you can calculate any one of them if you know the other three. Figure 12-3 shows a *nomogram* (also called an *alignment chart*) that lets you easily calculate any power, sample size, or effect size for an unpaired t test or a one-way ANOVA involving three, four, or five groups. It assumes a 0.05 alpha level (p < 0.05 is considered significant). You simply lay a ruler (or stretch a string) across the three scales, intersecting two scales at the values of the two design parameters you know, and then read the value of the third parameter where the string crosses the third scale. (Effect size is expressed as the ratio of the difference worth knowing about divided by the within-group standard deviation; this ratio is often called *delta/sigma*.) Here are some examples:

- ✔ **Find the sample size** needed to provide 80 percent power for a t test comparing two groups if the between-group difference you're interested in is equal to one-half the within-group standard deviation (a 0.5 delta/ sigma effect size). Lay the ruler across the 0.5 on the right-side scale (effect size), and across the 80 on the left side of the middle scale (for 80 percent power on a t test). The ruler crosses the left-side scale at the value 62, meaning that you need 62 analyzable subjects in each group (124 analyzable subjects altogether).

- ✔ **Find the effect size** (the true between-group difference) that would give you a 90 percent chance of getting a significant t test when comparing two groups of 40 subjects each, if the variable has a standard deviation of 25. Lay the ruler across 40 on the left scale and 90 on the left side of the middle scale. The ruler crosses the right scale at about 0.74, which means that the effect size (difference/SD) is 0.74, so the difference is 0.74 × 25, or about 18.

✔ **Find the power** of an ANOVA comparing four groups of 20 subjects each, when the true effect size (largest mean – smallest mean)/within-group SD is 0.6. Laying the ruler across 20 on the left scale and 0.6 on the right scale, read the value 47 on the right side of the middle scale (for an ANOVA). A study with four groups of 20 subjects is underpowered (providing only 47 percent power) to obtain a significant result in an ANOVA when the true means of the groups span a range of only 0.6 times the within-group SD.

Power/Sample size for t test and ANOVA (3–5 groups)

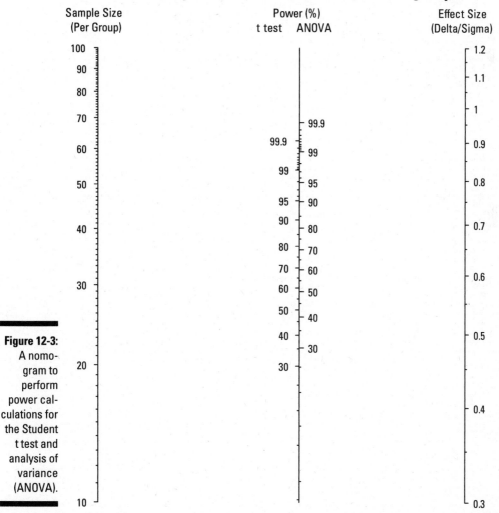

Figure 12-3: A nomogram to perform power calculations for the Student t test and analysis of variance (ANOVA).

Chapter 13

Comparing Proportions and Analyzing Cross-Tabulations

In This Chapter

▶ Testing for association between categorical variables with the Pearson chi-square and Fisher Exact tests

▶ Adjusting for confounders with the Mantel-Haenszel test for stratified fourfold tables

▶ Spotting trends across ordinal (sequenced) categories with the Kendall tau test

▶ Estimating sample sizes for tests of association

*S*uppose you're conducting a clinical trial of a new treatment for an acute disease with a high mortality rate, for which no effective treatment currently exists. You study 100 consecutive subjects with this condition and randomly assign 60 of them to receive the new treatment and 40 to receive a placebo or sham treatment. Then you record whether each subject lives or dies. Your data file has two dichotomous categorical variables: the treatment group (drug or placebo) and the outcome (lives or dies).

You find that 30 of the 40 untreated (placebo) subjects died (a 75 percent mortality rate), while only 27 of the 60 treated subjects died (45 percent mortality). The drug appears to reduce mortality by about 30 percentage points. But can you be sure this isn't just a random sampling fluctuation?

Data from two (possibly associated) categorical variables is generally summarized as a *cross-tabulation* (also called a *cross-tab* or a *two-way table*). The rows of the cross-tab represent the different categories (or *levels*) of one variable, and the columns represent the different levels of the other variable. The cells of the table contain the count of the number of subjects with the indicated levels for the row and column variables. If one variable can be thought of as the "cause" or "predictor" of the other, the cause variable becomes the rows, and the "outcome" or "effect" variable becomes the columns. If the cause and outcome variables are both dichotomous (have only two levels), as they are in this example, then the cross-tab has two rows and two columns (and therefore four cells of counts) and is referred to as a 2-by-2 (or 2x2) cross-tab, or a *fourfold table*. Cross-tabs are usually displayed with an extra row at the bottom and an extra column at the right to contain the sums of the cells in the rows and columns of the table. These sums are called *marginal totals,* or just *marginals*.

Comparing proportions based on a fourfold table is the simplest example of testing the association between two categorical variables. More generally, the variables can have any number of categories, so the cross-tab can be larger than 2x2, with many rows and many columns. But the basic question to be answered is always the same: Is the spread of numbers across the columns so different from one row to the next that the numbers can't be reasonably explained away as random fluctuations?

In this chapter, I describe a variety of tests you can use to answer this question: the Pearson chi-square test, the Fisher Exact test, the Mantel-Haenszel test, and the Kendall test. I also explain how to estimate power and sample sizes for the chi-square and Fisher Exact tests.

You can run all the tests in this chapter either from case-level data in a database (one record per subject) or from data that has already been summarized in the form of a cross-tab:

✔ Most statistical software is set up to work with case-level data. Your file needs to have two categorical variables representing the row and column variables whose relationship you want to test. If you're running a Mantel-Haenszel test, your file also needs to have another variable representing the *stratum* (see the Mantel-Haenszel section later in this chapter). You merely have to tell the software which test (or tests) you want to run and identify the variables to be used for the test. Flip to Chapter 4 for an introduction to statistical software.

✔ Most online calculators expect you to have already cross-tabulated the data. These calculators usually present a screen showing an empty table, and you enter the counts into the table's cells.

Examining Two Variables with the Pearson Chi-Square Test

The most commonly used statistical test of association between two categorical variables is called the *chi-square test of association*. This classic test was developed around 1900 by Karl Pearson and has been a mainstay of practical statistical analysis ever since. It's called the chi-square test because it involves calculating a number (a *test statistic*) that fluctuates in accordance with the chi-square distribution (see Chapter 25). Many other statistical tests also use the chi-square distribution, but the test of association is by far the most popular, so whenever I refer to a chi-square test without specifying which one, I'm referring to the Pearson chi-square test of association between two categorical variables.

In the following sections, I explain how the chi-square test works, list some pros and cons of the test, and describe a modification you can make to the test.

Understanding how the chi-square test works

You don't have to know the details of the chi-square test if you have a computer do the calculations for you (which I always recommend), so technically, you don't have to read this section. But you'll have a better appreciation for the strengths and limitations of this test if you know how it works. Here, I walk you through the steps of conducting a chi-square test.

Calculating observed and expected counts

All statistical significance tests start with a *null hypothesis* (H_0) that asserts that no real effect is present in the population, and any effect you think you see in your sample is due only to random fluctuations. (See Chapter 3 for more information.) The H_0 for the chi-square test asserts that there's no association between the row variable and the column variable, so you should expect the relative spread of cell counts across the columns to be the same for each row.

Figure 13-1 shows how this works out for the observed data taken from the example in this chapter's introduction. You can see from the marginal "Total" row that the overall mortality rate (for both treatment groups combined) is 57/100, or 57 percent.

Figure 13-1:
The observed results of a trial of a new drug for a high-mortality disease.

Observed Counts		Outcome		
		Lived	Died	Total
Treatment	Drug:	33	27	60
	Placebo:	10	30	40
	Total:	43	57	100

Illustration by Wiley, Composition Services Graphics

What if the true mortality rate for this condition is 57 percent, and the drug truly has no effect on mortality?

- ✔ In the drug-treated group, you'd expect about 34.2 deaths (57 percent of 60), with the remaining 25.8 subjects surviving. (Expected outcomes are usually not whole numbers.)

- ✔ In the placebo group, you'd expect about 22.8 deaths (57 percent of 40), with the remaining 17.2 subjects surviving.

These expected outcomes are displayed in Figure 13-2.

Figure 13-2:
Expected
cell counts
if the null
hypothesis
is true (the
drug does
not affect
survival).

Expected Counts if the Null Hypothesis Is True		Outcome		
		Lived	Died	Total
Treatment	Drug:	25.8	34.2	60
	Placebo:	17.2	22.8	40
	Total:	43	57	100

Illustration by Wiley, Composition Services Graphics

Notice that the expected counts table in Figure 13-2 has the same *marginal totals* (row totals and column totals) as the observed counts table in Figure 13-1; the difference is that under H_0 (no association between row variable and column variable), the relative spread of expected counts across the columns is the same for each row (and the relative spread of counts down the rows is the same for each column). In other words, the "expected" numbers in both rows (drug and placebo) have the same relative spread between lived and died.

Now that you have observed and expected counts, you're no doubt curious as to how they differ. You can subtract each expected count from the observed count in each cell to get a *difference table* (observed – expected), like Figure 13-3:

Because the observed and expected tables in Figures 13-1 and 13-2 always have the same marginal totals, the marginal totals in the difference table are all equal to zero. All four cells in the center of this difference table have the same absolute value (7.2), with a plus and a minus value in each row and each column.

The pattern just described is always the case for 2x2 tables. For larger tables, the difference numbers aren't all the same, but they always sum up to zero for each row and each column.

Figure 13-3:
Differences
between
observed
and
expected
cell counts
if the null
hypothesis
is true.

Differences between Observed and Expected Counts		Outcome		
		Lived	Died	Total
Treatment	Drug:	+7.2	−7.2	0
	Placebo:	−7.2	+7.2	0
	Total:	0	0	0

Illustration by Wiley, Composition Services Graphics

The values in the difference table in Figure 13-3 show how far off from H_0 your observed data is. The question remains: Are those difference values larger than what may have arisen from random fluctuations alone if H_0 is really true? You need some kind of "yardstick" by which to judge how unlikely those difference values are. Recall from Chapter 9 that the *standard error* (SE) expresses the general magnitude of random sampling , so the SE makes a good yardstick for judging the size of the differences you may expect to see from random fluctuations alone. It turns out that the SE of the differences is approximately equal to the square root of the expected counts. The rigorous proof of this is too complicated for most mortals to understand, but a pretty simple informal explanation is based on the idea that random event occurrences often follow the Poisson distribution, for which the SE of the event count equals the square root of the expected count (as I explain in Chapter 9).

Summarizing and combining scaled differences

For the upper-left cell in the cross-tab (drug-treated subjects who lived), you see the following:

✓ The observed count (Ob) is 33.

✓ The expected count (Ex) is 25.8.

✓ The difference (Diff) is 33 − 25.8, or +7.2.

✓ The SE of the difference is $\sqrt{25.8}$, or 5.08.

You can "scale" the Ob–Ex difference by dividing it by the SE yardstick, getting the ratio (Diff/SE) = +7.2/5.08, or 1.42. This means that the difference between the *observed* number of drug-treated subjects who lived and the number you would have *expected* if the drug had no effect on survival is about 1.42 times as large as you would have expected from random sampling fluctuations alone. You can do the same calculation for the other three cells and summarize these scaled differences, as shown in Figure 13-4.

Figure 13-4: Differences between observed and expected cell counts, scaled according to the estimated standard errors of the differences.

Scaled Differences (Ob − Ex)/Sqrt(Ex)		Outcome	
		Lived	Died
Treatment	Drug:	1.42	−1.23
	Placebo:	−1.74	1.51

Illustration by Wiley, Composition Services Graphics

The next step is to combine these individual scaled differences into an overall measure of the difference between what you observed and what you would have expected if the drug truly did not affect survival. You can't just add them up, because the negative and positive differences would tend to cancel each other out. You want all differences (positive and negative) to contribute to the overall measure of how far your observations are from what you expected under H_0. Statisticians love to sum the *squares* of differences (because squares are always positive), and that's exactly what's done in the chi-square test. Figure 13-5 shows the squared scaled differences, which are calculated from the observed and expected counts in Tables 13-1 and 13-2 using the formula $(Ob - Ex)^2/Ex$, not by squaring the rounded-off numbers in Table 13-4, which would be less accurate.

Figure 13-5:
Components of the chi-square statistic: squares of the scaled differences.

Squared Scaled Differences $(Ob - Ex)^2/Ex$		Outcome	
		Lived	Died
Treatment	Drug:	2.01	1.52
	Placebo:	3.01	2.27

Illustration by Wiley, Composition Services Graphics

You then add up these squared scaled differences: $2.01 + 1.52 + 3.01 + 2.27 = 8.81$. This sum is an excellent test statistic to measure the overall departure of your data from the null hypothesis:

- ✔ If the null hypothesis is true (the drug does not affect survival), this statistic should be quite small.

- ✔ The more effect the drug has on survival (in either direction), the larger this statistic should be.

Determining the p value

The only remaining task is to determine the *p value* — the probability that random fluctuations alone, in the absence of any true effect of the drug on survival, could lead to a value of 8.81 or greater for this test statistic. (I introduce p values in Chapter 3.) Once again, the rigorous proof is very complicated, but an informal explanation goes something like this:

When the expected cell counts are very large, the Poisson distribution becomes very close to a normal distribution (see Chapter 25 for more on the Poisson distribution). If the H_0 is true, each scaled difference should be (approximately) a normally distributed random variable with a mean of zero (because you subtract the expected value from the observed value) and a standard deviation of 1 (because you divide by the standard error). The sum of the squares of one or more normally distributed random numbers is a number that follows the chi-square distribution (also covered in Chapter 25). So the test statistic from this test should follow the chi-square distribution (which is why this is called the chi-square test), and you should be able to look up your 8.81 in a chi-square table to get the p value for the test.

Now, the chi-square distribution is really a family of distributions, depending on a number called the *degrees of freedom,* usually abbreviated d.f. or df, or by the Greek lowercase letter *nu* (ν), which tells how many *independent* normally distributed numbers were squared and added up.

What's the df for the chi-square test? It depends on the number of rows in the cross-tab. For the 2x2 cross-tab (fourfold table) in this example, you added up the four values in Figure 13-5, so you may think that you should look up the 8.81 chi-square value with 4 df. But you'd be wrong. Note the italicized word *independent* in the preceding paragraph. And keep in mind that the differences (Ob – Ex) in any row or column always add up to zero. The four terms making up the 8.81 total aren't independent of each other. It turns out that the chi-square test statistic for a fourfold table has only 1 df, not 4. In general, an *N*-by-*M* table, with *N* rows, *M* columns, and therefore $N \times M$ cells, has only $(N-1)(M-1)$ df because of the constraints on the row and column sums. Don't feel bad if this wrinkle caught you by surprise — even Karl Pearson (the guy who invented the chi-square test) got that part wrong!

So, referring to a chi-square table (or, better yet, having the computer calculate the p value for you in any statistical software package), the p value for chi-square = 8.81, with 1 df, is 0.003. This means that there's only a 0.003 probability, or about 1 chance in 333 (because 1/0.003 = 333), that random fluctuations could produce such an impressive apparent performance if the drug truly had no effect on survival. So your conclusion would be that the drug is associated with a significant reduction in mortality.

Putting it all together with some notation and formulas

The calculations of the Pearson chi-square test can be summarized concisely using the cell-naming conventions in Figure 13-6, along with the standard summation notation described in Chapter 2.

Figure 13-6: A general way of naming the cells of a cross-tab table.		Column 1	Column 2	Total
	Row 1 :	$Ob_{1,1}$	$Ob_{1,2}$	R_1
	Row 2 :	$Ob_{2,1}$	$Ob_{2,2}$	R_2
	Total:	C_1	C_2	T

Illustration by Wiley, Composition Services Graphics

Using these conventions, the basic formulas for the Pearson chi-square test are as follows:

- ✔ **Expected values:** $Ex_{i,j} = \dfrac{R_i \times C_j}{T}$, $i = 1, 2, \ldots N; j = 1, 2, \ldots M$

- ✔ **Chi-square statistic:** $\chi^2 = \sum\limits_{i=1}^{N}\sum\limits_{j=1}^{M} \dfrac{\left(Ob_{i,j} - Ex_{i,j}\right)^2}{Ex_{i,j}}$

- ✔ **Degrees of freedom:** df $= (N-1)(M-1)$

where i and j are array indices that indicate the row and column, respectively, of each cell.

Pointing out the pros and cons of the chi-square test

The Pearson chi-square test is so popular for several reasons:

- ✔ The calculations are fairly simple and can even be carried out by hand, although I'd never recommend that. They can easily be programmed in Excel; several web pages can perform the test; and it has been implemented on PDAs, smartphones, and tablets. Almost every statistical software package (including the ones in Chapter 4) can perform the chi-square test for cross-tabulated data.

- ✔ The test works for tables with any number of rows and columns, and it easily handles cell counts of any magnitude. The calculations are almost instantaneous on a computer for tables of any size and counts of any magnitude.

But the chi-square test has some shortcomings:

- ✔ It's not an exact test. The p value it produces is only approximate, so using $p < 0.05$ as your criterion for significance doesn't necessarily guarantee that your Type I error rate (the chance of falsely claiming significance) will be only 5 percent (see Chapter 3 for an introduction to Type I errors). It's quite accurate when all the cells in the table have large counts, but it becomes unreliable when one or more cell counts is very small (or zero). There are different suggestions as to how many counts you need in order to confidently use the chi-square test, but the simplest rule is that you should have at least five observations in each cell of your table (or better yet, at least five *expected* counts in each cell).

- ✔ The chi-square test isn't good at detecting small but steady progressive trends across the successive categories of an *ordinal* variable (see Chapter 4 if you're not sure what *ordinal* is). It may give a significant result if the trend is strong enough, but it's not designed specifically to work with ordinal categorical data.

Modifying the chi-square test: The Yates continuity correction

For the special case of fourfold tables, a simple modification to the chi-square test, called the *Yates continuity correction,* gives more reliable p values. The correction consists of subtracting 0.5 from the magnitude of the (Ob – Ex) difference before squaring it.

The Yates correction to the Pearson chi-square test should *always* be used for fourfold tables but should *not* be used for tables with more than two rows or more than two columns.

For the sample data in the earlier section "Understanding how the chi-square test works," the application of the Yates correction changes the 7.20 (or –7.20) difference in each cell to 6.70 (or –6.70). This lowers the chi-square value from 8.81 down to 7.63 and increases the p value from 0.0030 to 0.0057, which is still very significant — the chance of random fluctuations producing such an apparent effect in your sample is only about 1 in 175 (because 1/0.0057 = 175).

Focusing on the Fisher Exact Test

The Pearson chi-square test that I describe in the earlier section "Examining Two Variables with the Pearson chi-Square Test" isn't the only way to analyze cross-tabulated data. R. A. Fisher (probably the most famous statistician of all time) invented another test in the 1920s that gives the exact p value for tables with large or small cell counts (even cell counts of zero!). Not surprisingly, this test is called the *Fisher Exact* test. In the following sections, I show you how the Fisher Exact test works, and I note both its pros and cons.

Understanding how the Fisher Exact test works

You don't have to know the details of the Fisher Exact test if you have a computer do the calculations for you (which I always recommend), so you don't have to read this section. But you'll have a better appreciation for the strengths and limitations of this test if you know how it works.

This test is, conceptually, pretty simple. You look at every possible table that has the same marginal totals as your observed table. You calculate the exact probability (Pr) of getting each individual table using a formula that, for a fourfold table (using the notation for Figure 13-6), is

$$Pr = \frac{(R_1!)(R_2!)(C_1!)(C_2!)}{(Ob_{1,1}!)(Ob_{1,2}!)(Ob_{2,1}!)(Ob_{2,2}!)(T!)}$$

Those exclamation points indicate calculating the factorials of the cell counts (see Chapter 2). For the example in Figure 13-1, the observed table has a probability of

$$Pr = \frac{(60!)(40!)(43!)(57!)}{(33!)(27!)(10!)(30!)(100!)} = 0.00196$$

Other possible tables with the same marginal totals as the observed table have their own Pr values, which may be larger than, smaller than, or equal to the Pr value of the observed table. The Pr values for all possible tables with a specified set of marginal totals always add up to exactly 1.

The Fisher Exact test p value is obtained by adding up the Pr values for all tables that are at least as different from the H_0 as your observed table. For a fourfold table, that means adding up all the Pr values that are less than (or equal to) the Pr value for your observed table.

For the example in Figure 13-1, the p value comes out to 0.00385, which means that there's only 1 chance in 260 (because 1/0.00385 = 260) that random fluctuations could have produced such an apparent effect in your sample.

Noting the pros and cons of the Fisher Exact test

The big advantages of the Fisher Exact test are as follows:

✔ It gives the exact p value.

✔ It is exact for all tables, with large or small (or even zero) cell counts.

So why do people still use the chi-square test, which is approximate and doesn't work for tables with small cell counts? Why doesn't everyone always use the Fisher test? Nowadays many statisticians *are* recommending that everyone use the Fisher test instead of the chi-square test whenever possible. But there are several problems with the Fisher Exact test:

✔ The calculations are a *lot* more complicated, especially for tables larger than 2x2. Many statistical software packages either don't offer the Fisher Exact test or offer it only for fourfold tables. Several interactive web pages perform the Fisher Exact test for fourfold tables (including `StatPages.info/ctab2x2.html`), but at this time I'm not aware of any web pages that offer that test for larger tables. Only the major statistical software packages (like SAS, SPSS, and R, described in Chapter 4) offer the Fisher Exact test for tables larger than 2x2.

✔ The calculations can become numerically unstable for large cell counts, even in a 2x2 table. The equations involve the factorials of the cell counts and marginal totals, and these can get very large — even for modest sample sizes — often exceeding the largest number that a computer is capable of dealing with. Many programs and web pages that offer the Fisher Exact test for fourfold tables fail with data from more than 100 subjects. (The web page `StatPages.info/ctab2x2.html` works with cell counts of any size.)

✔ The exact calculations can become impossibly time consuming for larger tables and larger cell counts. Even if a program can, in theory, do the calculations, it may take hours — or even centuries — to carry them out!

✔ The Fisher Exact test is no better than the chi-square test at detecting gradual trends across ordinal categories.

Calculating Power and Sample Size for Chi-Square and Fisher Exact Tests

Note: The basic ideas of power and sample-size calculations are described in Chapter 3, and you should review that information before going further here.

Suppose you're planning a study to test whether giving a certain dietary supplement to a pregnant woman reduces her chances of developing morning sickness during the first trimester (the first three months) of pregnancy. This condition normally occurs in 80 percent of pregnant women, and if the supplement can reduce that incidence rate to only 60 percent, it's certainly worth knowing about. So you plan to enroll a group of pregnant women and randomize them to receive either the dietary supplement or a placebo that looks, smells, and tastes exactly like the supplement. You'll have them take the product during their first trimester, and you'll record whether they experience morning sickness during that time (using explicit criteria for what constitutes morning sickness). Then you'll tabulate the results in a 2x2 cross-tab (with "supplement" and "placebo" defining the two rows, and "did" and "did not" experience morning sickness heading the two columns). And you'll test for a significant effect with a chi-square or Fisher Exact test. How many subjects must you enroll to have at least an 80 percent chance of getting $p < 0.05$ on the test if the supplement truly can reduce the incidence from 80 percent to 60 percent?

TIP

You have several ways to estimate the required sample size. The quickest one is to refer to the sample-size table for comparison of proportions in this book's Cheat Sheet at www.dummies.com/cheatsheet/biostatistics. But the most general and most accurate way is to use power/sample-size software such as PS or GPower (see Chapter 4). Or, you can use the online sample-size calculator at StatPages.info/proppowr.html, which produces the same results. Using that web page, the calculation is set up as shown in Figure 13-7.

Figure 13-7:
The online
sample-size
calculator
for compar-
ing two
proportions
with a chi-
square or
Fisher Exact
test.

Significance Level (alpha):	0.05	(Usually 0.05)
Power (% chance of detecting):	80	(Usually 80)
Group 1 Population Proportion:	0.8	(Between 0.0 and 1.0)
Group 2 Population Proportion:	0.6	(Between 0.0 and 1.0)
Relative Sample Sizes Required (Group 2 / Group 1):	1.0	(For equal samples, use 1.0)

Compute

Sample Size Required

	Group 1	Group 2	Total
"Classical" Calculation:	81	81	162
With Continuity Correction:	91	91	182

Screenshot courtesy of John C. Pezzullo, PhD

You fill in the five parameters in the upper block, hit the Compute button, and see the results in the lower block. This web page provides two different calculations:

✔ **The classical calculation,** which applies to the uncorrected chi-square test, says that 81 analyzable subjects in each group (162 analyzable subjects altogether) are required.

✔ **The continuity-corrected calculation,** which applies to the Yates chi-square or Fisher Exact test, says that 91 analyzable subjects in each group (182 analyzable subjects altogether) are required.

You should base your planning on the larger value from the continuity-corrected calculation, just to be on the safe side.

You need to enroll additional subjects to allow for possible attrition during the study. If you expect x percent of the subjects to drop out, your enrollment should be:

Enrollment = $100 \times$ Analyzable Number/$(100 - x)$

So if you expect 15 percent of enrolled subjects to drop out and therefore be non-analyzable, you need to enroll $100 \times 182/(100 - 15)$, or about 214, subjects.

Analyzing Ordinal Categorical Data with the Kendall Test

Neither the chi-square nor the Fisher Exact test (I describe both earlier in this chapter) is designed for testing the association between two *ordinal* categorical variables — categories that can be put into a natural order. These tests are insensitive to the order of the categories; if you shuffle the columns (or rows) into some other sequence, they produce the same p value. This characteristic makes the chi-square and Fisher Exact tests insensitive to gradual trends across the ordinal categories.

As an example, consider a study in which you test a new drug for a chronic progressive disease (one that tends to get worse over time) at two different doses along with a placebo. You record the outcome after six months of treatment as a three-way classification: improved, unchanged, or worsened. You can think of treatment as an ordinal categorical variable — placebo < low-dose < high-dose — and outcome as an ordinal variable — worsened < unchanged < improved. A study involving 100 test subjects may produce the results shown in Figure 13-8.

Figure 13-8:
An association between two ordinal variables: dose level and response.

	Worsened	Unchanged	Improved	Total
Placebo	17	11	6	34
Low Dose	11	12	10	33
High Dose	8	11	14	33
Total	36	34	30	100

Illustration by Wiley, Composition Services Graphics

Notice that

- ✔ Most placebo subjects got worse, some stayed the same, and a few got better. This reflects the general downward course of an untreated progressive disease.

- ✔ The low-dose subjects didn't seem to change much, on average, with roughly equal numbers getting better, getting worse, and remaining the same. The low-dose drug may at least be showing some tendency to counteract the general progressive nature of the disease.

- ✔ The high-dose subjects seemed to be getting better more often than getting worse, indicating that at higher doses, the drug may be able to actually reverse the usual downward course of the disease.

So an encouraging pattern does appear in the data. But both the chi-square and Fisher Exact tests conclude that there's no significant association between dose level of the drug and outcome (p = 0.153 by chi-square test and 0.158 by Fisher Exact test). Why can't the tests see what you can see by looking at the table? Because both of these tests, by the way they calculate their p value, are unable to notice a progressive trend across the three rows and the three columns.

Fortunately, other tests are designed specifically to spot trends in ordinal data. One of the most common ones involves calculating a test statistic called Kendall's tau. The basic idea is to consider each possible pair of subjects, determining whether those two subjects are *concordant* or *discordant* with the hypothesis that the two variables are positively correlated. In this example, it's like asking whether the subject who received a higher dose of the drug also had a better outcome.

For example, if one subject in the pair received the placebo and was unchanged while the other subject received the low dose and got better, that pair would be concordant. But if one subject received a low dose and got better while another subject received a high dose and remained unchanged, that pair would be considered discordant.

The Kendall test counts how many pairs are concordant, discordant, or *noninformative* (where both subjects are in the same category for one or both variables). The test statistic is based on the difference between the number of concordant and discordant pairs divided by a theoretical estimate of the standard error of that difference. The test statistic is then looked up in a table of the normal distribution to obtain a p value.

For the sample data in Figure 13-8, the Kendall test (using the R statistical software package) gives p = 0.010, which, being less than 0.05, indicates a significant association between dose level and outcome. The Kendall test can spot the slight but consistent trend across the columns and down the rows of the table, whereas the chi-square and Fisher Exact tests can't.

Studying Stratified Data with the Mantel-Haenszel Chi-Square Test

All the tests I describe earlier in this chapter examine the relationship between *two* categorical variables. Sometimes, however, one or more "nuisance" variables can get in the way of your analysis. Building on the example I use at the beginning of this chapter, suppose you've tested your new drug in three countries. And suppose that because of differences in demographics, healthcare, climate, and so on, the mortality of the disease tends to be different in each of the three countries. Furthermore, suppose that there's a slight imbalance between the number of drug and placebo subjects in each country. The country would be considered a *confounder* of the relationship between treatment and survival. Confounding can obscure real effects or produce spurious apparent effects when none are truly present. So you want some way to *control* for this confounder (that is, mathematically compensate for any effect it might have on the observed mortality) in your analysis.

The most general way to handle confounding variables is with multivariate regression techniques that I describe in Chapter 19. Another way is by *stratification,* in which you split your data file into two or more *strata* on the basis of the values of the confounder so that cases within each stratum have the same (or nearly the same) value for the confounder (or confounders). You then analyze the data within each stratum and pool the results for all the strata.

When you analyze the relationship between two dichotomous categorical variables, you can control for one or more confounders using the *Mantel-Haenszel (MH)* chi-square test. This test is simple to set up, and the results are usually easy to interpret, so it's often the preferred way to analyze fourfold tables when you want to adjust for confounding variables.

To run an MH test, you first create a separate fourfold table for each stratum. Suppose that your data, broken down by country, looks like Figure 13-9.

Country	Treatment	Lived	Died	Total
USA	Drug:	10	8	18
	Placebo:	4	7	11
Canada	Drug:	11	9	20
	Placebo:	3	10	13
Mexico	Drug:	12	10	22
	Placebo:	3	13	16
All Three Countries	Drug:	33	27	60
	Placebo:	10	30	40

Figure 13-9: Results of a trial of a new drug for a high-mortality disease, stratified by country.

Illustration by Wiley, Composition Services Graphics

Conceptually, the MH test works by estimating an odds ratio for each country, pooling those estimates into an overall odds ratio for all countries, and testing whether the pooled odds ratio is significantly different from 1. (An *odds ratio* is a measure of how much the spread of counts across the columns differs between the rows, with a value of 1 indicating no difference at all; see Chapter 14 for details.)

Using the R statistical package, an MH test on the data in Figure 13-9 produces a p value of 0.0068, which indicates that there's only about 1 chance in 147 (because 1/0.0068 = 147) that random fluctuations could produce such an apparent effect in your sample.

Like the chi-square test, the Mantel-Haenszel test is only an approximation. It's most commonly used for 2x2 tables, although some software can run an extended form of the test for tables larger than 2x2, provided the categorical variables are ordinal (see the section "Analyzing Ordinal Categorical Data with the Kendall Test").

Chapter 14

Taking a Closer Look at Fourfold Tables

· ·

In This Chapter

▶ Beginning with the basics of fourfold tables

▶ Digging into sampling designs for fourfold tables

▶ Using fourfold tables in different scenarios

· ·

*I*n Chapter 13, I show you how to compare proportions between two or more groups with a cross-tab table. In general, a cross-tab shows the relationship between two categorical variables. Each row of the table represents one particular category of one variable, and each column of the table represents one particular category of the other variable. The table can have two or more rows and two or more columns, depending on the number of levels (different categories) present in each of the two variables. So a cross-tab between a treatment variable that has three levels (like old drug, new drug, and placebo) and an outcome variable that has five levels (like died, got worse, unchanged, improved, and cured) has three rows and five columns.

A special case occurs when both variables are *dichotomous* (or *binary*); that is, they both have only two values, like gender (male and female) and compliance (good and bad). The cross-tab of these two variables has two rows and two columns. Because a 2x2 cross-tab table has four cells, it's commonly called a *fourfold table*.

Everything in Chapter 13 applies to the fourfold table and to larger cross-tab tables. Because the fourfold table springs up in so many different contexts in biological research, and because so many other quantities are calculated from the fourfold table, it warrants a chapter all its own. In this chapter, I describe the various research scenarios in which fourfold tables often occur: comparing proportions, testing for association, evaluating risk factors, quantifying the performance of diagnostic tests, assessing the effectiveness of therapies, and measuring inter-rater and intra-rater reliability. I describe how to calculate several common measures (called *indices*) used in each scenario, along with their confidence intervals. And I describe different kinds of *sampling strategies* (ways of selecting subjects to study) that you need to be aware of.

Focusing on the Fundamentals of Fourfold Tables

The most obvious thing you can get from a fourfold table is a p value indicating whether a significant association exists between the two categorical variables from which the table was created. A *p value* is the probability that random fluctuations alone, in the absence of any real effect in the population, could have produced an observed effect at least as large as what you observed in your sample. If the p value is less than some arbitrary value (often set at 0.05), the effect is said to be *statistically significant* (see Chapter 3 for a more detailed discussion of p values and significance). Assessing significance is often the main reason (and sometimes the only reason) why someone creates a cross-tab of any size. But fourfold tables can yield other interesting numbers besides a p value.

In the rest of this chapter, I describe some of the many useful numbers that you can derive from the cell counts in a fourfold table. The statistical software that cross-tabulates your raw data often provides some of these indices (you may have to tell the software which ones you want; see Chapter 4 for software basics). The formulas for many of these indices are simple enough to do on a calculator after you get the four cell counts, but you can also use a web page (which I refer to throughout this chapter as the *fourfold table web page*) to calculate several dozen kinds of indices from a fourfold table, so you shouldn't have to do any calculations by hand: `StatPages.info/ctab2x2.html`.

Like any other number you calculate from your data, an index from a fourfold table is only a *sample statistic* — an estimate of the corresponding population parameter. So a good researcher always wants to quote the *precision* of that estimate. In Chapters 9 and 10, I describe how to calculate the standard error (SE) and confidence interval (CI) for simple sample statistics like means, proportions, and regression coefficients. And in this chapter, I show you how to calculate the SE and CI for the various indices you can get from a fourfold table.

Though an index itself may be easy to calculate, its SE or CI usually is not. Approximate formulas are available for some of the more common indices; these are usually based on the fact that the random sampling fluctuations of an index (or its logarithm) are often nearly normally distributed if the sample size isn't too small. I provide such formulas where they're available. Fortunately, the fourfold table web page provides confidence intervals for all the indices it calculates, using a general (but still approximate) method.

For consistency, all the formulas in this chapter refer to the four cell counts of the fourfold table, and the row totals, column totals, and grand total, in the same standard way, shown in Figure 14-1. This convention is used on the web page and in many other statistics books.

Figure 14-1:
These designations for cell counts and totals are used throughout this chapter.

	Column 1	Column 2	Total
Row 1	a	b	r1
Row 2	c	d	r2
Total	c1	c2	t

Illustration by Wiley, Composition Services Graphics

Choosing the Right Sampling Strategy

When designing a study whose objective involves two categorical variables that will be cross-tabulated into a fourfold table, you have to give thought to how you select your subjects. For example, suppose you're planning a simple research project to investigate the relationship between obesity and high blood pressure (*hypertension*, or HTN). You enroll a sample of subjects and prepare a fourfold table from your data, with obesity as the row variable (obese in the top row; non-obese in the bottom row) and HTN as the column variable (subjects with HTN in the left column; subjects without HTN in the right column). For the sake of the example, if an association exists, obesity is considered the cause and HTN the effect. How will you go about enrolling subjects for this study?

You have several ways to acquire subjects for a study of cause-and-effect relationships (like obesity and HTN), where the data will be cross-tabulated into a fourfold table:

- ✔ **You can enroll a certain number of subjects without knowing how many do or do not have the risk factor, or how many do or do not have the outcome.** You can decide to enroll, say, 100 subjects, not knowing in advance how many of these subjects are obese or how many have HTN. In terms of the cells in Figure 14-1, this means that you predetermine the value of *t* as 100, but you don't know what the values of *r1*, *r2*, *c1*, or *c2* will be until you determine the obesity and hypertension status of each subject. This is called a *natural sampling* design.

- ✔ **You can enroll a certain number of subjects with the risk factor, and a certain number without the risk factor.** You can decide to enroll, say, 50 obese and 50 non-obese subjects, not knowing what their HTN status is. You specify, in advance, that *r1* will be 50 and *r2* will be 50 (and therefore *t* will be 100), but you don't know what *c1* and *c2* are until you determine the HTN status of each subject. This is called a *cohort* or *prospective* study design — you select two cohorts of subjects based on the presence or absence of the risk factor (the cause) and then compare how many subjects in each cohort got the outcome (conceptually looking forward from cause to effect). Statisticians often use this kind of design when the risk factor is very rare, to be sure of getting enough subjects with the rare risk factor.

✔ **You can enroll a certain number of subjects who have the outcome and a certain number who do not have the outcome.** You can decide to enroll, say, 50 subjects with hypertension and 50 subjects without hypertension, without knowing what their obesity status is. You specify, in advance, that $c1$ will be 50 and $c2$ will be 50 (and therefore t will be 100), but you don't know what $r1$ and $r2$ are until you determine the obesity status of each subject. This is called a *case-control* or *retrospective* study design — you select a bunch of *cases* (subjects with the outcome of hypertension) and a bunch of *controls* (subjects without hypertension) and then compare the prevalence of the obesity risk factor between the cases and the controls (conceptually looking backward from effect to cause). Statisticians often use this kind of design when the outcome is very rare, to be sure of getting enough subjects with the rare outcome.

Why is this distinction among ways of acquiring subjects important? As you see in the rest of this chapter, some indices are meaningful only if the sampling is done a certain way.

Producing Fourfold Tables in a Variety of Situations

Fourfold tables can arise from a number of different scenarios, including the following:

✔ Comparing proportions between two groups (see Chapter 13)

✔ Testing whether two binary variables are associated

✔ Assessing risk factors

✔ Evaluating diagnostic procedures

✔ Evaluating therapies

✔ Evaluating inter-rater reliability

Note: These scenarios can also give rise to tables larger than 2x2. And fourfold tables can arise in other scenarios besides these.

Describing the association between two binary variables

Suppose you select a random sample of 60 adults from the local population. Suppose you measure their height and weight, calculate their body mass index, and classify them as obese or non-obese. You can also measure their blood pressure under various conditions and categorize them as hypertensive or non-hypertensive. This is a natural sampling strategy, as described in the earlier section "Choosing the Right Sampling Strategy." You can summarize your data in a fourfold table (see Figure 14-2).

This table indicates that most obese people have hypertension, and most non-obese people don't have hypertension. You can show that this apparent association is statistically significant in this sample using either a Yates chi-square or a Fisher Exact test on this table (as I describe in Chapter 13), getting $p = 0.016$ or $p = 0.013$, respectively.

But when you present the results of this study, just saying that a significant association exists between obesity and hypertension isn't enough; you should also indicate how strong this relationship is. For two continuous variables (such as weight or blood pressure, that are not restricted to whole numbers, but could, in theory at least, be measured to any number of decimal places), you can present the *correlation coefficient* — a number that varies from 0 (indicating no correlation at all) to plus or minus 1 (indicating perfect positive or perfect negative correlation). Wouldn't it be nice if there was a correlation coefficient designed for two binary categorical variables that worked the same way?

The *tetrachoric* correlation coefficient (R_{Tet}), also called the *terachoric* correlation coefficient, is based on the concept that a subject's category (like hypertensive or non-hypertensive) *could* have been derived from some continuous variable (like systolic blood pressure), based on an arbitrary "cut value" (like 150 mmHg). This concept doesn't make much sense for intrinsically dichotomous variables like gender, but it's reasonable for things like hypertension based on blood pressure or obesity based on body mass index.

Figure 14-2:
A fourfold table summarizing obesity and hypertension in a sample of 60 subjects.

	Hypertension	No Hypertension	Total
Obese	14 (a)	7 (b)	21 (r1)
Not Obese	12 (c)	27 (d)	39 (r2)
Total	26 (c1)	34 (c2)	60 (t)

Illustration by Wiley, Composition Services Graphics

The R_{Tet} calculated from two binary variables is an estimate of the ordinary correlation coefficient between the two original continuous variables. Recall that a correlation coefficient can be positive or negative, and can range from 0 (signifying no correlation at all) to 1 (signifying perfect correlation). You can calculate the R_{Tet} from all three kinds of sampling strategies described in the earlier "Choosing the Right Sampling Strategy" section: natural, cohort, and case-control. The exact formula is extremely complicated, but an approximate value can be calculated as

$$R_{Tet} = \cos\left(\pi \big/ \left(1 + \sqrt{ad/bc}\right)\right)$$

where *cos* is the cosine of an angle in radians.

For the data in Figure 14-2, $R_{Tet} = \cos\left(\pi \big/ \left(1 + \sqrt{(14 \times 27)/(7 \times 12)}\right)\right)$, which is about 0.53.

Note: No simple formulas exist for the standard error or confidence intervals for the tetrachoric correlation coefficient, but the fourfold-table web page (at StatPages.info/ctab2x2.html) can calculate them. For this example, the 95 percent CI is 0.09 to 0.81.

Assessing risk factors

How much does a suspected risk factor (cause) increase the chances of getting a particular outcome (effect)? For example, how much does being obese increase your chances of having hypertension? You can calculate a couple of indices from the fourfold table that describe this increase, as you discover in the following sections.

Relative risk (risk ratio)

The *risk* (or probability) of getting a bad outcome is estimated as the fraction of subjects in a group who had the outcome. You can calculate the risk separately for subjects with and without the risk factor. The risk for subjects with the risk factor is *a/r1*; for the example from Figure 14-2, it's 14/21, which is 0.667 (66.7 percent). And for those without the risk factor, the risk is *c/r2*; for this example, it's 12/39, which is 0.308 (30.8 percent).

The *relative risk* (RR), also called the *risk ratio*, is the risk of getting the outcome if you have the risk factor divided by the risk of getting the outcome if you don't have the risk factor. You calculate it as: *RR = (a/r1)/(c/r2)*.

For this example, the RR is (14/21)/(12/39), which is 0.667/0.308, which is 2.17. So in this sample, obese subjects are slightly more than twice as likely to have hypertension than non-obese subjects.

You can calculate RRs only from natural samples and cohort samples (described earlier in this chapter); you can't calculate them from case-control samples. This is because the risks are estimated from the number of people with and without the outcome, and in a case-control study, you arbitrarily dictate how many subjects with and without the risk factor you study. So the risks (and therefore the RR) calculated from a case-control study doesn't reflect the true RR in the whole population.

You can calculate an approximate 95 percent confidence interval around the observed RR using the following formulas, which are based on the assumption that the logarithm of the RR is normally distributed:

1. **Calculate the standard error of the log of RR using the following formula:**

$$SE = \sqrt{b/(a \times r1) + d/(c \times r2)}$$

2. **Calculate Q with the following formula: $Q = e^{1.96 \times SE}$ where Q is simply a convenient intermediate quantity, which will be used in the next part of the calculation, and e is the mathematical constant 2.718.**

3. **Find the lower and upper limits of the confidence interval with the following formula:**

$$95\% \ CI = \left(RR\!\Big/\!Q\right) \text{ to } (RR \times Q)$$

For other confidence levels, replace the 1.96 in Step 2 with the appropriate multiplier shown in Table 10-1 of Chapter 10. So for 50 percent CIs, use 0.67; for 80 percent, use 1.28; for 90 percent, use 1.64; for 98 percent, use 2.33; and for 99 percent, use 2.58.

So for the example in Figure 14-2, you calculate 95 percent CI around the observed relative risk as follows:

1. $SE = \sqrt{7/(14 \times 21) + 27/(12 \times 39)}$, **which is 0.2855.**

2. $Q = e^{1.96 \times 0.2855}$, **which is 1.75.**

3. **The** $95\% \ CI = \left(2.17\!\Big/\!1.75\right)$ to (2.17×1.75), **which is 1.24 to 3.80.**

Or, you can enter the four cell counts from Figure 14-2 into the fourfold table web page, and it will calculate the RR as 2.17, with 95 percent confidence limits of 1.14 to 3.71 (using a different formula).

Odds ratio

The *odds* of something happening is the probability of it happening divided by the probability of it not happening: $p/(1 - p)$. In a sample of data, you estimate the odds of having an outcome event as the number of subjects who had the event divided by the number of subjects who didn't have it.

The odds of having the outcome event for subjects with the risk factor are a/b; for the example in Figure 14-2, they're 14/7, which is 2.00. And for those without the risk factor, the odds are c/d; for this example they're 12/27, which is 0.444 (odds usually aren't expressed as percentages). See Chapter 3 for a more detailed discussion of odds.

The *odds ratio* (OR) is the odds of getting the outcome if you have the risk factor divided by the odds of getting the outcome if you don't have the risk factor. You calculate it as: $OR = (a/b)/(c/d)$.

For this example, the odds ratio is (14/7)/(12/27), which is 2.00/0.444, which is 4.50. So in this sample, obese subjects have 4.5 times the odds of having hypertension than non-obese subjects.

You can calculate odds ratios from all three kinds of sampling strategies: natural, cohort, and case-control. (See the earlier "Choosing the Right Sampling Strategy" section for more about these strategies.)

You can calculate an approximate 95 percent confidence interval around the observed odds ratio using the following formulas, which are based on the assumption that the logarithm of the OR is normally distributed:

1. **Calculate the standard error of the log of the OR with the following formula:**

$$SE = \sqrt{1/a + 1/b + 1/c + 1/d}$$

2. **Calculate Q with the following formula: $Q = e^{1.96 \times SE}$, where Q is simply a convenient intermediate quantity, which will be used in the next part of the calculation, and e is the mathematical constant 2.718.**

3. **Find the limits of the confidence interval with the following formula:**

$$95\% \ CI = \left(OR\Big/Q\right) \text{ to } (OR \times Q)$$

For other confidence levels, replace the 1.96 in Step 2 with the appropriate multiplier shown in Table 10-1 of Chapter 10. So for 50 percent CIs, use 0.67; for 80 percent, use 1.28; for 90 percent, use 1.64; for 98 percent, use 2.33; and for 99 percent, use 2.58.

So for the example in Figure 14-2, you calculate 95 percent CI around the observed odds ratio as follows:

1. $SE = \sqrt{1/14 + 1/7 + 1/12 + 1/27}$, **which is 0.5785.**

2. $Q = e^{1.96 \times 0.5785}$, **which is 3.11.**

3. $95\% \ CI = \left(4.50\Big/3.11\right)$ to (4.50×3.11), **which is 1.45 to 14.0.**

Or, you can enter the four cell counts from Figure 14-2 into the fourfold table web page, and it will calculate the OR as 4.5, with 95 percent confidence limits of 1.27 to 16.5 (using a different formula).

Evaluating diagnostic procedures

Many diagnostic procedures give a positive or negative test result, which, ideally, should correspond to the true presence or absence of the medical condition being tested for (as determined by some gold standard that's assumed to be perfectly accurate in diagnosing the condition). But gold standard diagnostic procedures can be time-consuming, expensive, and unpleasant for the patient, so quick, inexpensive, and relatively noninvasive screening tests are very valuable if they're reasonably accurate.

Most tests produce some *false positive* results (coming out positive when the condition is truly not present) and some *false negative* results (coming out negative when the condition truly is present). It's important to know how well a test performs.

You usually evaluate a proposed screening test for a medical condition by administering the proposed test to a group of subjects, whose true status has been (or will be) determined by the gold standard method. You can then cross-tabulate the test results against the true condition, producing a fourfold table like Figure 14-3.

Figure 14-3:
This is how data is summarized when evaluating a proposed diagnostic screening test.

		True Status, by the Gold Standard		
		Condition Present	Condition Not Present	Total
Test Result	**Positive**	a = TP (True Positive)	b = FP (False Positive)	r1 = All Positive
	Negative	c = FN (False Negative)	d = TN (True Negative)	r2 = All Negative
	Total	c1 = All Present	c2 = All Not Present	t

Illustration by Wiley, Composition Services Graphics

For example, consider a home pregnancy test that's administered to 100 randomly chosen women who suspect they may be pregnant. This is a natural sampling from a population defined as "all women who think they might be pregnant," which is the population to whom a home pregnancy test would be marketed. Eventually, their true status becomes known, so it's cross-tabulated against the test results, giving Figure 14-4.

Figure 14-4:
Results from
a test of a
proposed
home preg-
nancy test.

		True Status		
		Pregnant	Not Pregnant	Total
Pregnancy Test Result	Positive	33 (a)	12 (b)	45 (r1)
	Negative	4 (c)	51 (d)	55 (r2)
	Total	37 (c1)	63 (c2)	100 (t)

Illustration by Wiley, Composition Services Graphics

You can easily calculate at least five important characteristics of the home test from this table, as you find out in the following sections.

Accuracy, sensitivity, specificity, positive predictive value, and negative predictive value (see the next few sections) are simple proportions. I tell you how to calculate the SEs and CIs for these indices in Chapters 9 and 10.

Overall accuracy

Overall accuracy measures how often a test is right. A perfectly accurate test never produces false positive or false negative results. In Figure 14-4, cells *a* and *d* represent correct test results, so the overall accuracy of the home pregnancy test is $(a + d)/t$. Using the data in Figure 14-4, accuracy = (33 + 51)/100, which is 0.84, or 84 percent.

You can calculate overall accuracy only from a natural sample study design, and it applies only to the population from which that sample was selected.

Sensitivity and specificity

A perfectly *sensitive* test never produces a false negative result; if the condition is truly present, the test always comes out positive. (In other words, if it's there, you'll see it.) So when a perfectly sensitive test comes out negative, you can be sure the person doesn't have the condition. You calculate *sensitivity* by dividing the number of true positive cases by the total number of cases where the condition was truly present: $a/c1$ (that is, true positive/all present). Using the data in Figure 14-4, sensitivity = 33/37, which is 0.89; that means that the home test comes out positive in 89 percent of truly pregnant women.

A perfectly *specific* test never produces a false positive result; if the condition is truly absent, the test always comes out negative. (In other words, if it's not there, you won't see it.) So when a perfectly specific test comes out positive, you can be sure the person has the condition. You calculate *specificity* by dividing the number of true negative cases by the total number of cases where the condition was truly absent: *d/c2* (that is, true negative/all not present). Using the data in Figure 14-4, specificity = 51/63, which is 0.81; that means that the home test comes out negative in 81 percent of truly non-pregnant women.

Sensitivity and specificity are important characteristics of the test itself, but they don't answer the very practical question of, "How likely is a particular test result (positive or negative) to be correct?" That's because the answers depend on the prevalence of the condition in the population the test is applied to. (Positive predictive value and negative predictive value, explained in the following section, do answer that question, because their values do depend on the prevalence of the condition in the population.)

You can calculate sensitivity and specificity from a study that uses natural sampling or from a study where you predetermine the number of subjects who truly do and don't have the condition. You can't calculate sensitivity or specificity if you predetermine the number of subjects with positive and negative test results.

Positive predictive value and negative predictive value

The *positive predictive value* (PPV) is the fraction of all positive test results that are true positives (the woman is truly pregnant). If you see it, it's there! You calculate PPV as *a/r1*. For the data in Figure 14-4, the PPV is 33/45, which is 0.73. So if the pregnancy test comes out positive, there's a 73 percent chance that the woman is truly pregnant.

The *negative predictive value* (NPV) is the fraction of all negative test results that are true negatives (the woman is truly not pregnant). If you don't see it, it's not there! You calculate NPV as *d/r2*. For the data in Figure 14-4, the NPV is 51/55, which is 0.93. So if the pregnancy test comes out negative, there's a 93 percent chance that the woman is truly not pregnant.

You can calculate PPV and NPV from a study that uses natural sampling or from a study where you predetermine the number of subjects with positive and negative test results. But you can't calculate PPV or NPV if you predetermine the number of subjects who truly do and don't have the conditions; you must calculate them from groups having the same prevalence of the condition that you want the PPV and NPV values to be applicable to.

Investigating treatments

One of the simplest ways to investigate the effectiveness of some treatment (drug, surgical procedure, and so on) is to study a sample of subjects with the target condition (obesity, hypertension, diabetes, and so on) and randomly assign some of them to receive the proposed treatment and some of them to receive a placebo or sham treatment. Then observe whether the treatment helped the subject. Of course, placebos help many subjects, so you need to compare the fraction of successful outcomes between the two groups of subjects.

Suppose you study 200 subjects with arthritis, randomize them so that 100 receive an experimental drug and 100 receive a placebo, and record whether each subject felt that the product helped their arthritis. You tabulate the results in a fourfold table, like Figure 14-5.

	Patient Was Helped	Patient Not Helped	Total
Real Treatment	70 (a)	30 (b)	100 (r1)
Placebo or Sham	50 (c)	50 (d)	100 (r2)
Total	120 (c1)	80 (c2)	200 (t)

Figure 14-5: Comparing a treatment to a placebo.

Illustration by Wiley, Composition Services Graphics

Seventy percent of subjects taking the new drug report that it helped their arthritis, which is quite impressive until you see that 50 percent of subjects who received the placebo also reported improvement. (Pain studies are notorious for showing very strong placebo effects.) Nevertheless, a Yates chi-square or Fisher Exact test (see Chapter 13) shows that the drug helped a significantly greater fraction of the time than the placebo ($p = 0.006$ by either test).

But how do you quantify the amount of improvement? You can calculate a couple of useful effect-size indices from this fourfold table, as you find out in the following sections.

Difference in proportion

One very simple and obvious number is the *between-group difference* in the fraction of subjects helped: $a/r1 - c/r2$. For the numbers in Figure 14-5, the difference $= 70/100 - 50/100$, which is $0.7 - 0.5 = 0.2$, or a 20 percent superiority in the proportion of subjects helped by the drug relative to the placebo.

You can calculate (approximately) the standard error (*SE*) of the difference as: $SE = \sqrt{a(r1-a)/r1^3 + c(r2-c)/r2^3}$. For the data in Figure 14-5, $SE = \sqrt{70(100-70)/100^3 + 50(100-50)/100^3}$, which is 0.0678, so you'd report the difference in proportion helped as 0.20 ± 0.0678.

You obtain the 95 percent CI around the difference by adding and subtracting 1.96 times the SE, which gives 0.2 − 1.96 × 0.0678, and 0.2 + 1.96 × 0.0678, for a 95 percent CI of 0.067 to 0.333.

Number needed to treat

The *number needed to treat* (NNT) is an interesting number that physicians love. Basically, it answers the very practical question, "How many subjects would I have to treat with the new drug before helping, on average, one additional subject beyond those who would have been helped even by a placebo?" This number turns out to be simply the reciprocal of the difference in the proportions helped (ignoring the sign of the difference), which I describe in the preceding section: NNT = $1/|\text{Diff}|$. So for the example in Figure 14-5, NNT = 1/0.2, or 5 subjects.

The SE of the NNT isn't particularly useful because NNT has a very skewed sampling distribution. You can obtain the confidence limits around NNT by taking the reciprocals of the confidence limits for Diff (and swapping the lower and upper limits). So the 95 percent confidence limits for NNT are 1/0.333 and 1/0.067, which is 3.0 to 15, approximately.

Looking at inter- and intra-rater reliability

Many measurements in biological and sociological research are obtained by the subjective judgment of humans. Examples include the reading of X-rays, CAT scans, ECG tracings, ultrasound images, biopsy specimens, and audio and video recordings of subject behavior in various situations. The human may make quantitative measurements (like the length of a bone on an ultrasound image) or categorical ratings (like the presence or absence of some atypical feature on an ECG tracing).

You need to know how consistent such ratings are among different raters reading the same thing *(inter-rater reliability)* and how reproducible the ratings are for one rater reading the same thing multiple times *(intra-rater reliability)*.

When considering a binary reading (like *yes* or *no*) between two raters, you can estimate *inter*-rater reliability by having each rater read the same batch of, say, 50 specimens, and then cross-tabbing the results, as in Figure 14-6.

Cell *a* contains a count of how many specimens were rated *yes* by Rater 1 and *yes* by Rater 2; cell *b* counts how many specimens were rated *yes* by Rater 1 but *no* by Rater 2; and so on.

Figure 14-6:
Results of
two raters
reading the
same set
of 50 speci-
mens and
rating each
specimen
yes or *no.*

	Rated Yes by Rater 2	Rated No by Rater 2	Total
Rated Yes by Rater 1	22 (a)	5 (b)	27 (r1)
Rated No by Rater 1	7 (c)	16 (d)	23 (r2)
Total	29 (c1)	21 (c2)	50 (t)

Illustration by Wiley, Composition Services Graphics

You can construct a similar table for estimating *intra*-rater reliability by having one rater read the same batch of specimens on two separate occasions; in this case, you'd replace the word *Rater* with *Reading* in the row and column labels.

Ideally, all the specimens would be counted in cells *a* or *d* of Figure 14-6; cells *b* and *c* would contain zeros. *Cohen's Kappa* (signified by the Greek lowercase kappa: κ) is a measure of how close the data comes to this ideal. You calculate kappa as: $\kappa = 2(ad - bc)/(r1 \times c2 + r2 \times c1)$.

For perfect agreement, $\kappa = 1$; for completely random ratings (indicating no rating ability whatsoever), $\kappa = 0$. Random sampling fluctuations can actually cause κ to be negative. Like the student taking a true/false test, where the number of wrong answers is subtracted from the number of right answers to compensate for guessing, getting a score less than zero indicates the interesting combination of being stupid *and* unlucky!

There's no universal agreement as to what a "good" value of kappa is. One fairly common convention (but by no means the only one) is that values of κ less than 0.4 are poor, those between 0.4 and 0.75 are fair-to-good, and those more than 0.75 are excellent.

For the data in Figure 14-6: $\kappa = 2(22 \times 16 - 5 \times 7)/(27 \times 21 + 23 \times 29)$, which is 0.5138, indicating only fair agreement between the two raters.

You won't find any simple formulas for calculating SEs or CIs for kappa, but the fourfold table web page (`StatPages.info/ctab2x2.html`) provides approximate CIs for Cohen's Kappa. For the preceding example, the 95 percent CI is 0.202 to 0.735.

Chapter 15

Analyzing Incidence and Prevalence Rates in Epidemiologic Data

. . . .

In This Chapter

▶ Determining and expressing how prevalent a condition is

▶ Calculating incidence rates, rate ratios, and their standard errors

▶ Comparing incidence rates between two populations

▶ Estimating sample size needed to compare incidence rates

. . . .

*E*pidemiology studies the patterns, causes, and effects of health and diseases in defined populations (sometimes very large populations, like entire cities or countries, or even the whole world). This chapter describes two concepts, prevalence and incidence, that are central to epidemiology and are frequently encountered in other areas of biological research as well. I describe how to calculate incidence rates and prevalence proportions; then, concentrating on the analysis of incidence (because prevalence can be analyzed using methods described elsewhere in this book), I describe how to calculate confidence intervals around incidence rates and rate ratios, and how to compare incidence rates between two populations.

Understanding Incidence and Prevalence

Incidence and prevalence are two related but distinct concepts. In the following sections, I define each of these concepts and provide examples; then I describe the relationship between incidence and prevalence.

Prevalence: The fraction of a population with a particular condition

The *prevalence* of a condition in a population is the proportion of the population that has that condition at any given moment. It's calculated by dividing the number of people in a defined group who have the condition by the total number of people in that group.

Prevalence can be expressed as a decimal fraction, a percentage, or a "one out of so many" kind of number. For example, a 2011 survey found that 11.3 percent of the U.S. adult population has diabetes. So the prevalence of diabetes in U.S. adults can be expressed as the decimal 0.113, 11.3 percent, or roughly 1 out of 9.

Because prevalence is a simple proportion, it's analyzed in exactly the same way as any other proportion. The standard error of a prevalence can be estimated by the formulas in Chapter 9; confidence intervals can be obtained from exact methods based on the binomial distribution or from formulas based on the normal approximation to the binomial distribution (see Chapter 10); and prevalence can be compared between two or more populations using the chi-square or Fisher Exact test (see Chapter 13). For this reason, the remainder of this chapter focuses on how to analyze incidence rates.

Incidence: Counting new cases

The *incidence* of a condition is the rate at which new cases of that condition appear in a population. Incidence is generally expressed as an *incidence rate* (R), defined as the number of observed events (N) divided by the exposure (E): $R = N/E$. *Exposure* is the product of the number of subjects in the population times the interval of time during which new events are being counted. Exposure is measured in units of person-time, such as person-days or person-years, so incidence rates are expressed as the number of cases per unit of person-time. The unit of person-time is often chosen so that the incidence rate will be a "conveniently sized" number.

The incidence rate should be estimated by counting events over a narrow enough interval of time so that the number of observed events is a small fraction of the total population studied. One year is narrow enough for diabetes (only 0.02 percent of the population develops diabetes in a year), but it isn't narrow enough for something like the flu, which 30 percent of the population may come down with in a one-year period.

Suppose that last year, in my city with 300,000 adults, 30 adults were newly diagnosed with diabetes. The incidence of adult diabetes in my city would be calculated as 30 cases in 300,000 adults in one year, which works out to 0.0001 new cases per person-year. To avoid working with tiny fractional numbers like 0.0001 (humans usually prefer to work with numbers between

1 and 1,000 whenever possible), it's more convenient to express this incidence rate as 1 new case per 10,000 patient-years, or perhaps as 10 new cases per 100,000 person-years. Similarly, say that in my cousin's city, with 80,000 adults, 20 adults were newly diagnosed with diabetes. The incidence rate would be calculated as 24 cases in 80,000 people in one year, which works out to 24/80,000 or 0.0003 new cases per person-year and is expressed more conveniently as 30 new cases per 100,000 person-years. So the incidence rate in my cousin's city is three times as large as the incidence rate in my city.

Understanding how incidence and prevalence are related

From the definitions and examples in the preceding sections, you see that incidence and prevalence are two related but distinct concepts. The incidence rate tells you how fast new cases of some condition arise in a population, and prevalence tells you what fraction of the population has that condition at any moment.

You might expect that conditions with higher incidence rates would have higher prevalence than conditions with lower incidence rates, and that tends to be true when comparing conditions that last for about the same amount of time. But there are counter-examples — short-lasting conditions (such as acute infections) may have high incidence rates but low prevalence, whereas long-lasting conditions (diabetes, for example) may have low incidence rates but high prevalence.

Analyzing Incidence Rates

The preceding sections show you how to calculate incidence rates and express them in convenient units. But, as I emphasize in Chapter 9, whenever you report a number you've calculated, you should also indicate how precise that number is. So how precise are those incident rates? And is the difference between two incidence rates significant? The next sections show you how to calculate standard errors and confidence intervals for incidence rates and how to compare incidence rates between two populations.

Expressing the precision of an incidence rate

The precision of an incidence rate (R) is usually expressed by a confidence interval (CI). The standard error (SE) of R isn't often quoted, because the event rate usually isn't normally distributed; the standard error is usually calculated only as part of the confidence interval calculation.

Random fluctuations in R are usually attributed entirely to fluctuations in the event count (N), assuming the exposure (E) is known exactly — or at least much more precisely than N. So the confidence interval for the event rate is based on the confidence interval for N. Here's how you calculate the confidence interval for R:

1. **Calculate the confidence interval (CI) for N.**

   Chapters 9 and 10 provide approximate standard error and confidence interval formulas, based on the normal approximation to the Poisson distribution (see Chapter 25). These approximations are reasonably good when N is large (at least 50 events):

   $$95\% \text{ CI} = N - 1.96\sqrt{N} \text{ to } N + 1.96\sqrt{N}$$

   Better yet, you can get the exact Poisson confidence interval around an event count by using software, such as the online calculator at `StatPages.info/confint.html`.

2. **Divide the lower and upper confidence limits for N by the exposure (E).**

   The answer is the confidence interval for the incidence rate R.

For the example of 24 new diabetes cases in one year in a city with 80,000 adults, the event count (N) is 24, and the exposure (E) is 80,000 person-years (80,000 persons for one year). The incidence rate (R) is N/E, which is 24 per 80,000 person-years, or 30 per 100,000 person-years. How precise is the incidence rate?

First find the confidence limits for N. Using the approximate formula, the 95 percent confidence interval (CI) around the event count of 24 is $24 - 1.96\sqrt{24}$ to $24 + 1.96\sqrt{24}$, or 14.4 to 33.6 events. Dividing the lower and upper confidence limits of N by the exposure gives 14.4/80,000 to 33.6/80,000, which you can express as 18.0 to 42.0 events per 100,000 person-years — the confidence interval for the incidence rate.

Using the exact online calculator, you get 15.4 to 35.7 as the 95 percent confidence interval around 24 observed events. Dividing these numbers by the 80,000 person-years of exposure gives 19.2 to 44.6 events per 100,000 person-years as the exact 95 percent confidence interval around the incidence rate.

Comparing incidences with the rate ratio

When comparing incidence rates between two populations, you should calculate a *rate ratio* (RR) by dividing one incidence rate by the other. So for two groups with event counts N_1 and N_2, exposures E_1 and E_2, and incidence rates R_1 and R_2, respectively, you calculate the rate ratio for Group 2 relative to Group 1 as a reference, like this:

$$RR = \frac{R_2}{R_1} = \frac{N_2/E_2}{N_1/E_1}$$

For the example of diabetes incidence in the two cities, you have $N_1 = 30$, $E_1 = 300,000$, $N_2 = 24$, and $E_2 = 80,000$. The RR for my cousin's city relative to my city is $RR = (24/80,000)/(30/300,000)$, or 3.0, indicating that my cousin's city has three times the diabetes incidence that my city has.

You could calculate the difference $(R_2 - R_1)$ between two incidence rates if you wanted to, but in epidemiology, rate ratios are used much more often than rate differences.

Calculating confidence intervals for a rate ratio

Whenever you report a rate ratio you've calculated, you should also indicate how precise that ratio is. The exact calculation of a confidence interval (CI) around a rate ratio is quite difficult, but if your observed event counts aren't too small (say, ten or more), then the following approximate formula for the 95 percent CI around an RR works reasonably well:

$$95\% \text{ CI} = RR/Q \text{ to } RR \times Q$$

where $Q = e^{1.96\sqrt{1/N_1 + 1/N_2}}$.

For other confidence levels, replace the 1.96 in the Q formula with the appropriate critical z value for the normal distribution (see Chapter 26).

So for the diabetes example (where $N_1 = 30$, $N_2 = 24$, and $RR = 3.0$), $Q = e^{1.96\sqrt{1/24 + 1/30}} = 1.71$, so the 95 percent CI goes from 3.0/1.71 to 3.0 × 1.71, or from 1.75 to 5.13.

The calculations are even simpler if you use the nomogram in Figure 15-1. You lay a ruler (or stretch a string) between the values of N_1 and N_2 on the left and right scales, and then read off the two values from the left and right sides of the center scale. The right-side number is Q; the left-side number is $1/Q$. So, if you multiply the observed RR by these two numbers, you have the 95 percent confidence limits. It doesn't get much easier than that!

For the diabetes example, a ruler placed on 30 and 24 on the left and right scales crosses the center scale at the numbers 0.585 and 1.71, consistent with the preceding calculations.

Comparing two event rates

Two event rates (R_1 and R_2), based on N_1 and N_2 events and E_1 and E_2 exposures, can be tested for a significant difference by calculating the 95 percent confidence interval (CI) around the rate ratio (RR) and observing whether that CI crosses the value 1.0 (which indicates identical rates). If the 95 percent CI includes 1, the RR isn't significantly different from 1, so the two rates aren't significantly different from each other (p > 0.05). But if the 95 percent CI doesn't include 1, the RR is significantly different from 1, so the two rates are significantly different from each other (p < 0.05).

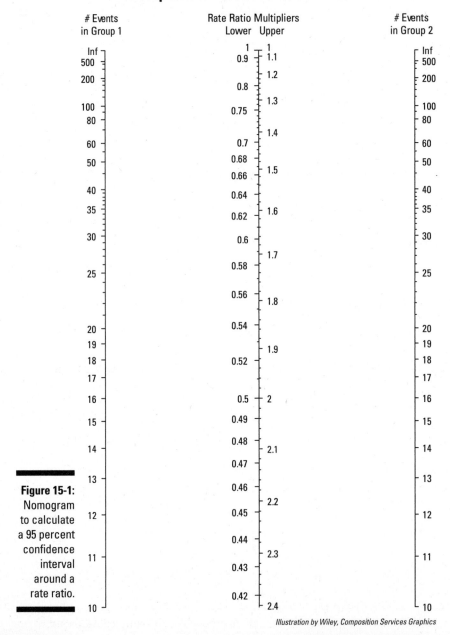

Multipliers for 95% CI around a Rate Ratio

Figure 15-1:
Nomogram to calculate a 95 percent confidence interval around a rate ratio.

For the diabetes example, the observed rate ratio was 3.0, with a 95 percent confidence interval of 1.75 to 5.13, which doesn't include the value 1. So the rate ratio is significantly greater than 1, and I would conclude that my cousin's city has a significantly higher diabetes incidence rate than my city ($p < 0.05$).

This test is very easy to do (requiring no calculations at all!) using the Figure 15-1 nomogram. Just lay the ruler across the N_1 and N_2 values on the left and right scales, and look at the numbers on the center scale. If your observed RR is lower than the left-side number or higher than the right-side number, the two event rates are significantly different from each other (the RR is significantly different from 1.0), at the $p < 0.05$ level.

For the diabetes example, a ruler placed on 30 and 24 on the left and right scales crosses the center scale at the numbers 0.585 and 1.71, so any observed rate ratio outside of this range is significantly different from 1, consistent with the foregoing calculations.

Comparing two event counts with identical exposure

If — and only if — the two exposures (E_1 and E_2) are identical, there's a *really* simple rule for testing whether two event counts (N_1 and N_2) are significantly different at the $p < 0.05$ level:

If $\dfrac{(N_1 - N_2)^2}{N_1 + N_2} > 4$, then the Ns are significantly different ($p < 0.05$).

If the square of the difference is more than four times the sum, then the numbers are significantly different ($p < 0.05$).

The value 4 appearing in this rule is an approximation to 3.84, the chi-square value corresponding to $p = 0.05$ (see Chapter 25 for more info).

For example, if there were 30 fatal auto accidents in your town last year and 40 this year, are things getting more dangerous, or was the increase just random fluctuations? Using the simple rule, you calculate $(30 - 40)^2/(30 + 40)$ = $100/70 = 1.4$, which is less than 4. Having 30 events isn't significantly different from 40 events (during equal time intervals), so the apparent increase could just be "noise." But had the number of events gone from 30 to 50 events, the jump would have been significant because $(30 - 50)^2/(30 + 50)$ = $400/80 = 5.0$, which is greater than 4.

Estimating the Required Sample Size

Sample-size calculations for rate comparisons are more difficult than you want to attempt by hand. Instead, you can use the Excel file SampleSizeCalcs.xls, available at www.dummies.com/extras/biostatistics. You may want to review Chapter 3 for a refresher on the concepts of power and sample size.

As in all sample-size calculations, you need to specify the desired statistical power (often set to 80 percent) and the alpha level for the test (often set to 0.05). When comparing event rates (R_1 and R_2) between two groups, considering R_1 to be the reference group, you must also specify

- ✔ The expected rate in the reference group (R_1)
- ✔ The effect size of importance, expressed as the rate ratio $RR = R_2/R_1$ and entered into the spreadsheet as the expected value of R_2
- ✔ The expected ratio of exposure in the two groups (E_2/E_1), entered into the GroupSize Ratio field of the spreadsheet

When you enter the necessary parameters into the spreadsheet, it will give you the required exposure for each group and the number of events you can expect to see in each group.

For example, suppose you're designing an experiment to test whether rotavirus gastroenteritis is more prevalent in inner cities than in the suburbs. You'll enroll an equal number of inner city and suburban residents and follow them for one year to see whether they come down with rotavirus. Say that the incidence of rotavirus in suburbia is known to be 1 case per 100 person-years (an incidence rate of 0.01 case per patient-year). You want to have an 80 percent chance of getting a significant result of p < 0.05 (that is, 80 percent power at 0.05 alpha) when comparing the incidence rates between the two areas if they differ by more than 25 percent (that is, a rate ratio of 1.25).

You'd fill in the fields of the spreadsheet, as shown in Figure 15-2.

The spreadsheet calculates that you need more than 28,000 person-years of observation in each group (a total of almost 57,000 subjects in a one-year study) in order to have enough observed events to have an 80 percent chance of getting a significant result when comparing rotavirus incidence between inner-city and suburban residents. This shockingly large requirement illustrates the difficulty of studying the incidence rates of rare illnesses.

Figure 15-2: Calculating the sample size required to compare two incidence rates.

	A	B
1	General Settings	
2	Alpha Level:	0.050
3	Power:	80%
4	Goupsize Ratio: Group2 / Group1:	1
5	Expected Attrition Rate:	0%
6		
51	Comparison of Event Rates:	
52	Even Rate for Group1:	0.01
53	Even Rate for Group2:	0.0125
54	Total Exposure Needed for Group1:	28281.6
55	Total Exposure Needed for Group2:	28281.6
56	Expected Events in Group1:	282.8
57	Expected Events in Group2:	353.5

Illustration by Wiley, Composition Services Graphics

Chapter 16

Feeling Noninferior (Or Equivalent)

In This Chapter

▶ Demonstrating the absence of an effect in your data

▶ Testing for bioequivalence, therapeutic noninferiority, and absence of harmful effects

*M*any statistical tests let you determine whether two things are different from each other, like showing that a drug is better than a placebo, or that the blood concentration of some enzyme is higher in people with some medical condition than in people without that condition. But sometimes you want to prove that two (or more) things are *not* different. Here are three examples I refer to throughout this chapter:

✔ **Bioequivalence:** You're developing a generic formulation to compete with a name-brand drug, so you have to demonstrate that your product is *bioequivalent* to the name-brand product; that is, that it puts essentially the same amount of active ingredient into the bloodstream.

✔ **Therapeutic noninferiority:** You want to show that your new treatment for some disease is no worse than the current best treatment for that disease.

✔ **Absence of harmful effects:** Your new drug must demonstrate that, compared to a placebo, it doesn't prolong the QT interval on an ECG (see Chapter 6 for more info on the role of QT testing during drug development).

This chapter describes how to analyze data from equivalence and noninferiority or nonsuperiority studies. Nonsuperiority studies are less frequently encountered than noninferiority studies, and the analysis is basically the same, so for the rest of this chapter, whatever I say about noninferiority also applies (in the reverse direction) to nonsuperiority.

Understanding the Absence of an Effect

Absence of proof is not proof of absence! Proving the *total* absence of an effect statistically is impossible. For example, you can't interpret a nonsignificant outcome from a t test as proving that no difference exists between two groups. The difference may have been real but small, or your sample size may have been too small, or your analytical method may not have been precise enough or sensitive enough. To demonstrate the absence of an effect, you need to test your data in a special way.

Defining the effect size: How different are the groups?

Before being able to test whether or not two groups are different, you first have to come up with a numerical measure that quantifies how different the two groups are. I call this the *effect size,* and it's defined in different ways for different kinds of studies:

- ✔ **Bioequivalence studies:** In bioequivalence (BE) studies, the amount of drug that gets into the bloodstream is usually expressed in terms of the *AUC* — the *area under the curve* of blood concentration of the drug versus time, as determined from a pharmacokinetic analysis (see Chapter 5). The effect size for BE studies is usually expressed as the ratio of the AUC of the new formulation divided by the AUC of the reference formulation (such as the brand-name drug). A ratio of 1.0 means that the two products are perfectly bioequivalent (that is, 1.0 is the no-effect value for a BE study).

- ✔ **Therapeutic noninferiority studies:** In a therapeutic trial, the effect size is often expressed as the difference or the ratio of the efficacy endpoint for that trial. So for a cancer treatment trial, it could be the between-group difference in any of the following measures of efficacy: median survival time, five-year survival rate, the percent of subjects responding to the treatment, or the hazard ratio from a survival regression analysis (see Chapter 24). For an arthritis treatment trial, it could be the between-group difference in pain score improvements or the percentage of subjects reporting an improvement in their condition. Often the effect size is defined so that a larger (or more positive) value corresponds to a better treatment.

- ✔ **QT safety studies:** In a QT trial, the effect size is the difference in QT interval prolongation between the drug and placebo.

Defining an important effect size: How close is close enough?

Instead of trying to prove *absolutely no difference* between two groups (which is impossible), you need only prove *no important difference* between the groups. To do the latter, you must first define exactly what you mean by an *important* difference — you must come up with a number representing the smallest effect size you consider to be clinically meaningful. If the true effect size (in the entire population) is less than that amount, then for all practical purposes it's like no difference at all between the groups. The minimal important effect size is referred to by several names, such as *allowable difference* and *permissible tolerance*.

Just how much of an effect is important depends on what you're measuring:

- ✔ **For bioequivalence studies:** The customary tolerance in the AUC ratio is 0.8 to 1.25; two drugs are considered equivalent if their true AUC ratio lies within this range.

- ✔ **For therapeutic noninferiority studies:** The tolerance depends on the disease and the chosen efficacy endpoint. It's usually established by consensus between expert clinicians in the particular discipline and the regulatory agencies.

- ✔ **For QT safety studies:** Current regulations say that the drug must not prolong the QT interval by more than 10 milliseconds, compared to placebo. If the true prolongation is less than 10 milliseconds, the drug is judged as not prolonging QT.

Recognizing effects: Can you spot a difference if there really is one?

When you're trying to prove the absence of some effect, you have to convince people that your methodology isn't oblivious to that effect and that you can actually spot the effect in your data when it's truly present in the population you're studying.

For example, I can always "prove" statistically that a drug doesn't prolong the QT interval simply by having the ECGs read by someone who hasn't the foggiest idea of how to measure QT intervals! That person's results will consist almost entirely of random "noise," and the statistical tests for a QT prolongation will come out nonsignificant almost every time.

Here the concept of *assay sensitivity* comes into the picture. I use the word *assay* here to refer to the entire methodology used in the study — not just a laboratory assay. To prove assay sensitivity, you need to show that you can recognize a difference if it's really there.

You demonstrate adequate assay sensitivity by using a *positive control.* In addition to the groups that you're trying to show are not different, you must also include in your study another group that definitely is different from the reference group:

✔ **In bioequivalence studies:** One simple and obvious choice is the brand-name product itself, but at a different dose than that of the reference group — perhaps half (or maybe twice) the standard dose. To prove assay sensitivity, you'd better get a significant result when comparing the positive control to the standard product.

✔ **For therapeutic noninferiority studies:** Noninferiority studies have a real problem with regard to assay sensitivity — there's usually no way to use a positive control (a truly inferior treatment) in the study because noninferiority studies are generally used in situations when it would be unethical to withhold effective treatment from people with a serious illness. So when a noninferiority trial comes out successful, you can't tell whether it was a well-designed trial on a treatment that's truly noninferior to the reference treatment or whether it was a badly designed trial on a truly inferior treatment.

✔ **For QT safety studies:** The drug *moxifloxacin* (known to prolong QT, but not by a dangerous amount) is often used as a positive control. Subjects given moxifloxacin had better show a statistically significant QT prolongation compared to the placebo.

Proving Equivalence and Noninferiority

After you understand the lack of meaningful differences (see the previous section), you can put all the concepts together into a statistical process for demonstrating that there's no important difference between two groups.

Equivalence and noninferiority can be demonstrated statistically by using significance tests in a special way or by using confidence intervals.

Using significance tests

Significance tests are used to show that an observed effect is unlikely to be due only to random fluctuations. (See Chapter 3 for a general discussion of hypothesis testing.) You may be tempted to test for bioequivalence by comparing the AUCs of the two drug formulations with a two-group Student t test or by comparing the ratio of the AUCs to the no-effect value of 1.0 using a one-group t test. Those approaches would be okay if you were trying to prove that the two formulations weren't *exactly* the same, but that's not what equivalence testing is all about.

Instead, you have to think like this:

- ✔ **Bioequivalence:** The rules for drug bioequivalence say that the *true* AUC ratio has to be between 0.8 and 1.25. That's like saying that the *observed* mean AUC ratio must be *significantly* greater than 0.8, *and* it must be significantly less than 1.25. So instead of performing one significance test (against the no-effect value of 1.0), you perform two tests — one against the low (0.8) limit and one against the high (1.25) limit. Each of these tests is one-sided, because each test is concerned only with differences in one direction, so this procedure is called the *two one-sided tests method* for equivalence testing.

- ✔ **Therapeutic noninferiority:** You use the same idea for noninferiority testing, but you have to show only that the new treatment is significantly better than the worst end of the permissible range for the reference treatment. So if a cancer therapy trial used a five-year survival rate as the efficacy variable, the reference treatment had a 40 percent rate, and the permissible tolerance was five percent, then the five-year survival rate for the new treatment would have to be significantly greater than 35 percent.

- ✔ **QT safety:** You have to show that the drug's true QT prolongation, relative to placebo, is less than 10 milliseconds (msec). So you have to show that the excess prolongation (drug minus placebo) is significantly less than 10 milliseconds.

If these significance-testing approaches sound confusing, don't worry — you can test for equivalence and noninferiority another way that's much easier to visualize and understand, and it always leads to exactly the same conclusions.

Using confidence intervals

In Chapter 10, I point out that you can use confidence intervals as an alternative to the usual significance tests by calculating the effect size, along with its confidence interval (CI), and checking whether the CI includes the no-effect value (0 for differences; 1 for ratios). It's always true that an effect is statistically significant if, and only if, its CI doesn't include the no-effect value. And confidence levels correspond to significance levels: 95 percent CIs correspond to $p = 0.05$; 99 percent CIs to $p = 0.01$, and so on.

Figure 16-1 illustrates this correspondence. The vertical line corresponds to the no-effect value (1 for a pharmacokinetic study, using the AUC ratio, in the left diagram; 0 for efficacy testing, using the difference in five-year survival, in the right diagram). The small diamonds are the observed value of the effect size, and the horizontal lines are the 95 percent CIs. When confidence intervals span across the no-effect value, the effect is not significant; when they don't, it is significant.

Figure 16-1:
Using 95 percent confidence intervals to test for significant effects for a pharmacokinetics trial and a cancer therapy trial.

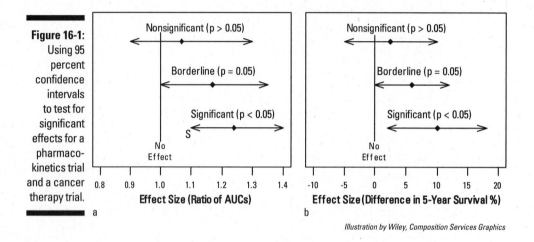

Illustration by Wiley, Composition Services Graphics

You can also use confidence intervals to analyze equivalence and noninferiority/nonsuperiority studies, as shown in Figure 16-2.

Figure 16-2:
Using confidence intervals to test for bioequivalence using the AUC ratio, and testing for noninferiority using the difference in five-year survival.

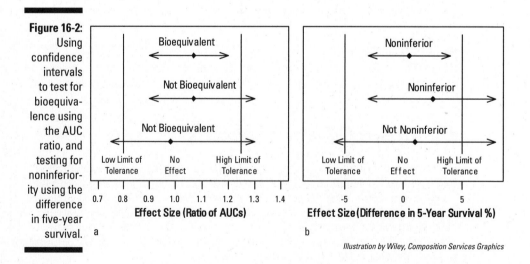

Illustration by Wiley, Composition Services Graphics

You can see two additional vertical lines, representing the lower and upper limits of the allowable tolerance. This time, you don't care whether the confidence interval includes the no-effect line (which is why I made it so light). Instead, you're interested in whether the line stays within the tolerance lines:

- ✔ **Equivalence:** You can conclude equivalence if, and only if, the entire CI fits *between* the two tolerance lines.

- ✔ **Noninferiority and nonsuperiority:** You can conclude noninferiority if, and only if, the entire CI lies to the *right* of the worst tolerance line. (It doesn't matter how high the CI extends.) You can conclude nonsuperiority if, and only if, the entire CI lies to the *left* of the better tolerance line. (It doesn't matter how low the CI extends.)

- ✔ **QT testing:** For a drug to be judged as not substantially prolonging the QT interval, the CI around the difference in QT prolongation between drug and placebo must never extend beyond 10 milliseconds.

When testing noninferiority or nonsuperiority at the 5 percent significance level, you should use 95 percent CIs, as you would expect. But when testing equivalence at the 5 percent level, you should use 90 percent CIs! That's because for equivalence, the 5 percent needs to be applied at both the high and low ends of the CI, not just at one end. And for QT testing, the 5 percent is applied only at the upper end.

Some precautions about noninferiority testing

Although noninferiority testing is sometimes necessary, it has a number of weaknesses that you should keep in mind:

- ✔ **No positive control:** In the earlier section "Recognizing effects: Can you spot a difference if there really is one?" I describe how noninferiority trials usually can't incorporate a truly ineffective treatment, for ethical reasons.

- ✔ **No true proof of efficacy:** Proving that a new drug isn't inferior to a drug that has been shown to be significantly better than placebo isn't really the same as proving that the new drug is significantly better than placebo. The new drug may be less effective than the reference drug (perhaps even significantly less effective) but still within the allowable tolerance for noninferiority.

✔ **Noninferiority creep:** If a new drug is tested against a reference drug that was, itself, approved on the basis of a noninferiority study, this new "third-generation" drug may be less effective than the reference drug, which may have been less effective than the first drug that was tested against placebo. Each successive generation of noninferior drugs may be less effective than the preceding generation. This so-called *noninferiority creep* (sometimes referred to as *bio-creep*) is a matter of considerable concern among researchers and regulatory agencies.

✔ **Estimating sample size:** Estimating the required sample size needed for equivalence and noninferiority or nonsuperiority studies has no simple rules of thumb; you need to use special software designed for these studies. Some web pages are available to estimate sample size for some of these studies; these are listed on the StatPages.info website.

Part IV
Looking for Relationships with Correlation and Regression

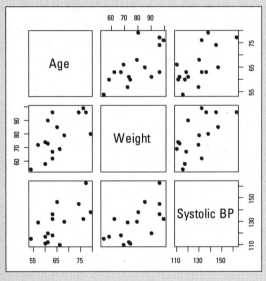

Illustration by Wiley, Composition Services Graphics

In this part . . .

- Understand what correlation and regression are. (Simply stated: *Correlation* refers to the strength of the relationship between two variables, and *regression* refers to a set of techniques for describing the relationship between two variables.)

- Get a handle on the simplest kind of regression — fitting a straight line to your data.

- Do regression analysis when there's more than one predictor variable. (As you may guess, this type of regression is called *multiple regression.*)

- Predict a yes-or-no outcome with logistic regression, and assess sensitivity and specificity with ROC curves.

- Find out about other useful kinds of regression you encounter in biological research, such as Poisson regression and non-linear regression.

Chapter 17

Introducing Correlation and Regression

. . . .

In This Chapter

▶ Getting a handle on correlation analysis

▶ Understanding the many kinds of regression analysis

. . . .

orrelation, regression, curve-fitting, model-building — these terms all describe a set of general statistical techniques dealing with the relationships among variables. This chapter provides an overview of the concepts and terminology that I use throughout Parts IV and V.

Introductory statistics courses usually present only the simplest form of correlation and regression, equivalent to fitting a straight line to a set of data. But in the real world, things are seldom that simple — more than two variables may be involved, and the relationship among them can be quite complicated. You can study correlation and regression for many years and not master all of it. In this chapter, I cover the kinds of correlation and regression most often encountered in biological research and explain the differences between them. I also explain some terminology — predictors and outcomes; independent and dependent variables; parameters; linear and nonlinear relationships; and univariate, bivariate, multivariate, and multivariable analysis.

The words *correlation* and *regression* are often used interchangeably, but they refer to two different things:

✔ **Correlation** refers to the strength of the relationship between two or more variables.

✔ **Regression** refers to a set of techniques for describing the relationship between two or more variables.

Correlation: How Strongly Are Two Variables Associated?

Correlation refers to the extent to which two variables are related. In the following sections, I describe a measurement called the *Pearson correlation coefficient,* and I discuss ways to analyze correlation coefficients.

The term *co-related* was first used by Francis Galton in 1888 in a paper describing the extent to which physical characteristics could be inherited from generation to generation. He said, "Two variable organs are said to be co-related when the variation of the one is accompanied on the average by more or less variation of the other, and in the same direction." Within ten years, Karl Pearson (the guy who invented the chi-square test that I describe in Chapter 13) had developed a formula for calculating the correlation coefficient from paired values of two variables (X and Y).

Lining up the Pearson correlation coefficient

The Pearson correlation coefficient (represented by the symbol r) measures the extent to which two variables (X and Y), when graphed, tend to lie along a straight line. If the variables have no relationship (if the points scatter all over the graph), r will be 0; if the relationship is perfect (if the points lie exactly along a straight line), r will be +1 or –1. Correlation coefficients can be positive (indicating upward-sloping data) or negative (indicating downward-sloping data). Figure 17-1 shows what several different values of r look like.

Figure 17-1:
100 data points, with varying degrees of correlation.

$r = 0.$ $r = 0.5$ $r = 0.8$ $r = 0.9$ $r = 0.99$

$r = 0$ $r = -0.5$ $r = -0.8$ $r = -0.9$ $r = -0.99$

Illustration by Wiley, Composition Services Graphics

Note: The Pearson correlation coefficient measures the extent to which the points lie along a *straight* line. If your data lies closely along a curved line, the r value may be quite low, or even zero, as seen in Figure 17-2. All three graphs in Figure 17-2 have the same amount of random scatter in the points, but they have quite different r values. So you shouldn't interpret *r* = 0 as evidence of independence (lack of association) between two variables; it could indicate only the lack of a *straight-line* relationship between the two variables.

Figure 17-2:
Pearson *r* is based on a straight-line relationship and is too small (or even zero) if the rela-tionship is nonlinear.

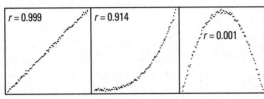

Illustration by Wiley, Composition Services Graphics

Analyzing correlation coefficients

The following are the common kinds of statistical analyses that are per-formed on correlation coefficients. I include formulas and examples here because the calculations aren't too difficult and because your software may not provide these calculations in a convenient form (see Chapter 4 for an introduction to statistical software).

Is r significantly different from zero?

Because your raw data (the *X* and *Y* values) always have random fluctuations (either sampling fluctuations or measurement imprecision, as I describe in Chapter 9), a calculated correlation coefficient is also subject to random fluctuations. Even when *X* and *Y* are completely independent in the popula-tion, your calculated r value is almost never exactly zero. One way to test for a significant association between *X* and *Y* is to test whether *r* is *significantly* different from zero by calculating a p value from the r value. (A *p value* is the probability that random fluctuations alone, in the absence of any real effect in the population, could have produced an observed effect (in this case, an observed r value) that's at least as large as what you observed in your sample; see Chapter 3 for more on p values.)

The correlation coefficient has a strange sampling distribution, but the quantity t — calculated from the observed correlation coefficient r, based on N observations, by the formula $t = r / \sqrt{\left(1-r^2\right)/\left(N-2\right)}$ — fluctuates in accordance with the Student t distribution (see Chapter 25) with $N-2$ degrees of freedom (df). You can get a p value from a t value by going to a table of the Student t distribution or by using an online calculator.

For example, if $r = 0.500$ for a sample of 12 subjects, then $t = 0.5 / \sqrt{\left(1-0.5^2\right)/\left(12-2\right)}$, which works out to $t = 1.8257$, with 10 degrees of freedom. Using the `StatPages.info/pdfs.html` web page and entering the t and df values, you get p = 0.098, which is greater than 0.05, so the r value of 0.500 is not significantly different from zero. (Over the years, p $\leq$ 0.05 has become accepted as a reasonable criterion for declaring significance.)

How precise is an r value?

You can calculate confidence limits around an observed r value using a somewhat roundabout process. The quantity z, calculated by the *Fisher z transformation* $z = \frac{1}{2}\log\left[\left(1+r\right)/\left(1-r\right)\right]$, is approximately normally distributed with a standard deviation of $1/\sqrt{N-3}$, so using the formulas for normal-based confidence intervals (see Chapter 10), you can calculate the low and high 95 percent confidence limits around z: $z_{Low} = z - 1.96/\sqrt{N-3}$ and $z_{High} = z + 1.96/\sqrt{N-3}$. You can turn these into the corresponding confidence limits around r by the reverse of the z transformation: $r = (e^{2z} - 1)/(e^{2z} + 1)$, for $z = z_{Low}$ and $z = z_{High}$.

Using the example from the preceding section of $r = 0.500$ for a sample of 12 subjects, you perform the following steps:

1. **Calculate the Fisher z transformation of the observed r value:**

   $$z = \tfrac{1}{2}\log\left(\left(1+0.5\right)/\left(1-0.5\right)\right) = 0.549$$

2. **Calculate the low and high 95 percent confidence limits for z:**

   $$z_{Low} = 0.549 - 1.96/\sqrt{12-3} = -0.104$$

   $$z_{High} = 0.549 + 1.96/\sqrt{12-3} = +1.203$$

3. **Calculate the low and high 95 percent confidence limits for r:**

   $$r_{Low} = (e^{2 \times (-0.104)} - 1)/(e^{2 \times (-0.104)} + 1) = -0.104$$

   $$r_{High} = (e^{2 \times 1.203} - 1)/(e^{2 \times 1.203} + 1) = 0.835$$

Notice that the 95 percent confidence interval goes from –0.104 to +0.835, a range that includes the value zero. This means that the true r value could indeed be zero, which is consistent with the nonsignificant p value of 0.098 that you obtained from the significance test of r in the preceding section.

Are two r values significantly different?

Suppose you have two correlation coefficients and you want to test whether they have a significant difference between them. Whether the two r values are based on the same variables or are from the same group of subjects doesn't matter. The significance test for comparing two correlation coefficient values (call them r_1 and r_2), obtained from N_1 and N_2 subjects, respectively, utilizes the Fisher z transformation to get z_1 and z_2. The difference $(z_2 - z_1)$ has a standard deviation of $SE_{z_2-z_1} = \sqrt{1/(N_1-3)+1/(N_2-3)}$. You obtain the test statistic for the comparison by dividing the difference by its standard error; you can convert this to a p value by referring to a table (or web page) of the normal distribution.

For example, if you want to compare an r value of 0.4, based on 100 subjects, with an r value of 0.6, based on 150 subjects, you perform the following steps:

1. **Calculate the Fisher z transformation of each observed r value:**

$$z_1 = \tfrac{1}{2}\log\left[(1+0.4)/(1-0.4)\right] = 0.424$$

$$z_2 = \tfrac{1}{2}\log\left[(1+0.6)/(1-0.6)\right] = 0.693$$

2. **Calculate the $(z_2 - z_1)$ difference:**

0.693 – 0.424 = 0.269

3. **Calculate the standard error of the $(z_2 - z_1)$ difference:**

$$SE_{z_2-z_1} = \sqrt{1/(100-3)+1/(150-3)} = 0.131$$

4. **Calculate the test statistic:**

0.269/0.131 = 2.05

5. **Look up 2.05 in a normal distribution table or web page such as** StatPages.info/pdfs.html, **which gives the p value of 0.039 for a two-sided test (where you're interested in knowing whether either r is larger than the other).**

The p value of 0.039 is less than 0.05, meaning that the two correlation coefficients are significantly different from each other.

What's the required sample size for a correlation test?

If you're planning a study whose main purpose is to determine whether two variables (call them X and Y) are significantly correlated, you want to make sure that you have a large enough sample size to give you a good chance of showing significance. (Find out more about power and sample size in Chapter 3.) To perform a sample-size calculation, you need to specify three things (the *design parameters* of the study):

✔ **The *alpha level* of the test:** The p value that's considered significant when you're testing the correlation coefficient. Usually this is set to 0.05, unless you have special considerations.

✔ **The desired *power* of the test:** The probability that the regression comes out significant. Often this is set to 0.8 (or 80%).

✔ **The *effect size of importance:*** The smallest r value that you consider "worth knowing about." If the true r is less than this value, then you don't care whether the test comes out significant, but if r is greater than this value, you want to get a significant result.

I can't tell you what value of r is worth knowing about; it depends on your research goals. If you're hoping to be able to estimate Y from a known value of X, then r has to be fairly high, perhaps 0.8 or higher. But in more pure science applications, where you're trying to discover cause-and-effect relationships in biological systems, you may be interested in knowing about even weak associations like $r = 0.1$ or 0.2. Figure 17-1 may help you choose the r value that's worth knowing about for your study.

You can use software like G*Power (see Chapter 4) to perform the sample-size calculation, but you also have some fairly simple formulas for getting a pretty good sample-size estimate. They all involve dividing a "magic number," which depends on the desired power and alpha level, by the square of the "important" r value. Here are the formulas for a few commonly used values of power and alpha:

✔ For 80 percent power at 0.05 alpha, the required $N = 8/r^2$.

✔ For 90 percent power at 0.05 alpha, the required $N = 10/r^2$.

✔ For 80 percent power at 0.01 alpha, the required $N = 11/r^2$.

✔ For 90 percent power at 0.01 alpha, the required $N = 14/r^2$.

For example, if you want to be 80 percent sure you'll get $p < 0.05$ when testing for a significant relationship when the true r is equal to 0.2, then you need about $8/0.2^2$, which is $8/0.04$, or about 200 data points. The exact answer, obtained from software like G*Power, is 194 data points. The preceding simple approximations slightly overestimate the required N, which is on the safe side (it's better to have slightly more subjects than you need than not to have enough subjects for adequate power).

Regression: What Equation Connects the Variables?

Regression analysis goes beyond just asking *whether* two (or more) variables are associated; it's concerned with finding out exactly *how* those variables are associated — what formula relates the variables together. In the following sections, I explain the purpose of regression analysis, note some terms and notation typically used, and describe common types of regression.

Understanding the purpose of regression analysis

You may be wondering why people would want to do regression analysis in the first place. Fitting a formula to a set of data can be useful in a lot of ways:

✔ You can test for a significant association or relationship between two or more variables. This is exactly equivalent to testing for a significant correlation between the variables but is more general. This is the main reason many researchers do regressions.

✔ You can get a compact representation of your data. This is especially useful in the more physical sciences, where you deal with precise measurements. If you measure the vapor pressure of a liquid at every degree from –100 degrees to +300 degrees, the resulting data could occupy several printed pages. But if you can find a formula that fits the data to within its measured precision, that formula may well fit on one printed line.

✔ You can make precise predictions, or prognoses. With a properly fitted survival function (see Chapter 24), you can generate a customized survival curve for a newly diagnosed cancer patient based on that patient's age, gender, weight, disease stage, tumor grade, and other factors. A bit morbid, perhaps, but you could certainly do it.

✔ You can do mathematical manipulations easily and accurately on a fitted function that may be difficult or inaccurate to do graphically on the raw data. For example, you can

  • Interpolate between two measured values.

  • Extrapolate beyond the measured range. Extrapolating a fitted formula beyond the range of observed data it was fitted to can be risky! There's no guarantee that the curve that fits your observed data closely will realistically describe the relationship outside the range of values you observed. Many outstanding "extrapolation failures" have occurred throughout the history of science.

- Smooth the data (estimate what the *Y* variable would be without the random fluctuations).

- Find minima, maxima, slopes, integrals (areas under the curve), and so on.

✔ If you're developing an *assay* (a laboratory analysis to determine the concentration of some substance) or an analytical instrument, you can prepare calibration curves, which you can then use to automatically calculate the result from the instrument's raw readings.

✔ You can test a theoretical model, such as a multicompartment kinetic model of a drug's absorption, distribution, metabolism, and elimination from the body. By fitting this model to observed data, you can validate (or perhaps invalidate) the proposed model.

✔ You can obtain numerical values for the parameters that appear in the model. If the model has a theoretical basis and isn't just an *empirical* formula (one that just happens to have a shape that resembles your data), then the parameters appearing in that model will probably have physical (or physiological) meaning. For example, one of the parameters in a dose-response model may be the ED_{50} — the dose that produces one-half the maximum effect.

Talking about terminology and mathematical notation

A *regression model* is usually a formula that describes how one variable (called the *dependent variable,* the *outcome,* or the *result*) depends on one or more other variables (called *independent variables,* or *predictors*) and on one or more parameters. (Regression models can have more than one dependent variable, as I describe below.) *Parameters* aren't variables; they're other terms that appear in the formula that make the function come as close as possible to the observed data. For simple regressions (one predictor and one outcome variable), you can think of the parameters as specifying the position, orientation, and shape of the fitted line on the scatter plot (like the *slope* and *Y-intercept* of a straight line).

If you have only one independent variable, it's often designated by *X,* and the dependent variable is designated by *Y.* If you have more than one independent variable, variables are usually designated by letters toward the end of the alphabet *(W, X, Y, Z).* Parameters are often designated by letters toward the beginning of the alphabet *(a, b, c, d).* There's no consistent rule regarding uppercase versus lowercase letters.

Sometimes a collection of predictor variables is designated by a subscripted variable (X_1, X_2, and so on) and the corresponding coefficients by another subscripted variable (b_1, b_2, and so on).

So in mathematical texts, you may see a regression model with three predictors written in one of several ways, such as

  ✔ $Z = a + bX + cY + dV$ (different letters for each variable and parameter)

  ✔ $Y = b_0 + b_1 X_1 + b_2 X_2$ (using a general subscript-variable notation)

In practical work, using the actual names of the variables from your data and using meaningful terms for parameters is easiest to understand and least error-prone. For example, consider the equation for the first-order elimination of an injected drug from the blood, $Conc = Conc_0 \times e^{-k_e \times Time}$. This form, with its short but meaningful names for the two variables, $Conc$ (blood concentration) and $Time$ (time after injection), and the two parameters, $Conc_0$ (concentration at $Time = 0$) and k_e (elimination rate constant), would probably be more meaningful to a reader than $Y = a \times e^{-b \times X}$.

Classifying different kinds of regression

Regression is a very broad topic, and you can devote many semesters to exploring its many varieties and subtleties. In the following sections, I list (and briefly describe) the regression techniques that are common in biological research. I describe these different kinds of regressions in much more detail in Chapters 18 through 21 and Chapter 24.

You can classify regression on the basis of

  ✔ How many outcomes (dependent variables) appear in the model

  ✔ How many predictors (independent variables) appear in the model

  ✔ What kind of data the outcome variable is

  ✔ What kind of mathematical form the model takes

Indicating the number of outcomes

Statisticians distinguish between regression models that have only one outcome variable and models that have two or more outcome variables:

  ✔ *Univariate* regression has only one outcome variable.

  ✔ *Multivariate* regression has two or more outcome variables. Multiple outcomes can be one kind of variable at two or more time points (like pain levels measured at one, two, and three hours after a surgical procedure) or two different kinds of variables (such as pain level and nausea level).

Indicating the number of predictors

Statisticians distinguish between regression models that have only one predictor and models that have two or more predictor variables:

- ✔ *Univariable* regression has only one predictor variable.
- ✔ *Multivariable* regression has two or more predictor variables.

Here's where things get bizarre. Notice the slight difference in spelling — *univariate* versus *univariable*, and *multivariate* versus *multivariable*. That difference is important when talking to statisticians — they use the "-variate" words when talking about the number of *outcomes,* and "-variable" words when talking about the number of *predictors*. But medical researchers almost never use the terms *univariable* or *multivariable;* they use *univariate* and *multivariate* when talking about the number of predictors, and they often refer to a regression model with multiple outcome variables simply as *multiple regression.*

And it gets worse! Sometimes, regression with only one predictor is referred to as *bivariate* regression because a total of two variables are involved — one predictor and one outcome. It's probably best to never use the term *bivariate regression* at all.

Fortunately, this confusion over nomenclature usually won't cause you any trouble when it comes time to analyze your data. Any software that can handle multiple predictors can also easily handle a model with only one predictor. But the distinction is still important to keep in mind, because as soon as you have two or more predictors, a lot of strange and unexpected things can happen. So I dedicate Chapter 19 to describing the situations you need to be aware of whenever you work with regression models with more than one predictor.

Examining the outcome variable's type of data

You can also classify regression based on what kind of data the outcome variable is:

- ✔ You use *ordinary* regression when the outcome is a continuous variable whose random fluctuations are governed by the normal distribution. (Chapters 18 and 19 deal with this kind of regression.)
- ✔ You use *logistic* regression when the outcome variable is a dichotomous category (like lived or died) whose fluctuations are governed by the binomial distribution. (See Chapter 20 for details.)
- ✔ You use *Poisson* regression when the outcome variable is the number of occurrences of a sporadic event whose fluctuations are governed by the Poisson distribution. (Chapter 21 has the scoop.)

✔ You use *survival* regression when the outcome is a *time to event,* often called a *survival time* (even when the event isn't death). Survival analysis is so important in biological research, and the techniques are so specialized, that I devote all of Part V to the methods of summarizing and analyzing survival data.

Figuring out what kind of function is being fitted

A third way to classify different types of regression analysis is according to whether the mathematical formula for the model is linear or nonlinear in the parameters.

In a *linear* function, you multiply each predictor variable by a parameter and then add these products to give the predicted value. You can also have one more parameter that isn't multiplied by anything — it's called the *constant term* or the *intercept.* Here are some linear functions:

✔ $Y = a + bX$

✔ $Y = a + bX + cX^2 + dX^3$

✔ $Y = a + bX + c\text{Log}(W) + dX/\text{Cos}(Z)$

In these examples, Y is the dependent variable (the outcome); X, W, and Z are the independent variables (predictors); and a, b, c, and d are parameters.

The predictor variables can appear in a formula in nonlinear form, like squared or cubed, inside functions like Log and Sin, and multiplied by each other; but as long as the coefficients appear only in a linear way (each coefficient multiplying a term involving predictor variables, with the terms added together), the function is still considered *linear in the parameters.*

A *nonlinear* function is anything that's not a linear function. For example:

$$Y = a/(b + e^{-c \times X})$$

is nonlinear in the parameters because the parameter b is in the denominator of a fraction, and the parameter c is in an exponent. The parameter a appears in a linear form, but if *any* of the parameters appear in a nonlinear way, the function is said to be nonlinear in the parameters.

Hardly anything is perfectly linear in the real world, but almost everything is linear to a first approximation. Physical scientists deal extensively with nonlinear regression because they're trying to accurately model relatively precise data and well-developed theoretical models. Social scientists, on the other hand, almost always use linear methods to deal with their much "softer" measurements (opinion surveys, subjective ratings, and so on) and empirical models. Biological researchers tend to occupy a middle ground, with more precise measurements and models that have at least some theoretical basis. So nonlinear regression does come up frequently in biological research.

Coming up with lots of different kinds of regression

The three different ways of "slicing the cake" — number of predictors, type of outcome variable, and linearity of the function — apply in all combinations. You can have

- A linear model with one predictor and a continuous outcome. This is the simplest kind of regression: the straight line (see Chapter 18).

- A linear model with many predictors of a continuous outcome. This is commonly referred to in medical research as *multiple regression*, although the proper name is *linear multivariable regression* (see Chapter 19).

- A model with one or more predictors of a dichotomous categorical outcome. This is univariate or multivariate logistic regression (see Chapter 20).

- A nonlinear model with one or more predictors of a continuous outcome. This is univariate or multivariate nonlinear regression (see Chapter 21).

Many other combinations are possible. Most of the remainder of this book deals with the kinds of regression that you may expect to encounter in your research.

Chapter 18

Getting Straight Talk on Straight-Line Regression

Chapter 17 talks about regression analyses in a general way. This chapter focuses on the simplest kind of regression analysis: *straight-line regression*. You can visualize it as "fitting" a straight line to the points in a scatter plot from a set of data involving just two variables. Those two variables are generally referred to as *X* and *Y*.

✔ The *X* variable is formally called the *independent variable* (or the *predictor* or *cause*).

✔ The *Y* variable is called the *dependent variable* (or the *outcome* or *effect*).

 You may see straight-line regression referred to in books and articles by several different names, including *linear regression, simple linear regression, linear univariate regression,* and *linear bivariate regression*. This abundance of references can be confusing, so I always use the term *straight-line regression*.

Knowing When to Use Straight-Line Regression

REMEMBER

Straight-line regression is the way to go when *all* of these things are true:

- ✔ You're interested in the relationship between two (and only two) numerical variables.

- ✔ You've made a scatter plot of the two variables and the data points seem to lie, more or less, along a straight line (as shown in Figures 18-1a and 18-1b). You shouldn't try to fit a straight line to data that appears to lie along a curved line (as shown in Figures 18-1c and 18-1d).

- ✔ The data points appear to scatter randomly around the straight line over the entire range of the chart, with no extreme outliers.

Figure 18-1:
Straight-line
regression
is appro-
priate for
both strong
and weak
linear rela-
tionships
(a and b),
but not for
nonlinear
(curved-line)
relationships
(c and d).

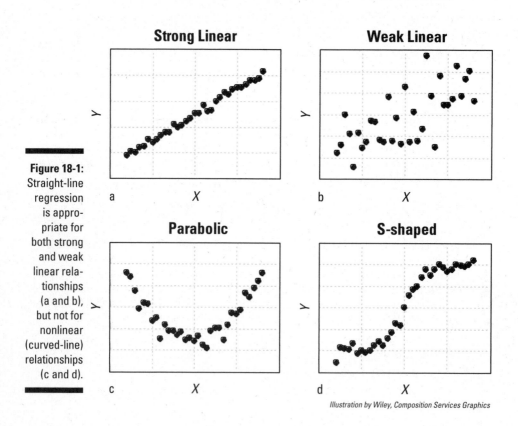

Illustration by Wiley, Composition Services Graphics

Straight-line regression is the way to go when one or more of these things are true:

- ✔ You want to test whether there's a significant association between the *X* and *Y* variables.
- ✔ You want to know the value of the slope or the intercept (or both).
- ✔ You want to be able to predict the value of *Y* for any value of *X*.

Understanding the Basics of Straight-Line Regression

The formula of a straight line can be written like this: $Y = a + bX$. This formula breaks down this way:

- ✔ *Y* is the dependent variable (or outcome).
- ✔ *X* is the independent variable (or predictor).
- ✔ *a* is the intercept (the value of *Y* when $X = 0$).
- ✔ *b* is the slope (the amount *Y* changes when *X* increases by 1).

The best line (in the least-squares sense) through a set of data is the one that minimizes the sum of the squares (SSQ) of the *residuals* (the vertical distances of each point from the fitted line), as shown in Figure 18-2.

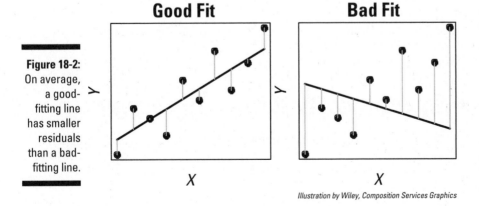

Figure 18-2: On average, a good-fitting line has smaller residuals than a bad-fitting line.

Good Fit   Bad Fit

For most types of curves, finding the best-fitting curve is a very complicated mathematical problem; the straight line is one of the very few kinds of lines for which you can calculate the least-squares parameters from explicit formulas. If you're interested (or if your professor says that you're interested), here's a general outline of how those formulas are derived.

For any set of data X_i and Y_i (in which i is an index that identifies each observation in the set, as described in Chapter 2), SSQ can be calculated like this:

$$SSQ = \sum_i (a + bX_i - Y_i)^2$$

If you're good at first-semester calculus, you can find the values of a and b that minimize SSQ by setting the partial derivatives of SSQ with respect to a and b equal to 0. If you stink at calculus, trust that this leads to these two simultaneous equations:

$a(N) + b(\Sigma X) = (\Sigma Y)$

$a(\Sigma X) + b(\Sigma X^2) = (\Sigma XY)$

where N is the number of observed data points.

These equations can be solved for a and b:

$$a = \frac{(\sum Y)(\sum X^2) - (\sum X)(\sum XY)}{(N)(\sum X^2) - (\sum X)^2}$$

$$b = \frac{(\sum XY) - (a)(\sum X)}{(\sum X^2)}$$

See Chapter 2 if you don't feel comfortable reading the mathematical notations or expressions in this section.

Running a Straight-Line Regression

Never try to do regression calculations by hand (or on a calculator). You'll go crazy trying to evaluate all those summations and other calculations, and you'll almost certainly make a mistake somewhere in your calculations.

Fortunately, every major statistical software package (and most minor ones) can do straight-line regression. Excel has built-in functions for the slope and intercept of the least-squares straight line. You can find straight-line regression web pages (several are listed at StatPages.info), and you can download apps to do this task on a smartphone or tablet. (See Chapter 4 for an introduction to statistical software.)

In the following sections, I list the basic steps for running a straight-line regression, complete with an example.

Taking a few basic steps

The exact steps you take to run a straight-line regression depend on what software you're using, but here's the general approach:

1. **Get your data into the proper form.**

   Usually, the data consists of two columns of numbers, one representing the independent variable and the other representing the dependent variable.

2. **Tell the software which variable is the independent variable and which one is the dependent variable.**

   Depending on the software, you may type the variable names or pick them from a menu or list in your file.

3. **If the software offers output options, tell it that you want these results:**

   - Graphs of observed and calculated values
   - Summaries and graphs of the residuals
   - Regression table
   - Goodness-of-fit measures

4. **Press the Go button (or whatever it takes to start the calculations).**

   You should get your answers in the blink of an eye.

Walking through an example

To see how to run and interpret the output of a simple straight-line regression, I use the following example throughout the rest of this chapter.

Consider how blood pressure (BP) is related to body weight. It may be reasonable to suspect that people who weigh more have higher BP. If you test this hypothesis on people and find that there really is an association between weight and BP, you may want to quantify that relationship. Maybe you want to say that every extra kilogram of weight tends to be associated with a certain amount of increased BP. The following sections take you through the steps of gathering data, creating a scatter plot, and interpreting the results.

Gathering the data

Suppose that you get a group of 20 representative adults from some population. Say you stand outside the college bookstore and recruit students as they pass by. You weigh them and measure their BP. To keep your study simple, you consider just the systolic blood pressure. Table 18-1 shows some actual weight and BP data from 20 people. Weight is recorded in kilograms (kg), and BP is recorded in the strange-sounding units of *millimeters of mercury* (mmHg). For clarity, I omit that rather cumbersome notation when a sentence reads better without it and when I'm obviously talking about a BP value.

Table 18-1	Weight and Blood Pressure	
Subject	*Body Weight (kg)*	*Systolic BP (mmHg)*
001	74.4	109
002	85.1	114
003	78.3	94
004	77.2	109
005	63.8	104
006	77.9	132
007	78.9	127
008	60.9	98
009	75.6	126
010	74.5	126
011	82.2	116
012	99.8	121
013	78.0	111
014	71.8	116
015	90.2	115
016	105.4	133
017	100.4	128
018	80.9	128
019	81.8	105
020	109.0	127

Creating a scatter plot

It's usually hard to spot patterns and trends in a table like Table 18-1, but you get a clearer picture of what's happening if you make a scatter plot of the 20 subjects, with weight (the independent variable) on the X axis and systolic BP (the dependent variable) on the Y axis. See Figure 18-3.

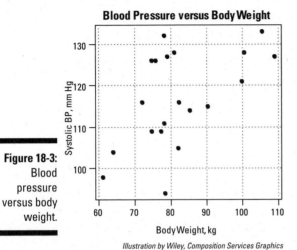

Figure 18-3:
Blood
pressure
versus body
weight.

Illustration by Wiley, Composition Services Graphics

Examining the results

In Figure 18-3, you can see a possible pattern. There seems to be a tendency for the following:

- **Low-weight people have low BP** (represented by the points near the lower-left part of the graph).

- **Higher-weight people have higher BP** (represented by the points near the upper-right part of the graph).

There aren't any really heavy people with really low BP; the lower-right part of the graph is pretty empty. But the agreement isn't completely convincing. Several people in the 70- to 80-kilogram range have BPs over 125.

A correlation analysis (described in Chapter 17) will tell you how strong the association is and let you decide whether or not it could be due solely to random fluctuations. A regression analysis will, in addition, give you a math-ematical formula that expresses the relationship between the two variables (weight and BP, in this example).

Interpreting the Output of Straight-Line Regression

In the following sections, I take you through the printed and graphical output of a typical straight-line regression run. Its looks will vary depending on your software (this output was generated by the R statistical software), but you should be able to find the following parts of the output:

✔ A simple statement of what you asked the program to do

✔ A summary of the residuals, including graphs that display the residuals and help you assess whether they're normally distributed

✔ The regression table

✔ Measures of goodness-of-fit of the line to the data

Seeing what you told the program to do

In Figure 18-4, the first two lines produced by the statistical software say that you wanted to fit a simple formula: BP ~ Weight to your observed BP and weight values.

```
Call:
lm (formula = BPs ~ Wgt)

Residuals:
    Min      IQ    Median      3Q       Max
 -20.999  -4.720   -3.403     6.528    17.196

Coefficients:
               Estimate Std. Error t value Pr (>|t|)
(Intercept)     76.8602    14.6552   5.245  5.49e-05 ***
Wgt              0.4871     0.1760   2.767    0.0127 *
---
Signif. codes:    0 `***'  0.001  `**'  0.01  `*'  0.05  `.'  0.1  ` ' 1

Residual standard error:  9.838 on 18 degrees of freedom
Multiple R-squared:  0.2984,        Adjusted R-squared:   0.2594
F-statistic:  7.656 on 1 and 18 DF,  p-value:  0.01271
```

Figure 18-4:
Typical
regression
output looks
like this.

Illustration by Wiley, Composition Services Graphics

The tilde in an expression like $Y \sim X$ is a widely used shorthand way of saying that you're fitting a model in which Y depends only on X. Read a tilde aloud as *depends only on* or *is predicted by* or *is a function of.* So in Figure 18-4, the tilde means you're fitting a model in which BP depends only on weight.

The actual equation of the straight line is BP = $a + b \times weight$, but the a (intercept) and b (slope) parameters have been left out of the model shown in Figure 18-4 for the sake of conciseness. This shorthand is particularly useful in Chapter 19, which deals with formulas that have lots of independent variables.

Looking at residuals

Most regression software gives several measures of how the data points scatter above and below the fitted line. The "residuals" section in Figure 18-4 provides information about how the observed data points scatter around the fitted line.

The *residual* for a point is the vertical distance of that point from the fitted line. It's calculated as *Residual* = $Y - (a + b \times X)$, where a and b are the intercept and slope of the fitted straight line. The residuals for the sample data are shown in Figure 18-5.

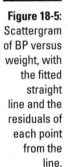

Figure 18-5:
Scattergram of BP versus weight, with the fitted straight line and the residuals of each point from the line.

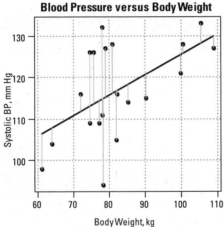

Blood Pressure versus Body Weight

Illustration by Wiley, Composition Services Graphics

Summary statistics for the residuals

If you read about summarizing data in Chapter 8, you know the distribution of a set of numbers is often summarized by quoting the mean, standard deviation, median, minimum, maximum, and quartiles. That's exactly what you find in the "residuals" section of your software's output. Here's what you see in Figure 18-4:

✔ **The Min and Max values** are the two largest residuals (the two points that lie farthest away from the line). One data point actually lies about 21 mmHg below the line, and one point lies about 17 above the line. (The sign of a residual is positive or negative, depending on whether the point lies above or below the fitted line, respectively.)

✔ **The first and third quartiles** (denoted 1Q and 3Q, respectively) tell you that about a quarter of the points (that is, 5 of the 20 points) lie more than 4.7 mmHg *below* the fitted line, a quarter of them lie more than 6.5 mmHg *above* the fitted line, and the remaining half of the points lie within those two quartiles.

✔ **The Median value** of –3.4 tells you that half of the residuals (that is, the residuals of 10 of the 20 points) are less than –3.4 and half are greater than –3.4 mmHg.

Note: The mean residual isn't included in these summary numbers because the mean of the residuals is always exactly 0 for any kind of regression that includes an intercept term.

The *residual standard error,* often called the *root-mean-square (RMS) error* in regression output, is a measure of how tightly or loosely the points scatter above or below the fitted line. You can think of it as the *standard deviation (SD)* of the residuals, although it's computed in a slightly different way from the usual SD of a set of numbers: RMS uses $N-2$ instead of $N-1$ in the denominator of the SD formula. The R program shows the RMS value near the bottom of the output, but you can think of it as another summary statistic for residuals.

For this data, the residuals have a standard deviation of about 9.8 mmHg.

Graphs of the residuals

Most regression programs will produce several graphs of the residuals if you ask them to. You can use these graphs to assess whether the data meets the criteria for doing a least-squares straight-line regression. Figure 18-6 shows two of the more common types of residual graphs, commonly called "residuals versus fitted" and "normal Q-Q" graphs.

A *residuals versus fitted* graph has the values of the residuals (observed Y minus predicted Y) plotted along the Y axis and the predicted Y values from the fitted straight line plotted along the X axis. A *normal Q-Q* graph shows the *standardized residuals* (residuals divided by the RMS value) along the Y axis and theoretical quantiles along the X axis. *Theoretical quantiles* are what you'd expect the standardized residuals to be if they were exactly normally distributed.

Together, the two kinds of graphs shown in Figure 18-6 give some insight into whether your data conforms to assumptions for straight-line regression:

✔ Your data must lie randomly above and below the line across the whole range of data.

✔ The average amount of scatter must be fairly constant across the whole range of data.

✔ The residuals should be approximately normally distributed.

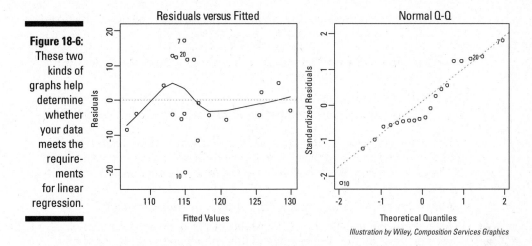

Figure 18-6: These two kinds of graphs help determine whether your data meets the requirements for linear regression.

You'll need some experience with residual graphs (maybe 10 or 20 years' worth) before you can interpret them confidently, so don't feel too discouraged if you can't tell at a glance whether your data complies with the requirements for straight-line regression. Here's how I interpret them (though other statisticians may disagree with me):

✔ The residuals versus fitted chart in Figure 18-6 indicates that points seem to lie equally above and below the fitted line, and that's true whether you're looking at the left, middle, or right part of the graph.

✔ Figure 18-6 also indicates that most of the points lie within ±10 mmHg of the line. But a lot of larger residuals for points appear to be where the BP is around 115 mmHg. This seems a little suspicious, and I should probably look at my raw data and see whether there's something unusual about these subjects.

✔ If the residuals are normally distributed, then in the normal Q-Q chart in Figure 18-6, the points should lie close to the dotted diagonal line and shouldn't display any overall curved shape. These points seem to follow the dotted line pretty well, so I'm not concerned about lack of normality in the residuals.

Making your way through the regression table

The table of regression coefficients is arguably the most important part of the output for any kind of regression; it's probably where you look first and where you concentrate most of your attention. Nearly all straight-line statistics programs produce a table of regression coefficients that looks much like the one in Figure 18-4.

For straight-line regression, the coefficients table has two rows that correspond to the two parameters of the straight line:

- ✔ **The intercept row:** You may find this row labeled at the far left by the term *Intercept* or *Constant.*

- ✔ **The slope row:** This row may be labeled as *Slope,* but it's more frequently labeled with the name of the independent variable (in this case, *Wgt*).

The table usually has about four columns (more or less, depending on the software). The names of the columns vary from one software package to another. The columns are discussed in the following sections.

The values of the coefficients (the intercept and the slope)

The first column usually shows the values of the slope and intercept of the fitted straight line. The heading of this column in the table might be *Coefficient, Estimate,* or perhaps (more cryptically) the single letter *B* or *C* (in uppercase or lowercase), depending on the software.

The intercept is the predicted value of *Y* when *X* is equal to 0 and is expressed in the same units of measurement as the *Y* variable. The slope is the amount the predicted value of *Y* changes when *X* increases by exactly one unit of measurement and is expressed in units equal to the units of *Y* divided by the units of *X*.

In the example shown in Figure 18-4, the estimated value of the intercept is 76.8602 mmHg, and the estimated value of the slope is 0.4871 mmHg/kilogram.

- ✔ The intercept value of 76.9 mmHg means that a person who weighs 0 kilograms should have a BP of about 77 mmHg. But nobody weighs 0 kilograms! The intercept in this example (and in many straight-line relations in biology) has no physiological meaning at all, because 0 kilograms is totally outside the range of possible human weights.

- ✔ The slope value of 0.4871 mmHg/kilogram *does* have a real-world meaning. It means that every additional 1 kilogram of weight is associated with a 0.4871 mmHg increase in systolic BP. Or, playing around with the decimal points, every additional 10 kilograms of body weight is associated with almost a 5 mmHg BP increase.

The standard errors of the coefficients

The second column in the regression table usually has the standard errors of the estimated parameters (sometimes abbreviated SE, Std. Err., or something similar). I use SE for standard error in the rest of this chapter.

Because your observed data always have random fluctuations, anything you calculate from your observed data also has random fluctuations (whether it's a simple average or something more complicated, like a regression coefficient). The SE tells you how precisely you were able to estimate the parameter from your data, which is very important if you plan to use the value of the slope (or the intercept) in some subsequent calculation. (See Chapter 11 to read how random fluctuations in numbers propagate through any calculations you may perform with those numbers.)

Keep these things in mind about SE:

- ✔ **Standard errors always have the same units as the coefficients themselves.** In the example shown in Figure 18-4, the SE of the intercept has units of mmHg, and the SE of the slope has units of mmHg/kg.

- ✔ **Round off the estimated values.** Quoting a lot of meaningless digits when you report your results is pointless. In this example, the SE of the intercept is about 14.7, so you can say that the estimate of the intercept in this regression is about 77 ± 15 mmHg. In the same way, you can say that the estimated slope is 0.49 ± 0.18 mmHg/kg.

    When quoting regression coefficients in professional publications, you may include the SE like this: "The predicted increase in systolic blood pressure with weight (± 1 SE) was 0.49 ± 0.18 mmHg/kg."

If you have the SE, you can easily calculate a *confidence interval* (CI) around the estimated parameter. (See Chapter 10 for more info.) To a very good approximation, the 95 percent confidence limits, which mark the low and high ends of the confidence interval around a coefficient, are given by these expressions:

Lower 95% CL = Coefficient – 2 × SE

Upper 95% CL = Coefficient + 2 × SE

More informally, these are written as *95% CI = coefficient ± 2 × SE*.

So the 95-percent CI around the slope is calculated as $0.49 \pm 2 \times 0.176$, which works out to 0.49 ± 0.35, which becomes 0.14 to 0.84 mmHg. If you submit a manuscript for publication, you may express the precision of the results in terms of CIs instead of SEs, like this: "The predicted increase in systolic blood pressure as a function of body weight was 0.49 mmHg/kg (95% CI: 0.14 – 0.84)." Of course, you should always follow the guidelines specified by the journal you're writing for.

 To be more precise, multiply the SE by the critical two-sided Student t value for the confidence level you want and the appropriate number of degrees of freedom (which, for *N* data points, is equal to $N - 2$). You can estimate critical t values from this book's online Cheat Sheet at www.dummies.com/cheatsheet/biostatistics or get them from more extensive tables, statistical software, or web pages. For a 95 percent CI and a set of 30 data points (28 degrees of freedom), the critical t value is 2.0484. The approximate value of 2 is fine for most practical work; you probably won't have to look up critical t values unless you have fewer than 20 data points.

The Student t value

In many statistical programs, the third column in a regression table shows the ratio of the coefficient divided by its standard error. This column can go by different names, but it's most commonly referred to as *t* or *t value.* You can think of this column as an intermediate quantity in the calculation of what you're really interested in: the p value for the coefficient.

The t values appearing in the regression table are *not* the "critical t values" that you use to construct confidence intervals, as described earlier.

The p value

The next (and usually last) column of the regression table contains the p value, which indicates whether the regression coefficient is significantly different from 0. Depending on your software, this column may be called p value, p, Signif, or $Pr(>|t|)$, as shown in Figure 18-4.

Note: In Chapter 19, I explain how to interpret this peculiar notation, but just keep in mind that it's only another way of designating the column that holds the p values.

In Figure 18-4, the p value for the intercept is shown as $5.49e - 05$, which is equal to 0.0000549 (see the description of scientific notation in Chapter 2). This value is much less than 0.05, so the intercept is significantly different from zero. But recall that in this example the intercept doesn't have any real-world importance (it's the expected BP for a person who doesn't weigh anything), so you probably don't care whether it's different from zero or not.

But the p value for the slope is very important — if it's less than 0.05, it means that the slope of the fitted straight line is significantly different from zero. In turn, that means that the X and Y variables are significantly associated with each other. A p value greater than 0.05 indicates that the true slope may be equal to zero, so there's no conclusive evidence for a significant association between X and Y. In Figure 18-4, the p value for the slope is 0.0127, which means that the slope is significantly different from zero, and this tells you that body weight is significantly associated with systolic BP.

If you want to test for a significant correlation between two variables, simply look at the p value for the slope of the least-squares straight line. If it's less than 0.05, then the X and Y variables are significantly correlated. The p value for the significance of the slope in a straight-line regression is always exactly the same as the p value for the correlation test of whether r is significantly different from zero, as described in Chapter 17.

Wrapping up with measures of goodness-of-fit

The last few lines of output in Figure 18-4 contain several indicators of how well a straight line represents the data. The following sections describe this part of the output.

The correlation coefficient

Most straight-line regression programs provide the classic Pearson r correlation coefficient between X and Y (see Chapter 17 for details). But the program may give you the correlation coefficient in a roundabout way: as r^2 rather than r itself. The software I use for this example shows r^2 on the line that begins with "Multiple R-squared: 0.2984." Just get out your calculator and take the square root of 0.2984 to get 0.546 for Pearson r.

R squared is always positive — the square of anything is always positive — but the correlation coefficient can be positive or negative, depending on whether the fitted line slopes upward or downward. If the fitted line slopes downward, make your r value negative.

Why did the program give you R squared instead of r in the first place? It's because R squared is a useful number in its own right. It's sometimes called the *coefficient of determination,* and it tells you what percent of the total variability in the Y variable can be explained by the fitted line.

- ✔ An R-squared value of 1 means that the points lie exactly on the fitted line, with no scatter at all.

- ✔ An R-squared value of 0 means that your data points are all over the place, with no tendency at all for the X and Y variables to be associated.

- ✔ An R-squared value of 0.3 (as in this example) means that 30 percent of the variance in the dependent variable is explainable by the straight-line model.

Note: I talk about the adjusted R-squared value in Chapter 19 when I explain multiple regression. For now, you can just ignore it.

The F statistic

The last line of the sample output addresses this question: Is the straight-line model any good at all? How much better is the straight-line model (which has an intercept and a predictor) compared to the *null model?*

The *null model* is a model that contains only a single parameter representing a constant term (such as an intercept), with no predictor variables at all.

If the p value associated with the F statistic is less than 0.05, then adding the predictor variable to the model makes it significantly better at predicting BPs.

For this example, the p value is 0.013, indicating that knowing a person's weight makes you significantly better at predicting that person's BP than not knowing the weight (and therefore having to quote the same overall mean BP value from your data [117 mmHg] as your guess every time).

Scientific fortune-telling with the prediction formula

As I describe in Chapter 17, one reason for doing regression analysis is to develop a prediction formula (or, if you want to sound fancy, a *predictive model*) that lets you guess the value of the dependent variable if you know the values of the independent variables.

Some statistics programs show the actual equation of the best-fitting straight line. If yours doesn't, don't worry. Just substitute the coefficients of the intercept and slope for *a* and *b* in the straight-line equation: $Y = a + bX$.

With the output shown in Figure 18-4, where the intercept (*a*) is 76.9 and the slope (*b*) is 0.487, you can write the equation of the fitted straight line like this: BP = 76.9 + 0.487 Weight.

Then you can use this equation to predict someone's BP if you know his weight. So, if a person weighs 100 kilograms, you can guess that that person's BP may be about $76.9 + 100 \times 0.487$, which is 76.9 + 48.7, or about 125.6 mmHg. Your guess won't be exactly on the nose, but it will probably be better than if you didn't know that BP increases with increasing weight.

How far off may your guess be? The residual standard error provides a yard-stick of your guessing prowess. As I explain in the earlier section "Summary statistics for the residuals," the residual standard error indicates how much the individual points tend to scatter above and below the fitted line. For the BP example, this number is ±9.8, so you can expect your prediction to be within about ±10 mmHg most of the time (about 68 percent of the time if the residuals are truly normally distributed with a standard deviation of ±10) and within ±20 mmHg about 95 percent of the time.

Recognizing What Can Go Wrong with Straight-Line Regression

Fitting a straight line to a set of data is a pretty simple task for any piece of software, but you still have to be careful. A computer program happily does whatever you tell it to, even if it's something you shouldn't do.

People frequently slip up on the following things when doing straight-line regression:

- ✔ **Fitting a straight line to curved data:** Examining the pattern of residuals in the *residuals versus fitted* chart in Figure 18-5 can alert you to this problem.

- ✔ **Ignoring outliers in the data:** Outliers can mess up all the classical statistical analyses, and regression is no exception. One or two data points that are way off the main trend of the points will tend to drag the fitted line away from the other points. That's because the strength with which each point tugs at the line is proportionate to the square of its distance from the line.

Always look at a scatter plot of your data to make sure outliers aren't present. Examine the residuals to make sure they seem to be distributed normally above and below the fitted line.

Figuring Out the Sample Size You Need

To figure out how many data points you need for a regression analysis, first ask yourself why you're doing the regression in the first place.

- ✔ **Do you want to show that the two variables are significantly associated?** Then you want to calculate the sample size required to achieve a certain statistical *power* for the significance test (see Chapter 3 for an introduction to statistical power).

- ✔ **Do you want to estimate the value of the slope (or intercept) to within a certain margin of error?** Then you want to calculate the sample size required to achieve a certain *precision* in your estimate.

Testing the significance of a slope is exactly equivalent to testing the significance of a correlation coefficient, so the sample-size calculations are also the same for the two types of tests. If you haven't already, check out Chapter 17, which has simple formulas for the number of subjects you need to test for any specified degree of correlation.

If you're doing the regression to estimate the value of a regression coefficient — for example, the slope of the straight line — then the calculations get more complicated. The precision of the slope depends on several things:

- **The number of data points:** More data points give you greater precision. Standard errors vary inversely as the square root of the sample size. Or, the required sample size varies inversely as the square of the desired SE. So, if you quadruple the sample size, you cut the SE in half. This is a very important, and very generally applicable, principle.

- **Tightness of the fit of the observed points to the line:** The closer the data points hug the line, the more precisely you can estimate the regression coefficients. The effect is directly proportional — twice as much Y-scatter of the points produces twice as large a SE in the coefficients.

- **How the data points are distributed across the range of the X variable:** This effect is hard to quantify, but in general, having the data points spread out evenly over the entire range of X produces more precision than having most of them clustered near the middle of the range.

How, then, do you intelligently design a study to acquire data for a linear regression where you're mainly interested in estimating a regression coefficient to within a certain precision? One practical approach is to first conduct a small pilot study of, say, 20 subjects and look at the SE of the regression coefficient. If you're really lucky, the SE may be as small as you wanted, or even smaller — then you're all done!

But the SE probably isn't small enough (unless you're a lot luckier that I've ever been). That's when you reach for the square-root law. Follow these steps to get the total sample size you need to get the precision you want:

1. **Divide the SE that you *got* from your pilot run by the SE you *want* your full study to achieve.**

2. **Square the ratio.**

3. **Multiply the square of the ratio by the sample size of your pilot study.**

Say you want to estimate the slope to a precision (standard error) of ±5. If a pilot study of 20 subjects gives you a SE of ±8.4 units, then the ratio is 8.4/5 (or 1.68). Squaring this ratio gives you 2.82, which tells you that to get an SE of 5, you need 2.82 × 20, or about 56 subjects. And of course, because you've already acquired the first 20 subjects for your pilot run — you took my advice, right? — you need only another 36 subjects to have a total of 56.

This estimation is only approximate. But at least you have a ballpark idea of how big a sample you need to achieve the desired precision.

Chapter 19

More of a Good Thing: Multiple Regression

. . . .

In This Chapter

▶ Understanding what multiple regression is

▶ Preparing your data for a multiple regression and interpreting the output

▶ Understanding how synergy and collinearity affect regression analysis

▶ Estimating the number of subjects you need for a multiple regression analysis

. . . .

Chapter 17 introduces the general concepts of *correlation* and *regression,* two related techniques for detecting and characterizing the relationship between two or more variables. Chapter 18 describes the simplest kind of regression — fitting a straight line to a set of data consisting of one *independent variable* (the *predictor*) and one *dependent variable* (the *outcome*). The *model* (the formula relating the predictor to the outcome) is of the form $Y = a + bX$, where Y is the outcome, X is the predictor, and a and b are *parameters* (also called *regression coefficients*). This kind of regression is usually the only one you encounter in an introductory statistics course, but it's just the tip of the regression iceberg.

This chapter extends simple straight-line regression to more than one predictor — to what's called the *ordinary multiple linear regression* model (or *multiple regression,* to say it simply).

Understanding the Basics of Multiple Regression

In Chapter 18, I outline the derivation of the formulas for determining the parameters (slope and intercept) of a straight line so that the line comes *as close as possible* to all the data points. The term *as close as possible,* in the least-squares sense, means that the sum of the squares of vertical distances of each point from the fitted line is smaller for the least-squares line than for any other line you could possibly draw.

The same idea can be extended to multiple regression models containing more than one predictor (and more than two parameters). For two predictor variables, you're fitting a plane (a flat sheet) to a set of points in three dimensions; for more than two predictors, you're fitting a "hyperplane" to points in four-or-more-dimensional space. Hyperplanes in multidimensional space may sound mind-blowing, but the formulas are just simple algebraic extensions of the straight-line formulas.

The most compact way to describe these formulas is by using matrix notation, but because you'll never have to do the calculations yourself (thanks to the software packages that I describe in Chapter 4), I'll spare you the pain of looking at a bunch of matrix formulas. If you really want to see the formulas, you can find them in almost any statistics text or in the Wikipedia article on regression analysis: http://en.wikipedia.org/wiki/Regression_analysis.

In the following sections, I define some basic terms related to multiple regression and explain when you should use it.

Defining a few important terms

Multiple regression is formally known as the *ordinary multiple linear regression model*. What a mouthful! The terms mean:

- **Ordinary:** The outcome variable is a continuous numerical variable whose random fluctuations are normally distributed (see Chapter 25 for more about normal distributions).

- **Multiple:** The model has more than two predictor variables.

- **Linear:** Each predictor variable is multiplied by a parameter, and these products are added together to give the predicted value of the outcome variable. You can also have one more parameter thrown in that isn't multiplied by anything — it's called the *constant term* or the *Intercept*. The following are some linear functions:

  - $Y = a + bX$ (the simple straight-line model; X is the predictor variable, Y is the outcome, and a and b are parameters)

  - $Y = a + bX + cX^2 + dX^3$ (the variables can be squared or cubed, but as long as they're multiplied by a coefficient and added together, the function is still considered linear in the parameters)

  - $Y = a + bX + cZ + dXZ$ (the XZ term, often written as $X*Z$, is called an *interaction*)

In textbooks and published articles, you may see regression models written in various ways:

- A collection of predictor variables may be designated by a subscripted variable and the corresponding coefficients by another subscripted variable, like this: $Y = b_0 + b_1X_1 + b_2X_2$.

- In practical research work, the variables are often given meaningful names, like *Age, Gender, Height, Weight, SystolicBP*, and so on.

- Linear models may be represented in a shorthand notation that shows only the variables, and not the parameters, like this:

    $Y = X + Z + X * Z$ instead of $Y = a + bX + cZ + dX * Z$

    or $Y = 0 + X + Z + X * Z$ to specify that the model has no intercept.

    And sometimes you'll see a "~" instead of the "="; read the "~" as "is a function of," or "is predicted by."

Knowing when to use multiple regression

Chapter 17 lists a number of reasons for doing regression analysis — testing for significant association, getting a compact representation of the data, making predictions and prognoses, performing mathematical operations on the data (finding the minimum, maximum, slope, or area of a curve), preparing calibration curves, testing theoretical models, and obtaining values of parameters that have physical or biological meaning. All these reasons apply to multiple regression.

Being aware of how the calculations work

Basically, fitting a linear multiple regression model involves creating a set of simultaneous equations, one for each parameter in the model. The equations involve the parameters from the model and the sums of various products of the dependent and independent variables, just as the simultaneous equations for the straight-line regression in Chapter 18 involve the slope and intercept of the straight line and the sums of X, Y, X^2, and XY. You then solve these simultaneous equations to get the parameter values, just as you do for the straight line, except now you have more equations to solve. As part of this process you can also get the information you need to estimate the standard errors of the parameters, using a very clever application of the law of propagation of errors (which I describe in Chapter 11).

As the number of predictors increases, the computations get much more laborious, but the computer is doing all the work, so who cares? Personal computers can easily fit a model with 100 predictor variables to data from 10,000 subjects in less than a second!

Running Multiple Regression Software

With so many programs available that can do multiple regression, you'll never have to run this procedure by hand, but you may need to do a little prep work on your data first. In the following sections, I explain how to handle categorical variables (if you have them) and make a few charts before you run a multiple regression.

Preparing categorical variables

The predictors in a multiple regression model can be either numerical or categorical. (For more info, flip to Chapter 7, which deals with different kinds of data.) The different categories that a variable can have are called *levels*. If a variable, like *Gender,* can have only two levels, like *Male* or *Female,* then it's called a *dichotomous* or a *binary* categorical variable; if it can have more than two levels, I call it a *multilevel* variable.

Using categorical predictors in a multiple regression model is never a no-brainer. You have to set things up the right way or you'll get results that are either wrong or difficult to interpret properly. Here are two important things to be aware of.

Having enough cases in each level of each categorical variable

Before using a categorical variable in a multiple regression model, you (or, better yet, your computer) should tabulate how many cases are in each level. You should have at least two cases (and preferably more) in each level. Usually, the more evenly distributed the cases are spread across all the levels, the more precise and reliable the results will be. If a level doesn't contain enough cases, the program may ignore that level, halt with a warning message, produce incorrect results, or crash.

So if you tally a Race variable and get: White: 73, Black: 35, Asian: 1, and Other: 10, you may want to create another variable in which Asian is lumped together with Other (which would then have 11 subjects). Or you may want to create a binary variable with the levels: White: 73 and Non-White: 46 (or perhaps Black: 35 and Non-Black: 84, depending on the focus of your research).

Similarly, if your model has two categorical variables with an interaction term (like Gender + Race + Gender * Race), prepare a two-way cross-tabulation of Gender by Race first. You should have at least two subjects (and preferably many more) in each distinct combination of Gender and Race. (See Chapter 13 for details about cross-tabulations.)

Choosing the reference level wisely

For each categorical variable in a multiple regression model, the program considers one of the categories to be the *reference level,* and evaluates how each of the other levels affects the outcome, relative to that reference level. Some software lets you specify the reference level for a categorical variable; other software chooses it for you, sometimes in a way you may not like (like the level whose description comes first in the alphabet).

Choose your reference level wisely, or the results won't be very meaningful or useful.

- ✔ For a variable representing the presence or absence of some condition (like a risk factor), the reference level should represent the *absence* of the condition.

- ✔ For a variable representing treatment groups, the reference level should be the placebo, or the standard treatment, or whatever treatment you want to compare the other treatments to.

- ✔ For a variable representing a subject characteristic, like Gender or Race, the reference level is arbitrary. Sometimes the appropriate choice may be implicit in the objectives of the study (one group may be of special interest). If there's no compelling reason to select one level over the others, you can choose the level with the most cases (which in the preceding Race example would be White, with 73 subjects).

Recoding categorical variables as numerical

If your statistics software lets you enter categorical variables as character data (like Gender coded as Male or Female), then you don't have to read this section; you just have to make sure that, for each categorical variable, you have enough cases in each level, and that you've chosen the reference level wisely (and told the software what that level was). But if your regression program accepts only numerical variables as predictors, then you have to recode your categorical variables from descriptive text to numeric codes.

Binary categorical predictors can be recoded to numbers very simply; just recode the reference level to 0, and the other level to 1.

For categorical variables with more than two levels, it's more complicated. You can't just code the different categories as different numbers, like 0, 1, 2, 3, and so on, because then the computer will think that it's a numerical (quantitative) variable, and give completely wrong answers. Instead, you have to split up the one multilevel variable into a set of binary *dummy variables* — one for each level in the original variable. For example, a variable called Race, with the levels White, Black, Asian, and Other, would be split up into four dummy variables, which could be called WhiteRace, BlackRace, AsianRace, and OtherRace. Each dummy variable would be coded as 1 if the subject is of that race or as 0 if the subject isn't of that race, as shown in Table 19-1.

Table 19-1		Coding a Multilevel Category into a Set of Binary Dummy Variables			
Subject	*Race*	*WhiteRace*	*BlackRace*	*AsianRace*	*OtherRace*
1	White	1	0	0	0
2	Black	0	1	0	0
3	Asian	0	0	1	0
4	Other	0	0	0	1
5	Black	0	1	0	0

Then instead of including the variable Race in the model, you'd include the dummy variables for all levels of Race *except the reference level.* So if the reference level for Race was White, you'd include BlackRace, AsianRace, and OtherRace into the regression, but would *not* include WhiteRace.

Leave the reference-level dummy variable out of the regression.

Creating scatter plots before you jump into your multiple regression

One common mistake many researchers make is immediately running a regression (or some other statistical analysis) before taking a look at their data. As soon as you put your data into a computer file, you should run certain error-checks and generate summaries and histograms for each variable to assess the way the values of the variables are distributed, as I describe in Chapters 8 and 9. And if you plan to analyze your data by multiple regression, you also should do some other things first. Namely, you should chart the relationship between each predictor variable and the outcome variable, and also the relationships *between the predictor variables themselves.*

Table 19-2 shows a small data file that I use throughout the remainder of this chapter. It contains the age, weight, and systolic blood pressure of 16 subjects from a small clinical study. You might be interested in whether systolic blood pressure is associated with age or body weight (or both). Research questions involving the association between numerical variables are often handled by regression methods.

Table 19-2	Sample Age, Weight, and Blood Pressure Data for a Multiple Regression Analysis		
Subject Number	Age (years)	Weight (kg)	Systolic BP (mm Hg)
1	60	58	117
2	61	90	120
3	74	96	145
4	57	72	129
5	63	62	132
6	68	79	130
7	66	69	110
8	77	96	163
9	63	96	136
10	54	54	115
11	63	67	118
12	76	99	132
13	60	74	111
14	61	73	112
15	65	85	147
16	79	80	138

If you're planning to run a regression model like this: SystolicBP ~ Age + Weight (in the shorthand notation described in the earlier section "Defining a few important terms"), you should first prepare several scatter charts: one of SystolicBP (outcome) versus Age (predictor), one of SystolicBP versus Weight (predictor), and one of Age versus Weight. For regression models involving many predictors, that can be a lot of scatter charts, but fortunately many statistics programs can automatically prepare a set of small "thumbnail" scatter charts for all possible pairings between a set of variables, arranged in a matrix like Figure 19-1.

These charts can give you an idea of what variables are associated with what others, how strongly they're associated, and whether your data has outliers. The scatter charts in Figure 19-1 indicate that there are no extreme outliers in the data. Each scatter chart also shows some degree of positive correlation (as described in Chapter 17). In fact, referring to Figure 17-1, you may guess that the charts in Figure 19-1 correspond to correlation coefficients between 0.5 and 0.8. You can have your software calculate correlation coefficients (r values) between each pair of variables, and you'd get values of $r = 0.654$ for Age versus Weight, $r = 0.661$ for Age versus SystolicBP, and $r = 0.646$ for Weight versus SystolicBP.

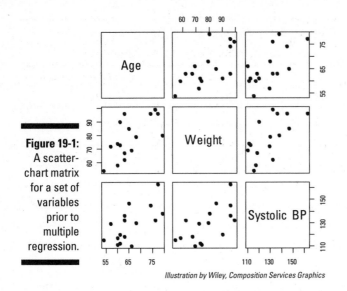

Figure 19-1:
A scatter-chart matrix for a set of variables prior to multiple regression.

Illustration by Wiley, Composition Services Graphics

Taking a few steps with your software

The exact steps you take to run a multiple regression depend on your software, but here's the general approach:

1. **Assemble your data into a file with one row per subject and one column for each variable you want in the model.**

2. **Tell the software which variable is the outcome and which are the predictors.**

3. **If the software lets you, specify certain optional output — graphs, summaries of the *residuals* (observed minus predicted outcome values), and other useful results.**

   Some programs, like SPSS (see Chapter 4), may offer to create new variables in the data file for the predicted outcome or the residuals.

4. **Press the Go button (or whatever it takes to start the calculations).**

   You should see your answers almost instantly.

Interpreting the Output of a Multiple Regression

The output from a multiple regression run is usually laid out much like the output from the simple straight-line regression run in Chapter 18.

Examining typical output from most programs

Figure 19-2 shows the output from a multiple regression run on the data in Table 19-2, using the R statistical software that I describe in Chapter 4. (Other software would produce generally similar output, but arranged and formatted differently.)

```
Call: lm(formula = SystolicBP ~ Age + Weight )

Residuals:
      Min       1Q   Median       3Q      Max
  -15.3596  -9.6585   0.0242   6.7305  17.8369

Coefficients:
                Estimate Std. Error t value Pr(>|t|)
(Intercept)     42.7498    25.7325    1.661    0.121
Age              0.8446     0.5163    1.636    0.126
Weight           0.3894     0.2659    1.464    0.167

Residual standard error: 11.23 on 13 degrees of freedom
Multiple R-squared: 0.5171,     Adjusted R-squared: 0.4428
F-statistic: 6.959 on 2 and 13 DF,  p-value: 0.008817
```

Figure 19-2: Output from a multiple regression on the data from Table 19-2.

Illustration by Wiley, Composition Services Graphics

The components of the output are

- A *description of the model* to be fitted: In Figure 19-2, this description is SystolicBP ~ Age + Weight.

- A *summary of the residuals* (observed minus predicted values of the outcome variable): For this example, the Max and Min Residuals indicate that one observed systolic BP value was 17.8 mmHg greater than predicted by the model, and one was 15.4 mmHg smaller than predicted.

- The *regression table,* or *coefficients table,* with a row for each parameter in the model, and columns for the following:

    - The estimated *value* of the parameter, which tells you how much the outcome variable changes when the corresponding variable increases by exactly 1.0 units, *holding all the other variables constant.* For example, the model predicts that every additional year of age increases systolic BP by 0.84 mmHg, *holding weight constant* (as in a group of people who all weigh the same).

- The *standard error* (precision) of that estimate. So the estimate of the Age coefficient (0.84 mmHg per year) is uncertain by about ± 0.52 mmHg per year.

- The *t value* (value of the parameter divided by its SE). For Age, the t value is 0.8446/0.5163, or 1.636.

- The *p value*, designated "Pr($>$|t|)" in this output, indicating whether the parameter is significantly different from zero. If $p < 0.05$, then the predictor variable is significantly associated with the outcome after compensating for the effects of all the other predictors in the model. In this example, neither the Age coefficient nor the Weight coefficient is significantly different from zero.

✔ Several numbers that describe the overall *ability of the model to fit the data:*

- The *residual standard error,* which, in this example, indicates that the observed-minus-predicted residuals have a standard deviation of 11.23 mmHg.

- The *multiple R-squared* is the square of an overall correlation coefficient for the multivariate fit.

- The *F statistic* and associated p value indicate whether the model predicts the outcome significantly better than a *null model,* which has only the intercept term and no predictor variables at all. The highly significant p value (0.0088) indicates that age and weight together predict SystolicBP better than the null model.

Checking out optional output available from some programs

Depending on your software, you may also be able to get several other useful results from the regression:

✔ **Predicted values** for the dependent variable (one value for each subject), either as a listing or as a new variable placed into your data file.

✔ **Residuals** (observed minus predicted value, for each subject), either as a listing or as a new variable placed into your data file.

✔ **The parameter error-correlations matrix,** which is important if two parameters from the same regression run will be used to calculate some other quantity (this comes up frequently in pharmacokinetic analysis). The Propagation of Errors web page (`http://StatPages.info/erpropgt.html`) asks for an error-correlation coefficient when calculating how measurement errors propagate through an expression involving two variables.

Deciding whether your data is suitable for regression analysis

Before drawing conclusions from any statistical analysis, make sure that your data fulfilled assumptions on which that analysis was based. Two assumptions of ordinary linear regression include the following:

✔ The amount of variability in the residuals is fairly constant and not dependent on the value of the dependent variable.

✔ The residuals are approximately normally distributed.

Figure 19-3 shows two kinds of optional diagnostic graphs that help you determine whether these assumptions were met.

✔ Figure 19-3a provides a visual indication of variability of the residuals. The important thing is whether the points seem to scatter evenly above and below the line, and whether the amount of scatter seems to be the same at the left, middle, and right parts of the graph. That seems to be the case in this figure.

✔ Figure 19-3b provides a visual indication of the normality of the residuals. The important thing is whether the points appear to lie along the dotted line or are noticeably "curved." In this figure, most of the points are reasonably consistent with a straight line, except perhaps in the lower-left part of the graph.

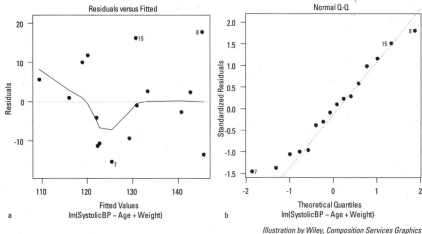

Figure 19-3: Diagnostic graphs from a regression.

a

b

Illustration by Wiley, Composition Services Graphics

Determining how well the model fits the data

Several numbers in the standard regression output relate to how closely the model fits your data:

- ✔ The residual standard error is the average scatter of the observed points from the fitted model (about ± 11 mm Hg in the example from Figure 19-2); the smaller that number is, the better.

- ✔ The larger the multiple R^2 value is, the better the fit (it's 0.44 in this example, indicating a moderately good fit).

- ✔ A significant F statistic indicates that the model predicts the outcome significantly better than the null model (p = 0.009 in this example).

Figure 19-4 shows another way to judge how well the model predicts the outcome. It's a graph of observed and predicted values of the outcome variable, with a superimposed *identity line* (Observed = Predicted). Your program may offer this "Observed versus Predicted" graph, or you can generate it from the observed and predicted values of the dependent variable. For a perfect prediction model, the points would lie exactly on the identity line. The correlation coefficient of these points is the multiple R value for the regression.

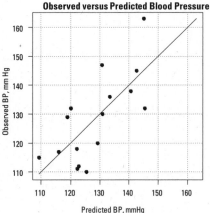

Figure 19-4:
Observed versus predicted outcomes for the model SystolicBP ~ Age + Weight, for the data in Table 19-2.

Observed versus Predicted Blood Pressure

Illustration by Wiley, Composition Services Graphics

Watching Out for Special Situations that Arise in Multiple Regression

Here I describe two topics that come up in multiple regression: interactions (both synergistic and anti-synergistic) and collinearity. Both relate to how the simultaneous behavior of two predictors can influence an outcome.

Synergy and anti-synergy

It sometimes happens that two predictor variables exert a *synergistic effect* on an outcome. That is, if both predictors were to increase by one unit, the outcome would change by more than simply the sum of the two increases you'd expect from changing each value individually by one unit. You can test for synergy between two predictors on an outcome by fitting a model that contains an *interaction term* (the product of those two variables):

SystolicBP = Age + Weight + Age * Weight

In some software, if you include the Age*Weight term, you don't have to include the separate Age and Weight terms; the program will do that for you.

If the interaction coefficient has a significant p value ($p < 0.05$), then the two variables have significant synergy between them. The sign of the coefficient indicates whether the synergy is positive or negative *(anti-synergy)*.

Collinearity and the mystery of the disappearing significance

After you get into multiple regression analysis, it won't be long before you encounter the puzzling/disturbing/exasperating phenomenon of "disappearing significance." It happens this way: First you run a bunch of simple straight-line regressions on each predictor separately versus the outcome, as a first look at your data. You may find that several predictors are each significantly associated with the outcome. Then you run a multiple regression, using all the predictors, only to find (to your shock and dismay) that one or more (maybe even all) of the formerly significant variables have lost their significance!

Model building

One of the reasons (but not the only reason) for running a multiple regression analysis is to come up with a prediction formula for some outcome variable, based on a set of available predictor variables. Ideally, you want this formula to be *parsimonious* — to have as few variables as possible but still make good predictions. So how do you select, from among a big bunch of predictor variables, the smallest subset needed to make a good prediction model? This is called the "model building" problem, which is a topic of active research by theoretical statisticians. See www.dummies.com/extras/bio statistics for an article that discusses model building.

In the example from Table 19-2, there's a significant association between Age and SystolicBP (p = 0.005), and between Weight and Systolic BP (p = 0.007). (You can run straight-line regressions, with the help of Chapter 18, on the data in that table if you don't believe me.) But the multiple regression output in Figure 19-2 shows that neither Age nor Weight has regression coefficients that are significantly different from zero! What happened?

You've just been visited by the *collinearity* fairy. In the regression world, the term *collinearity* (also called *multicollinearity*) refers to a strong correlation between two or more of the predictor variables. And, sure enough, if you run a straight-line regression on Age versus Weight, you'll find that they're significantly correlated with each other (p = 0.006).

The good news is that collinearity doesn't make the model any worse at predicting outcomes. The bad news is that collinearity between two variables can make it hard to tell which variable was *really* influencing the outcome and which one was getting a free ride (was associated with the outcome only because it was associated with another variable that was really influencing the outcome). This problem isn't trivial — it can be difficult, if not impossible, to discern the true cause-and-effect relationships (if there are any) among a set of associated variables. The nearby sidebar "Model building" describes a technique that may be helpful.

There's a good discussion of multicollinearity (what it is, what its consequences are, how to detect it, and what to do about it) in the Wikipedia article at http://en.wikipedia.org/wiki/Multicollinearity.

ny Subjects You Need

ould have a large enough sample to ensure that you
he test of your primary research hypothesis when
that hypothesis is large enough to be of clinical
hypothesis of your study is going to be tested by a
hould do some kind of power calculation, specifically
essions, to determine the sample size you need.

bly won't be able to do that. Programs are available
requirements for multiple regression (both PS and
pter 4, can handle some simple multivariate models),
ou for input that you almost certainly can't provide.

gh textbooks, you'll find many rules of thumb for
ding the following:

- ✔ You need 4 subjects for every predictor variable in your model.

- ✔ You need 10 subjects for every predictor variable in your model.

- ✔ You need 100 subjects, plus one more for every predictor variable.

- ✔ 100 is adequate; 200 is good; 400 or more is great.

These rules don't even remotely agree with each other, and they have no
real theoretical justification, so they're probably no better than the obvious
advice that "more subjects give more statistical power."

For practical purposes, you can probably make do with a simple, sample-size
estimate based on what you consider to be a clinically meaningful correlation
coefficient between the most important predictor and the outcome. The simple
formula from Chapter 26 — $N = 8/r^2$, where N is the number of observations
(subjects you need) and r is the clinically meaningful correlation coefficient —
is probably as good as anything else.

Chapter 20

A Yes-or-No Proposition: Logistic Regression

. . . .

In This Chapter

▶ Figuring out when to use logistic regression

▶ Getting a grip on the basics of logistic regression

▶ Running a logistic regression and making sense of the output

▶ Watching for things that can go wrong

▶ Estimating the sample size you need

. . . .

*Y*ou can use *logistic regression* to analyze the relationship between one or more predictor variables (the *X* variables) and a categorical outcome variable (the *Y* variable). Typical categorical outcomes include the following:

✔ Lived or died

✔ Did or didn't rain today

✔ Did or didn't have a stroke

✔ Responded or didn't respond to a treatment

✔ Did or did not vote for Joe Smith (in an exit poll)

In this chapter, I explain logistic regression — when to use it, the important concepts, how to run it with software, and how to interpret the output. I also point out the pitfalls and show you how to determine the sample sizes you need.

Using Logistic Regression

You can use logistic regression to do any (or all) of the following:

✔ Test whether the predictor and the outcome are significantly associated; for example, whether age or gender influenced a voter's preference for a particular candidate.

✔ Overcome the limitations of the 2-x-2 cross-tab method (described in Chapter 14), which can analyze only one predictor at a time that has to be a two-valued category, such as the presence or absence of a risk factor. With logistic regression, you can analyze any number of predictor variables, each of which can be a numeric variable or a categorical variable having two or more categories.

✔ Quantify the *extent* of an association between the predictor and the outcome (the amount by which a predictor influences the chance of getting the outcome); for example, how much a smoker's chance of developing emphysema changes with each additional cigarette smoked per day.

✔ Develop a formula to predict the probability of getting the outcome from the values of the predictor variables. For example, you may want to predict the probability that a patient will benefit from a certain kind of therapy, based on the patient's age, gender, severity of illness, and perhaps even genetic makeup.

✔ Make *yes* or *no* predictions about the outcome that take into account the consequences of false-positive and false-negative predictions. For example, you can generate a tentative cancer diagnosis from a set of observations and lab results, using a formula that balances the different consequences of a false-positive versus a false-negative diagnosis.

✔ See how one predictor influences the outcome after adjusting for the influence of other variables; for example, how the number of minutes of exercise per day influences the chance of having a heart attack, adjusting for the effects of age, gender, lipid levels, and other patient characteristics.

✔ Determine the value of a predictor that produces a certain probability of getting the outcome; for example, find the dose of a drug that produces a favorable clinical response in 80 percent of the patients treated with it (called the ED_{80}, or *80 percent effective dose*).

Understanding the Basics of Logistic Regression

In this section, I explain the concepts underlying logistic regression using a simple example involving data on mortality due to radiation exposure. This example illustrates why straight-line regression wouldn't work and what you have to use instead.

Gathering and graphing your data

As in the other chapters in Part IV, here you see a simple real-world problem and its data, which I use throughout this chapter to illustrate what I'm talking about. This example examines exposure to gamma-ray radiation, which is deadly in large-enough doses, looking only at the short-term lethality of acute large doses, not long-term health effects such as cancer or genetic damage.

In Table 20-1, "dose" is the radiation exposure expressed in units called *Roentgen Equivalent Man (REM)*. Looking at the "Dose" and "Outcome" columns, you can get a rough sense of how survival depends on dose. For low doses almost everyone lives, and for high doses almost everyone dies.

Table 20-1   Radiation Dose and Survival Data for 30 Subjects (Sorted by Dose Level)

Dose in REMs	Outcome (0 = Lived; 1 = Died)	Dose in REMS	Outcome (0 = Lived; 1 = Died)
0	0	433	0
10	0	457	1
31	0	559	1
82	0	560	1
92	0	604	1
107	0	632	0
142	0	686	1
173	0	691	1
175	0	702	1
232	0	705	1
266	0	774	1
299	0	853	1
303	1	879	1
326	0	915	1
404	1	977	1

How can you analyze this data? First, graph the data: Plot the dose received on the X axis (because it's the predictor). Plot the outcome (0 if the person lived; 1 if he died) on the Y axis. This plotting gives you the graph in Figure 20-1a. Because the outcome variable is *binary* (having only the values 0 or 1), the points are restricted to two horizontal lines, making the graph difficult to interpret. You can get a better picture of the dose-lethality relationship by grouping the doses into intervals (say, every 200 REM) and plotting the fraction of people in each interval who died, as shown in Figure 20-1b. Clearly, the chance of dying increases with increasing dose.

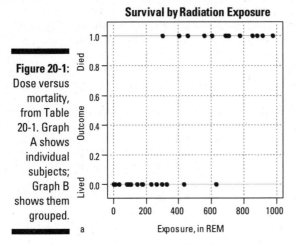

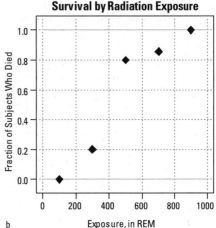

Figure 20-1: Dose versus mortality, from Table 20-1. Graph A shows individual subjects; Graph B shows them grouped.

Illustration by Wiley, Composition Services Graphics

Fitting a function with an S shape to your data

Don't try to fit a straight line to binary-outcome data. The true dose-lethality curve is almost certainly not a straight line. For one thing, the fraction of subjects dying can never be smaller than 0 nor larger than 1, but a straight line (or a parabola or any polynomial) very happily violates those limits for very low and very high doses. That can't be right!

Instead, you need to fit a function that has an S shape — a formula giving Y as some expression involving X that, by its very nature, can never produce a Y value outside of the range from 0 to 1, no matter how large or small X may become.

Of the many mathematical expressions that produce S-shaped graphs, the *logistic* function is ideally suited to this kind of data. In its simplest form, the logistic function is written like this: $Y = 1/(1 + e^{-X})$, where e is the mathematical constant 2.718 (which is what e represents throughout the rest of this chapter). Figure 20-2 shows the shape of the logistic function.

This function can be *generalized* (made more versatile for representing observed data) by adding two adjustable parameters (a and b) like this: $Y = 1/(1 + e^{-(a + bX)})$.

Notice that the $a+bX$ part looks just like the formula for a straight line (see Chapter 18); the rest of the logistic function is what bends that straight line into its characteristic S shape. The middle of the S (where $Y = 0.5$) always occurs when $X = -b/a$. The steepness of the curve in the middle region is determined by b, as follows:

✔ **If *b* is positive,** the logistic function is an upward-sloping S-shaped curve, like the one shown in Figure 20-2.

✔ **If *b* is 0,** the logistic function is a horizontal straight line whose *Y* value is equal to $1/(1 + e^a)$, as shown in Figure 20-3.

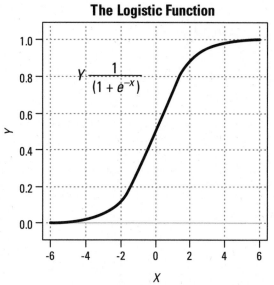

Figure 20-2: The logistic function looks like this.

Illustration by Wiley, Composition Services Graphics

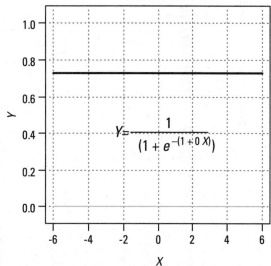

Figure 20-3: When *b* is 0, the logistic function becomes a horizontal straight line.

Illustration by Wiley, Composition Services Graphics

✔ **If _b_ is negative,** the curve is flipped upside down, as shown in Figure 20-4. Logistic curves don't have to slope upward.

✔ **If _b_ is a very large number (positive or negative),** the logistic curve is so steep that it looks like what mathematicians call a _step function,_ as shown in Figure 20-5.

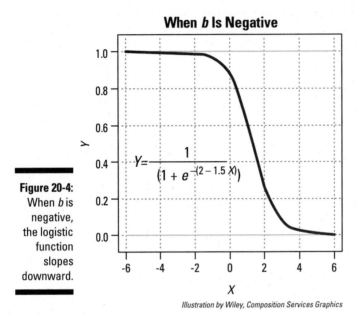

When _b_ Is Negative

$$Y = \frac{1}{(1 + e^{-(2 - 1.5\,X)})}$$

Figure 20-4:
When _b_ is negative, the logistic function slopes downward.

Illustration by Wiley, Composition Services Graphics

When _b_ Gets Very Large

$$Y = \frac{1}{(1 + e^{-(-20 + 10\,X)})}$$

Figure 20-5:
When _b_ is very large, the logistic function becomes a "step function."

Illustration by Wiley, Composition Services Graphics

Because the logistic curve approaches the limits 0.0 and 1.0 for extreme values of the predictor(s), you should not use logistic regression in situations where the fraction of subjects having the outcome does not approach these two limits. Logistic regression is fine for the radiation example because no one dies from a radiation exposure of zero REMs, and everyone dies from an extremely large dose (like 10,000 REMs). But logistic regression wouldn't be appropriate for analyzing the response of patients to a drug if very high doses of the drug don't produce a 100% cure (or if some subjects spontaneously get better even if given no drug at all).

Logistic regression fits the logistic model to your data by finding the values of *a* and *b* that make the logistic curve come as close as possible to all your plotted points. With this fitted model, you can then predict the probability of the outcome event (in this example, dying). See the later section "Predicting probabilities with the fitted logistic formula" for more details.

Getting into the nitty-gritty of logistic regression

You don't need to know all the theoretical and computation details for logistic regression, because computers do all that work. You should have a general idea of what's involved, though. The calculations are much more complicated than those for ordinary straight-line or multivariate least-squares regression. In fact, it's impossible to write down a set of formulas that give the logistic regression coefficients in terms of the observed *X* and *Y* values; you have to obtain them by a complicated iterative procedure that no sane human being would ever try to do by hand.

Logistic regression determines the values of the regression coefficients that are most consistent with the observed data, using what's called the *maximum likelihood* criterion. The likelihood of any statistical model is the probability, based on the model, of getting what you actually observed. There's a likelihood value for each case in the data set, and a total likelihood (*L*) for the entire data set. The likelihood value for each data point is just the predicted probability of getting the observed result. For subjects who died (refer to Table 20-1), the likelihood is the probability of dying (*Y*) predicted by the logistic formula. For subjects who lived, the likelihood

is the predicted probability of living, which is (1 − *Y*). The total likelihood (*L*) for the whole set of subjects is the product of all the calculated likelihoods for each subject.

To find the values of the coefficients that maximize *L*, it is sufficient (and computationally easier) to find the values that minimize the quantity −2 times the natural logarithm of *L*, which is sometimes designated as *−2LL*. Statisticians call *−2LL* the *deviance* — the closer the curve comes to the observed points, the smaller this deviance number will be. The actual numeric value of a deviance number for a logistic regression doesn't mean much by itself, but the difference in deviance between two different models is very important.

The final step is to find the values of the coefficients that will minimize the deviance of the observed *Y* values from the fitted logistic curve. This may sound like a hopelessly difficult task, but computer scientists have developed elegant and efficient ways to minimize a complicated function of several variables, and a logistic regression program uses one of these methods to get the coefficients.

Handling multiple predictors in your logistic model

The data in Table 20-1 has only one predictor variable, but you may have several predictors of a *yes* or *no* outcome. For example, a person's chance of dying from radiation exposure may depend not only on the radiation dose received, but also on age, gender, weight, general health, radiation wavelength, and the amount of time over which the radiation is received. In Chapter 19, I describe how the simple straight-line regression model can be generalized to handle multiple predictors. You can generalize the simple logistic formula to handle multiple predictors in the same way.

Suppose the outcome variable Y is dependent on three predictors, called X, V, and W. Then the multivariate logistic model looks like this:

$$Y = 1/(1 + e^{-(a + bX + cV + dW)}).$$

Logistic regression finds the best values of the parameters a, b, c, and d so that for any particular set of values for X, V, and W, you can predict Y — the probability of getting a *yes* outcome.

Running a Logistic Regression with Software

The logistic regression theory is difficult, and the calculations are complicated (see the earlier sidebar "Getting into the nitty-gritty of logistic regression" for details). However, the great news is that most general statistics programs (like those in Chapter 4) can run logistic regression, and it isn't any more difficult than running a simple straight-line or multiple linear regression (see Chapters 18 and 19). Here's all you have to do:

1. **Make sure your data set has a column for the outcome variable and that this column has only two different values.**

   You can code it as 1 or 0, according to whether the outcome is *yes* or *no,* or your software may let you record the data as *yes* or *no* (or as *Lived* or *Died,* or any other dichotomous classification), with the program doing the 0 or 1 recoding behind the scenes. (Check out Table 20-1 for an example.)

2. **Make sure your data set has a column for each predictor variable and that these columns are in a format that your software accepts.**

The predictors can be quantitative (such as age or weight; Table 20-1 uses dose amount) or categorical (like gender or treatment group), just as with ordinary least-squares regression. See Chapter 19, where I describe how to set up categorical predictor variables.

3. **Tell your program which variables are the predictors and which variable is the outcome.**

   Depending on the software, you may do this by typing the variable names or by selecting the variables from a menu or list.

4. **Tell your program that you want as many of the following outputs as it can give you:**

   - A summary of information about the variables

   - Measures of goodness-of-fit

   - A table of regression coefficients, including odds ratios and their confidence intervals

   - Predicted probabilities of getting the outcome (which, ideally, the program puts into a new column that it creates in the database)

   - If there's only one predictor, a graph of predicted probabilities versus the value of the predictor (this will be a graph of the fitted logistic curve)

   - A classification table of observed outcomes versus predicted outcomes

   - Measures of prediction accuracy (overall accuracy, sensitivity, and specificity)

   - An ROC curve

5. **Press the Go button and stand back!**

   The computer does all the work and presents you with the answers.

Interpreting the Output of Logistic Regression

Figure 20-6 shows the kind of printed output that a typical logistic regression program may produce from the data in Table 20-1. The following sections explain the output's different sections.

Seeing summary information about the variables

The program may provide some summary descriptive information about the variables: means and standard deviations of predictors that are numerical variables, and a count of how many subjects did or did not have the outcome event. In the "Descriptives" section of Figure 20-6, you see that 15 of the 30 subjects lived and 15 died. Some programs may also provide the mean and standard deviation of each numerical predictor variable.

Outcome: Died; Predictors: Dose	Dose	Died	Pr Death	Predict
	0	0	0.0079	0
Descriptives:	10	0	0.0089	0
15 cases Died=0; 15 cases Died=1.	31	0	0.0113	0
	82	0	0.0201	0
Deviance (= -2 Log Likelihood) :	92	0	0.0225	0
Null Model: 41.589	107	0	0.0266	0
Final Model: 15.747	142	0	0.0391	0
Chi Square= 25.842; df=1; p<0.0001	173	0	0.0549	0
	175	0	0.0561	0
Hosmer-Lemeshow Goodness of Fit Test:	232	0	1.1025	0
Chi Square= 4.161; df=8; p<0.842	266	0	0.1443	0
	299	0	0.1976	0
Cox/Snell R-square= 0.577	303	1	0.2049	0
Nagelkerke R-square= 0.770	326	0	0.2512	0
AIC= 19.747	404	1	0.4505	0
	433	0	0.5334	1
Coefficients and Standard Errors...	457	1	0.6008	1
Variable Coeff. StdErr p-value	559	1	0.8289	1
Intercept -4.8276 1.7521 0.0038	560	1	0.8305	1
Dose 0.0115 0.0040 0.0038	604	1	0.8902	1
	632	0	0.9179	1
Odds Ratios and 95% Confidence Intervals:	686	1	0.9540	1
Variable O.R. Low High	691	1	0.9565	1
Dose 1.0115 1.0037 1.0194	702	1	0.9614	1
	705	1	0.9627	1
Fitted Logistic Formula:	774	1	0.9827	1
Prob (Death) =	853	1	0.9929	1
1 / (1 + Exp (- (-4.828 + 0.01146 * Dose)))	879	1	0.9947	1
	915	1	0.9965	1
	977	1	0.9983	1

Figure 20-6: Typical output from a logistic regression.

Illustration by Wiley, Composition Services Graphics

Assessing the adequacy of the model

The program indicates how well the fitted function represents the data *(goodness-of-fit),* and it may provide several such measures, most of which have an associated p value. (A *p value* is the probability that random fluctuations alone, in the absence of any real effect in the population, could've produced an observed effect at least as large as what you observed in your sample; see Chapter 3 for a refresher.) It's easy to misinterpret these because they measure subtly different types of goodness-of-fit.

You may see the following, depending on your software:

- **A p value associated with the drop-in deviance ($-2LL$) between the null model (intercept-only) and the final model (with the predictor variables):** (See the earlier sidebar "Getting into the nitty-gritty of logistic regression" for the definition of $-2LL$.) If this p value is less than 0.05, it indicates that adding the predictor variables to the null model significantly improves its ability to predict the outcome. In Figure 20-6, the p value for the reduction in deviance is less than 0.0001, which means that adding radiation dose to the model makes it significantly better at predicting an individual person's chance of dying than the null model (which, in essence, always predicts a death probability equal to the observed fraction of subjects who died).

- **A p value from the Hosmer-Lemeshow (H-L) test:** If this p value is less than 0.05, your data isn't consistent with the logistic function's S shape. Perhaps it doesn't approach a 100 percent response rate for large doses. (Most treatments aren't 100 percent effective, even at large doses.) Perhaps the response rises with increasing dose up to some optimal dose and then declines with further dose increases. In Figure 20-6, the H-L p value is 0.842, which means that the data is consistent with the shape of a logistic curve.

- **One or more pseudo–R-square values:** *Pseudo–R-square values* indicate how much of the total variability in the outcomes is explainable by the fitted model, analogous to how R-square is interpreted in ordinary least-squares regression, as described in Chapter 19. In Figure 20-6, two such values are provided: the Cox/Snell and Nagelkerke R-square. These values (0.577 and 0.770, respectively) indicate that a majority of the variability in the outcomes is explainable by the logistic model.

- **Akaike's Information Criterion (AIC):** AIC is related to the final model deviance, adjusted for how many predictor variables are in the model. Like deviance, AIC is a "smaller is better" number. It's very useful for choosing between different models (for example, deciding which predictors to include in a model). For an excellent description of the AIC, and its use in choosing between competing models, go to `www.graphpad. com/guides/prism/6/curve-fitting`, click on "Comparing fits of nonlinear models" in the lefthand menu, and then choose "How the AIC computations work."

Checking out the table of regression coefficients

The most important output from a logistic regression program is the table of regression coefficients, which looks much like the coefficients table from ordinary straight-line or multivariate least-squares regression (see Chapters 18 and 19).

✔ Every predictor variable appears on a separate row.

✔ There's one row for the constant (or intercept) term.

✔ The first column is almost always the fitted value of the regression coefficient.

✔ The second column is usually the standard error (SE) of the coefficient.

✔ A p value column (perhaps called *Sig* or *Signif* or *Pr(>|z|)*) indicates whether the coefficient is significantly different from 0.

For each predictor variable, the logistic regression should also provide the odds ratio and its 95 percent confidence interval, either as additional columns in the coefficients table or as a separate table. You can see these items in Figure 20-6.

But don't worry if the program doesn't provide them: You can calculate them simply by exponentiating the corresponding coefficients and their confidence limits. The confidence limits for the coefficients are easily calculated by adding or subtracting 1.96 times the standard error from the coefficient. The formulas follow:

Odds ratio = $e^{Coefficient}$

Lower 95 percent confidence limit = $e^{Coefficient - 1.96 \times SE}$

Upper 95 percent confidence limit = $e^{Coefficient + 1.96 \times SE}$

Predicting probabilities with the fitted logistic formula

The program may show you the fitted logistic formula. In Figure 20-6, the formula is shown as:

Prob(Death) = 1/(1 + Exp(−(−4.828 + 0.01146 * Dose)))

If the software doesn't provide the formula, just substitute the regression coefficients from the regression table into the logistic formula.

The final model produced by the logistic regression program from the data in Table 20-1 and the resulting logistic curve are shown in Figure 20-7.

With the fitted logistic formula, you can predict the probability of having the outcome if you know the value of the predictor variable. For example, if a subject receives 500 REM of radiation, the probability of death is given by this formula: Probability of Death = $1/(1 + e^{-(-4.828 + 0.01146 \times 500)})$, which equals 0.71. A person who receives 500 REM of radiation has about a 71 percent chance of dying shortly thereafter.

You can also calculate some special points on a logistic curve, as you find out in the following sections.

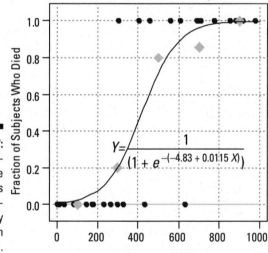

Survival by Radiation Exposure

$$Y = \frac{1}{(1 + e^{-(-4.83 + 0.0115\,X)})}$$

Exposure, in REM

Illustration by Wiley, Composition Services Graphics

Figure 20-7: The logistic curve that fits the dose-mortality data from Table 20-1.

Be careful with your algebra when evaluating these formulas! The *a* coefficient in a logistic regression is often a negative number, and subtracting a negative number is like adding its absolute value.

Calculating effective doses on a logistic curve

When logistic regression is applied to dose-response data, the dose (X) that produces a 50 percent response $(Y = 0.5)$ is called the *median effective dose* (ED_{50}). Similarly, the X value that makes $Y = 0.8$ is called the *80 percent effective dose* (ED_{80}), and so on. It's pretty easy to calculate these special dose levels from the a and b parameters of the fitted logistic model in the preceding section.

If you remember high-school algebra, you can solve the logistic formula $Y = 1/(1 + e^{-(a + bX)})$ for X as a function of Y; if you don't remember, here's the answer:

$$X = \frac{\log\left(\frac{Y}{1-Y}\right) - a}{b}$$

where *log* stands for natural logarithm. Substituting 0.5 for Y in the preceding equation gives the ED_{50} as simply $-a/b$. Similarly, substituting 0.8 for Y gives the ED_{80} as $\frac{1.39 - a}{b}$.

So if, for example, a drug produces a therapeutic response that's represented by a logistic model with $a = -3.45$ and $b = 0.0204$ dL/mg, the 80 percent effective dose (ED_{80}) would be equal to $(1.39 - (-3.45))/0.0234$, which works out to about 207 mg/dL.

Calculating lethal doses on a logistic curve

When death is the outcome event, the corresponding terms are *median lethal dose* (LD_{50}), *80 percent lethal dose* (LD_{80}), and so on. So, for the data in Table 20-1, $a = -4.83$ and $b = 0.0115$, so $-a/b = -(-4.83)/0.0115$, which works out to 420 REMs. Someone who receives a 420 REMs dose of radiation has a 50-50 chance of dying shortly thereafter.

Making yes or no predictions

A logistic model, properly fitted to a set of data, lets you calculate the predicted probability of having the outcome. But sometimes you'd rather make a *yes* or *no* prediction instead of quoting a probability. You can do this by comparing the calculated probability of getting a *yes* outcome to some arbitrary cut value (such as 0.5) that separates a *yes* prediction from a *no* prediction. That is, you can say, "If the predicted probability for a subject is greater than 0.5, I'll predict *yes;* otherwise, I'll predict *no.*"

In the following sections, I talk about *yes* or *no* predictions — what they can tell you about the predicting ability of the logistic model and how you can select the cut value that gives you the best tradeoff between wrongly predicting *yes* and wrongly predicting *no*.

Measuring accuracy, sensitivity, and specificity with classification tables

The logistic regression program provides several goodness-of-fit outputs (described earlier in this chapter), but these outputs may not be very easy to interpret. One other indicator, which is very intuitive, is the extent to which your *yes* or *no* predictions match the actual outcomes. You can cross-tabulate the predicted and observed outcomes into a fourfold classification table. Most statistical software can do all of this for you; it's often as simple as selecting a check box to indicate that you want the program to generate a classification table based on some particular cut value. Most software assumes a cut value of 0.5 unless you tell it to use some other value. Figure 20-8 shows the classification table for the radiation example, using 0.5 as the cut value.

Figure 20-8: A classification table of observed versus predicted outcomes from radiation exposure, using a cut value of 0.5 predicted probability.

		Observed Outcome		
		Died	**Lived**	**Total**
Predicted Outcome from Logistic Model	**Died**	13	2	15
	Lived	2	13	15
	Total	15	15	30

Illustration by Wiley, Composition Services Graphics

From the classification table, you can calculate several useful measures of the model's predicting ability for any specified cut value. (I define and describe these measures in more detail in Chapter 14.)

✔ **Overall accuracy:** Predicting correctly. The upper-left and lower-right cells correspond to correct predictions. Of the 30 subjects in the data set from Table 20-1, the logistic model predicted correctly (13 + 13)/30, or about 87 percent of the time; the model would make a wrong prediction only about 13 percent of the time.

✓ **Sensitivity:** Predicting a *yes* outcome when the actual outcome is *yes*. The logistic model predicted 13 of the 15 observed deaths (the upper-left box of Figure 20-8), so the sensitivity is 13/15, or about 87 percent; the model would make a false-negative prediction only about 13 percent of the time.

✓ **Specificity:** Predicting a *no* outcome when the actual outcome is *no*. The logistic model predicted survival in 13 of the 15 observed survivors (the lower-right box of Figure 20-8), so the specificity is 13/15, or about 87 percent; the model would make a false-positive prediction only about 13 percent of the time.

Sensitivity and specificity are especially relevant to screening tests for diseases. An ideal test would have 100 percent sensitivity and 100 percent specificity (and, therefore, 100 percent overall accuracy). But no test meets this ideal in the real world.

By judiciously choosing the cut-point for converting a probability into a *yes* or *no* decision, you can often achieve high sensitivity or high specificity, but not both simultaneously. Depending on the test and on what happens if it produces a false-positive or false-negative result, you have to consider whether high sensitivity or high specificity is more important.

For example, consider screening tests for two different diseases: colon cancer and prostate cancer.

✓ A false-positive result from a colon cancer screening test may induce a lot of anxiety for a while, until a follow-up colonoscopy reveals that no cancer is present. But a false-negative result can give an unwarranted sense of security that may cause other symptoms to go ignored until the cancer has progressed to an incurable stage.

✓ A false-positive result from a prostate cancer screening test may result in an unnecessary prostatectomy, an operation with many serious side effects. A false-negative result can cause prostate cancer to go untreated, but in most instances (especially in older men), prostate cancer is slow growing and usually not the ultimate cause of death. (It has been said that many men die *with* prostate cancer, but relatively few die *from* it.)

Some people may say that high sensitivity is more important than high specificity for a colon cancer test, while the reverse is true for a prostate cancer test. But other people may disagree. And nobody is likely to agree on just how to best balance the conflicting goals. This isn't an abstract or hypothetical issue — the appropriate diagnosis and treatment of prostate cancer is currently the subject of very vigorous debate centering around these very issues.

A logistic model fitted to a set of data can yield any sensitivity (between 0 and 100 percent) and any specificity (between 0 and 100 percent), depending on what cut value you select. The trick is to pick a cut value that gives the optimal combination of sensitivity and specificity, striking the best balance between false-positive and false-negative predictions, in light of the different consequences of the two types of false predictions. To find this optimal cut value, you need to know precisely how sensitivity and specificity play against each other — that is, how they simultaneously vary with different cut values. And there's a neat way to do exactly that, which I explain in the following section.

Rocking with ROC curves

A special kind of graph displays the sensitivity/specificity tradeoff for any fitted logistic model. It has the rather peculiar name *Receiver Operator Characteristics* (ROC) graph, which comes from its original use during World War II to analyze the performance characteristics of people who operated RADAR receivers. Nowadays it's used for all kinds of things that have nothing to do with RADAR, but the original name has stuck.

An ROC graph has a curve that shows you the complete range of sensitivity and specificity that can be achieved for any fitted logistic model, based on the selected cut value. The program generates an ROC curve by effectively trying all possible cut values between 0 and 1, calculating the predicted outcomes, cross-tabbing them against the observed outcomes, calculating sensitivity and specificity, and then graphing sensitivity versus specificity.

The ROC curve always runs from the lower-left corner of the graph (0 percent sensitivity and 100 percent specificity) to the upper-right corner (100 percent sensitivity and 0 percent specificity). Most programs also draw a diagonal straight line between the lower-left and upper-right corners (representing the formula: sensitivity = 1 – specificity) to indicate the total absence of any predicting ability at all.

Figure 20-9 shows the ROC curve for the data in Table 20-1, produced by the R statistical system. A conventional ROC graph has sensitivity (displayed either as fractions between 0 and 1 or as percentages between 0 and 100) running up the *Y* axis, and 1 – specificity running across the *X* axis. Alternatively, the specificity can run backwards (from right to left) across the *X* axis, as shown in Figure 20-9.

ROC curves almost always lie in the upper-left part of the graph area, and the farther away from the diagonal line they are, the better the predictive model is. For a nearly perfect model, the ROC curve runs up along the *Y* axis from the lower-left corner to the upper-left corner, then along the top of the graph from the upper-left corner to the upper-right corner.

Because of how sensitivity and specificity are calculated, the graph appears as a series of steps, with more data producing more and smaller steps. For clarity, I show the cut values for predicted probability as a scale along the ROC curve itself; sadly, most statistical software doesn't do this for you.

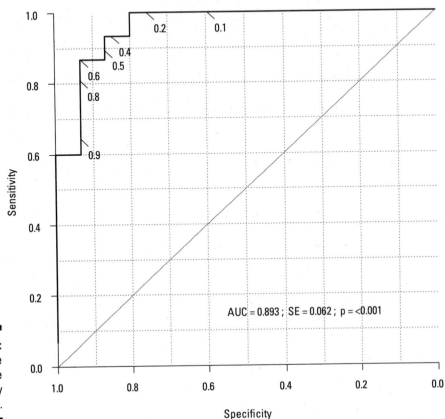

ROC Curve

AUC = 0.893 ; SE = 0.062 ; p = <0.001

Figure 20-9:
ROC curve
from dose
mortality
data.

Illustration by Wiley, Composition Services Graphics

The ROC curve helps you choose a cut value that gives the best tradeoff
between sensitivity and specificity:

✔ **To have very few false positives:** Choose a higher cut value to give a
high specificity. Figure 20-9 shows that by setting the cut value to 0.6,
you can simultaneously achieve about 93 percent specificity and 87 percent sensitivity.

✔ **To have very few false negatives:** Choose a lower cut value to give higher
sensitivity. Figure 20-9 shows you that if you set the cut value to 0.3, you
can have almost perfect sensitivity (almost no false negatives), but your
specificity will be only about 75 percent (about 25 percent false positives).

The software may optionally display the *area under the ROC curve* (ROC AUC), along with its standard error and a p value. This is another measure of how good the predictive model is. The diagonal line has an AUC of 0.5; the p value indicates whether the AUC is significantly greater than 0.5 (that is, whether your predictive model is better than a null model).

Heads Up: Knowing What Can Go Wrong with Logistic Regression

Logistic regression presents many of the same potential pitfalls as ordinary least-squares regression (see Chapters 18 and 19), as well as several that are specific to logistic regression. Watch out for some of the more common pitfalls, explained in the following sections.

Don't fit a logistic function to nonlogistic data

Don't use logistic regression to fit data that doesn't behave like the logistic S curve. Plot your grouped data (as shown in Figure 20-1b), and if it's clear that the fraction of *yes* outcome subjects isn't leveling off at $Y = 0$ or $Y = 1$ for very large or very small X values, then logistic regression isn't the way to go. And pay attention to the Hosmer-Lemeshow p value (described earlier) produced by the regression software. If this value is much less than 0.05, it indicates that your data is not consistent with a logistic model. In Chapter 21, I describe a more generalized logistic model that contains other parameters for the upper and lower leveling-off values.

Watch out for collinearity and disappearing significance

All regression models with more than one predictor variable can be plagued with problems of *collinearity* (when two or more predictor variables are strongly correlated with each other), and logistic regression is no exception. I describe this problem, and the troubles it can cause, in Chapter 19.

Check for inadvertent reverse-coding of the outcome variable

The outcome variable should always be 1 for a *yes* outcome and 0 for a *no* outcome (refer to Table 20-1 for an example). Some programs may let you record the outcome variable in your data file as descriptive terms like *Lived* and *Died;* then the program translates these terms to 0 and 1 behind the scenes. But the program may translate them as the opposite of what you want — it may translate Lived to 1 and Died to 0, in which case the fitted formula will predict the probability of living rather than dying. This reversal won't affect any p values, but it will cause all odds ratios and their confidence intervals to be the reciprocals of what they would have been, because they will now refer to the odds of living rather than the odds of dying.

Don't misinterpret odds ratios for numerical predictors

The value of a regression coefficient depends on the units in which the corresponding predictor variable is expressed. So the coefficient of a height variable expressed in meters is 100 times larger than the coefficient of height expressed in centimeters. In logistic regression, odds ratios are obtained by exponentiating the coefficients, so switching from centimeters to meters corresponds to raising the odds ratio (and its confidence limits) to the 100th power. The odds ratio always represents the factor by which the odds of getting the outcome event increases when the predictor increases by exactly one unit of measure (whatever that unit may be).

Sometimes you may want to express the odds ratio in more convenient units than what the data was recorded in. For the example in Table 20-1, the odds ratio for dose as a predictor of death is 1.0115 per REM. This isn't too meaningful because one REM is a very small increment of radiation. By raising 1.0115 to the 100th power (get out your calculator), you get the equivalent odds ratio of 3.1375 per 100 REMs, and you can express this as, "Every additional 100 REMs of radiation more than triples the odds of dying."

Don't misinterpret odds ratios for categorical predictors

Categorical predictors should be coded numerically as I describe in Chapter 7. If you express categories as text, the computer may not translate them the way you want it to, and the resulting odds ratios may be the reciprocal of what you want or may be different in other ways.

Check the software manual to see whether there's a way to force the program to code categorical variables the way you want. As a last resort, you can create one or more new numeric variables and do the recoding yourself.

Beware the complete separation problem

The complete separation problem, also called the *perfect predictor problem,* is a particularly nasty (and surprisingly frequent) problem that's unique to logistic regression. As incredible as it may sound, it's a sad fact that a logistic regression will fail if the data is too good!

If your predictor variable completely separates the *yes* outcomes from the *no* outcomes, the maximum likelihood method will try to make the coefficient of that variable infinite (although most regression software will give up before getting quite that far). The odds ratio also wants to be infinity if the coefficient is positive, or 0 if the coefficient is negative. The standard error wants to be infinite too, so your confidence interval may have a lower bound of 0, an upper bound of infinity, or both. Also, if you're doing multiple logistic regression, the perfect predictor problem will rear its ugly head if any of your predictor variables completely separates the outcomes.

Check out the problem shown in Figure 20-10. The regression is trying to make the curve come as close as possible to all the data points. Usually it has to strike a compromise, because (especially in the middle part of the data) there's a mixture of 1s and 0s. But with perfectly separated data, no compromise is necessary. As *b* becomes infinitely large, the logistic function morphs into a step function that touches all the data points.

Take the time to examine your data and see whether any individual variables may be perfect predictors:

1. **Pick each predictor variable, one by one.**

2. **Sort your data file by that variable.**

3. **Run down the listing looking at the values in the outcome column to see whether they are completely separated (all *nos* followed by all *yeses*).**

The perfect predictor problem may bite you even if each variable passes this test, because it can arise if a combination of two or more variables acting together can completely separate the outcome. Unfortunately, there's no easy way to detect this situation by sorting or graphing your data.

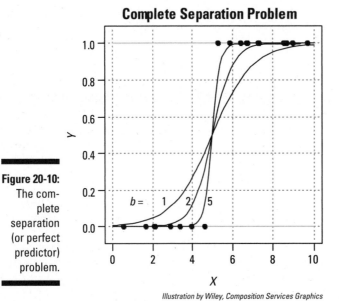

Complete Separation Problem

$b =$ 1 2 5

Figure 20-10:
The complete separation (or perfect predictor) problem.

Illustration by Wiley, Composition Services Graphics

Now for the really bad news: No really good solution to the complete separation problem exists. You may be able to add more data points — this sometimes introduces enough random variability to break the complete separation. Or you can remove the variable(s) responsible for complete separation from your model, but that's not very satisfying: Why would you want to throw away your best predictors? Some advanced logistic software will at least come up with a finite lower confidence limit for an infinite odds ratio (or a finite upper limit for a zero odds ratio), but that's about the best you can hope for.

Figuring Out the Sample Size You Need for Logistic Regression

Estimating the required sample size for a logistic regression (even a simple one-predictor regression) can be a pain. Specifying the desired power and alpha level is easy enough (see Chapter 3 for more about these items), and you can state the effect size of importance as an odds ratio.

But the required sample size also depends on a couple of other things:

  ✔ The relative frequencies of *yes* and *no* outcomes
  ✔ How the predictor variable is distributed

And with multiple predictors in the model, determining sample size is even more complicated. There can be a separate effect size of importance and desired power for each predictor, and the predictors themselves may be correlated.

Some programs and web pages calculate sample size for various logistic models involving one or more than one predictor and for dichotomous or continuous predictors. But these programs are likely to ask you for more information than you're able to provide. You can use simulation methods if data from an earlier, similar study is available, but this is no task for the amateur. For a rigorous sample-size calculation, you may have no choice but to seek the help of a professional statistician.

Here are two simple approaches you can use if your logistic model has only one predictor. In each case, you replace the logistic regression with another analysis that's sort of equivalent to it, and then do a sample-size calculation based on that other kind of analysis. It's not ideal, but it can give you an answer that's close enough for planning purposes.

- ✔ **If the predictor is a dichotomous category** (like gender), logistic regression gives the same p value you get from analyzing a fourfold table. Therefore, you can use the sample-size calculations I describe in Chapter 13.

- ✔ **If the predictor is a continuous numerical quantity** (like age), you can pretend that the outcome variable is the predictor and age is the outcome. I know this gets the cause-and-effect relationship backwards, but if you make that conceptual flip, then you can ask whether the two different outcome groups have different mean values for the predictor. You can test that question with an unpaired Student t test, so you can use the sample-size calculations I describe in Chapter 12.

Chapter 21

Other Useful Kinds of Regression

*T*his chapter covers some other kinds of regression you're likely to encounter in biostatistical work. They're not quite as ubiquitous as the types described in Chapters 18–20 (straight-line regression, multiple regression, and logistic regression), but you should be aware of them, so I collect them here. I don't go into a lot of detail, but I describe what they are, when you may want to use them, how to run them and interpret the output, and what special situations you should watch out for.

Note: I don't cover survival regression in this chapter, even though it's one of the most important kinds of regression analysis in biostatistics. It has its own chapter (Chapter 24), in Part V of this book, which deals with the analysis of survival data.

Analyzing Counts and Rates with Poisson Regression

Statisticians often have to analyze outcomes consisting of the number of occurrences of an event over some interval of time, like the number of fatal highway accidents in a city in a year. If the occurrences seem to be getting more numerous as time goes on, you may want to perform a regression analysis to see whether the upward trend is statistically significant and to estimate the annual rate of increase (with its standard error and confidence interval).

Although they're often analyzed by ordinary least-squares regression, event counts don't really meet the least-squares assumptions — they aren't well approximated as continuous, normally distributed data unless the counts are very large. Also, their variability is neither constant nor proportional to the counts themselves. So event-count outcomes aren't best analyzed by straight-line or multiple least-squares regression.

Because independent random events (like highway accidents) should follow a Poisson distribution (see Chapter 25), they should be analyzed by a kind of regression designed for Poisson outcomes. And there is indeed just that kind of specialized regression, called (you never would've guessed this) *Poisson regression.* The following sections provide the basics on the model used for this regression, how to run and interpret its output, and a few extra tasks it can handle.

Introducing the generalized linear model

Most statistical software packages don't offer anything explicitly called Poisson regression; instead, they have a more general regression technique called the *generalized linear model* (GLM).

Don't confuse the *generalized* linear model with the very similarly named *general* linear model that I describe in Chapter 12. It's unfortunate that these two names are almost identical, because they describe two very different things. The *general* linear model used to be abbreviated GLM before the *generalized* linear model came on the scene in the 1970s, but the former is now usually abbreviated as LM in a (not very successful) attempt to avoid confusion.

GLM is similar to LM only in that the predictor variables usually appear in the model as the familiar linear combination:

$$c_0 + c_1x_1 + c_2x_2 + c_3x_3 + \ldots$$

where the x's are the predictor variables, and the c's are the regression coefficients (with c_0 being called a *constant term,* or *intercept*).

But GLM extends the capabilities of LM in two important ways:

- ✔ With LM, the linear combination becomes the predicted value of the outcome, but with GLM, you can specify a transformation (called a *link function*) that turns the linear combination into the predicted value. As I note in Chapter 20, logistic regression applies exactly this kind of transformation: The linear combination (call it V) goes through the logistic function $1/(1 + e^{-V})$ to convert it into a predicted probability of having the outcome event, and you can use GLM to perform logistic regression.

✔ With LM, the outcome is assumed to be a continuous, normally distributed variable, but with GLM, the outcome can be continuous or integer, obeying any of several different distribution functions, like normal, exponential, binomial, or Poisson. (For example, as I explain in Chapter 20, logistic regression is used when the outcome is a binomial variable indicating whether the event did or did not occur.)

GLM is the Swiss army knife of regression — it can do ordinary least-squares regression, logistic regression, Poisson regression, and a whole lot more. Most of the advanced statistical software systems (SAS, SPSS, R) offer GLM so that they don't have to program a lot of other specialized regressions. So if your software package doesn't offer logistic or Poisson regression, check to see whether it offers GLM; if so, then you're all set. (Flip to Chapter 4 for an introduction to statistical software.)

Running a Poisson regression

Suppose you want to study the number of fatal highway accidents per year in a city. Table 21-1 shows some made-up fatal-accident data over the course of 12 years. Figure 21-1 shows a graph of this data, created using the R statistical software package.

Table 21-1   Yearly Data on Fatal Highway Accidents in One City

Calendar Year	*Fatal Accidents*
2000	10
2001	12
2002	15
2003	8
2004	8
2005	15
2006	4
2007	20
2008	20
2009	17
2010	29
2011	28

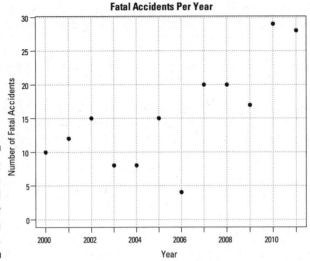

Figure 21-1:
Yearly data
on fatal
highway
accidents in
one city.

Illustration by Wiley, Composition Services Graphics

Running a Poisson regression is similar in many (but not all) ways to running the other common kinds of regression:

1. **Assemble the data for Poisson regression just as you would for any kind of regression.** For this example, you have a row of data for each year, a column containing the outcome values (the number of accidents each year), and a column for the predictor (the year).

2. **Tell the software what the predictor and outcome variables are, either by name or by picking from a list of variables, depending on the software.**

3. **Tell the software what kind of regression you want it to carry out by specifying the *family* of the dependent variable's distribution and the *link function*.**

   Step 3 is not obvious, and you have to consult your software's manual. The R program, for instance, has everything specified in a single instruction, which looks like this:

   glm(formula=Accidents ~ Year, family = poisson(link = "identity"))

   This tells R everything it needs to know: The outcome is the variable called Accidents, the predictor is the variable called Year, and the outcome variable follows the Poisson distribution. The link = "identity" tells R that you want to fit a model in which the true event rate rises in a linear fashion; that is, it increases by a constant amount each year.

4. **Press the Go button and get ready!**

   The computer does all the work and presents you with the answers.

Interpreting the Poisson regression output

After you follow the steps for running a Poisson regression in the preceding section, the program produces output like that shown in Figure 21-2.

Figure 21-2:
Poisson regression output from R's generalized linear model function (glm).

```
Call:
glm(formula=Accidents~Year,family=poisson(link="identity"))

Coefficients:
               Estimate   Std. Error    z value   Pr  (>|z|)
(Intercept)  -2651.4569     635.1064      -4.175  2.98e-05  ***
Year            1.3298        0.3169      -4.197  2.71e-05  ***

AIC: 81.72
```

Illustration by Wiley, Composition Services Graphics

This output has the same general structure as the output from other kinds of regression. The most important parts of it are the following:

✔ In the Coefficients table, the estimated regression coefficient for Year is 1.3298, indicating that the annual number of fatal accidents is increasing by about 1.33 accidents per year.

✔ The standard error (SE) of 0.3169 (or about 0.32) indicates the precision of the estimated rate increase per year. From the SE, using the rules given in Chapter 10, the 95 percent confidence interval (CI) around the estimated annual increase is approximately $1.3298 \pm 1.96 \times 0.3169$, which gives a 95 percent CI of 0.71 to 1.95.

✔ The z value column contains the value of the regression coefficient divided by its standard error. It's used to calculate the p value that appears in the last column of the table.

✔ The last column, $Pr(>|z|)$, is the p value for the significance of the increasing trend. The Year variable has a p value of $2.71e\text{-}05$, which is scientific notation (see Chapter 2) for 0.0000271, so the apparent increase in rate over the 12 years is highly significant. (Over the years, the value of 0.05 has become accepted as a reasonable criterion for declaring significance; don't declare significance unless the p value is less than 0.05. See Chapter 3 for an introduction to p values.)

✔ AIC (Akaike's Information Criterion) indicates how well this model fits the data. The value of 81.72 isn't useful by itself, but it's very useful when choosing between two alternative models, as I explain later in this chapter.

The R program can also provide the predicted annual event rate for each year, from which you can add a "trend line" to the scatter graph, indicating how you think the true event rate might vary with time (see Figure 21-3).

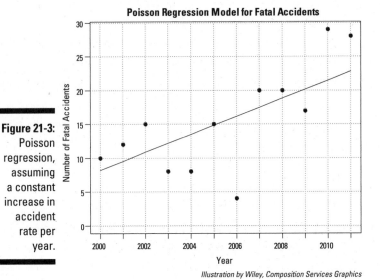

Figure 21-3: Poisson regression, assuming a constant increase in accident rate per year.

Illustration by Wiley, Composition Services Graphics

Discovering other things that Poisson regression can do

The following sections describe some additional things you can do with your data, using R's GLM function to perform Poisson regression.

Examining nonlinear trends

The straight line in Figure 21-3 doesn't seem to reflect the fact that the accident rate remained low for the first few years and then started to climb rapidly after 2006. Perhaps the true trend isn't a straight line (where the rate increases by the same *amount* each year); it may be an *exponential* rise (where the rate increases by a certain *percentage* each year). You can have R fit an exponential rise by changing the link option from "identity" to "log" in the statement that invokes the Poisson regression:

glm(formula=Accidents ~ Year, family=poisson(link="="log"))

This produces the output shown in Figure 21-4 and graphed in Figure 21-5.

Figure 21-4:
Output from
an exponen-
tial trend
Poisson
regression.

```
Call:
glm(formula=Accidents~Year,family=poisson(link="=log"))

Coefficients:
                 Estimate   Std. Error   z value  Pr (>|z|)
 (Intercept)   -206.18249     44.29432    -4.655   3.24e-06 ***
Year              0.10414      0.02207    -4.718   2.38e-06 ***

AIC: 78.476
```

Illustration by Wiley, Composition Services Graphics

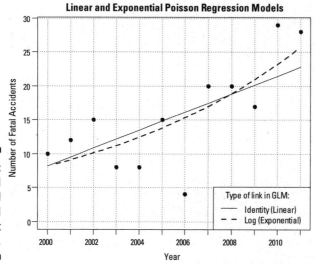

Linear and Exponential Poisson Regression Models

Figure 21-5:
Linear and
exponential
trends fitted
to accident
data.

Illustration by Wiley, Composition Services Graphics

Because of the "log" link used in this regression run, the coefficients are related to the logarithm of the event rate. So the relative rate of increase per year is obtained by taking the antilog of the regression coefficient for Year. This is done by raising e (the mathematical constant 2.718…) to the power of the regression coefficient for Year: $e^{0.10414}$, which is about 1.11. So according to an exponential increase model, the annual accident rate increases by a factor of 1.11 (that is, an 11 percent relative increase) each year. The dashed-line curve in Figure 21-4 shows this exponential trend, which appears to accommodate the steeper rate of increase seen after 2006.

Comparing alternative models

The AIC value for the exponential trend model is 78.476, which is about 3.2 units lower than for the linear trend model (AIC = 81.72). Smaller AIC values indicate better fit, so the true trend is more likely to be exponential rather than linear. But you can't conclude that the model with the lower AIC is really better unless the AIC is about six units better, so in this example you can't say for sure whether the trend is linear or exponential (or something else). But the exponential curve does seem to predict the high accident rates seen in 2010 and 2011 better than the linear trend model.

Working with unequal observation intervals

In this fatal accident example, each of the 12 data points represents the accidents observed during a one-year interval. But in other applications (like analyzing the frequency of ER visits after a treatment for emphysema, where there is one data point per person), the width of the observation interval may vary from one person to another. GLM lets you provide, for each data point, an interval width along with the event count. For arcane reasons, many statistical programs refer to this interval-width variable as the *offset*.

Accommodating clustered events

The Poisson distribution applies when the observed events are all independent occurrences. But this assumption isn't met if events occur in clusters. So, for example, if you count individual highway *fatalities* instead of fatal highway *accidents,* the Poisson distribution doesn't apply, because one fatal accident may kill several people.

The standard deviation (SD) of a Poisson distribution is equal to the square root of the mean of the distribution. But if clustering is present, the SD of the data is larger than the square root of the mean, a situation called *overdispersion.* GLM can accommodate overdispersion; you just tell R to make the distribution family *quasipoisson* rather than *poisson,* like this:

```
glm(formula=Accidents ~ Year, family=quasipoisson(link="="log"))
```

Anything Goes with Nonlinear Regression

No treatment of regression would be complete without discussing the most general (and potentially the most challenging) of all kinds of least-squares regression — general nonlinear least-squares regression, or nonlinear curve-fitting. In the following sections, I explain how nonlinear regression is different from other kinds, I describe how to run and interpret a nonlinear regression (with the help of a drug research example), and I show you some tips involving equivalent functions.

Distinguishing nonlinear regression from other kinds

In the kinds of regression I describe earlier in this chapter and in Chapters 18–20, the predictor variables and regression coefficients always appear in the model as a linear combination: $c_0 + c_1x_1 + c_2x_2 + c_3x_3 + \ldots + c_nx_n$. But in nonlinear regression, the coefficients no longer have to appear paired up with predictor variables (like c_2x_2); they now have a more independent existence and can appear on their own, anywhere in the formula. In fact, the name *coefficient,* which implies a number that's multiplied by a variable, is too limited to describe how they can be used in nonlinear regression; instead, they're referred to as *parameters.*

The formula for a nonlinear regression model may be any algebraic expression, involving sums and differences, products and ratios, and powers and roots, together with any combination of logarithmic, exponential, trigonometric, and other advanced mathematical functions (see Chapter 2 for an introduction to these items). The formula can contain any number of predictor variables and any number of parameters (and these formulas often contain many more parameters than predictor variables).

Table 21-2 shows a few of the many nonlinear functions you may encounter in biological research.

Table 21-2	Some Examples of Nonlinear Functions
Function	*Description*
$Conc = C_0 e^{-k \times Time}$	Concentration versus time: Exponential (first-order) decline from C_0 at time 0 to zero at infinite time
$Conc = C_0 e^{-k \times Time} + C_\infty$	Concentration versus time: Exponential (first-order) decline from C_0 at time 0 to some non-zero leveling-off value
$Y = Y_0 + \dfrac{Y_\infty - Y_0}{1 + e^{-(a+bX)}}$	An S-shaped, logistic-type curve with arbitrary leveling-off values (not necessarily 0 and 100 percent)
$Y = aX^b$	A power curve in which the power isn't necessarily a whole number
$Y = ae^{-b/(T+273)}$	Arrhenius equation for temperature dependence of rate constants and many other physical/chemical properties

Unlike other types of regression that I describe earlier in this chapter and book, in which you give the statistical software your data, click the Go button, and wait for the answer to appear, full-blown nonlinear regression is never such a no-brainer. First, you have to decide what function you want to fit to your data (out of the infinite number of possible functions you could dream up). Sometimes the general form of the function is determined (or at least suggested) by a scientific theory (this would be called a *theoretical* or *mechanistic* function and is more common in the physical sciences than in the life sciences). Other times, you may simply pick a function that has the right general shape (this would be called an *empirical* function). You also have to provide starting guesses for each of the parameters appearing in the function. The regression software tries to refine these guesses, using an iterative process that may or may not converge to an answer, depending on the complexity of the function you're fitting and how close your initial guesses are to the truth.

In addition to these special problems, all the other complications of multivariate regression (like collinearity; see Chapter 19) can appear in nonlinear problems, often in a more subtle and hard-to-deal-with way.

Checking out an example from drug research

One common nonlinear regression problem arises in drug development research. As soon as scientists start testing a promising new compound, they want to determine some of its basic pharmacokinetic (PK) properties; that is, to learn how the drug is absorbed, distributed, modified, and eliminated by the body. Some clinical trials are designed specifically to characterize the pharmacokinetics of the drug accurately and in great detail, but even the earliest Phase I trials (see Chapter 6) usually try to get at least some rudimentary PK data as a secondary objective of the trial.

Raw PK data often consists of the concentration of the drug in the blood at various times after administering a dose of the drug. Consider a simple experiment, in which 10,000 micrograms (μ g) of a new drug is given as a single *bolus* (a rapid injection into a vein). Blood samples are drawn at predetermined times after dosing and are analyzed for the drug. Hypothetical data from one subject is shown in Table 21-3 and graphed in Figure 21-6. The drug concentration in the blood is expressed in units of micrograms per deciliter (μg/dL); a *deciliter* is one-tenth of a liter.

Table 21-3	Blood Drug Concentration versus Time
Time after Dosing (In Hours)	*Drug Concentration in Blood (μ g/dL)*
0.25	57.4
0.5	54.0
1	44.8
1.5	52.7
2	43.6
3	40.1
4	27.9
6	20.6
8	15.0
12	10.0

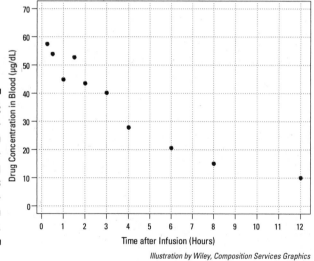

Figure 21-6: The concentration of an intravenous drug declines as it is eliminated from the body.

Illustration by Wiley, Composition Services Graphics

Several basic PK parameters (maximum concentration, time of maximum concentration, area under the curve) are usually calculated directly from the concentration-versus-time data, without having to fit any curve to the points. But two important parameters are usually obtained from a regression analysis:

✔ **The volume of distribution (V_d):** The effective volume of fluid or tissue through which the drug distributes. This effective volume could be equal to the blood volume but could be greater if the drug also spreads through fatty tissue or other parts of the body. If you know how much drug you infused *(Dose),* and you know the plasma concentration at the moment of infusion (C_0), before any of the drug had been eliminated, you can calculate the volume of distribution as $V_d = \text{Dose}/C_0$. But you can't directly measure C_0 — by the time the drug has distributed evenly through the bloodstream, some of it has already been eliminated from the body. So C_0 has to be estimated by extrapolating the measured concentrations backward in time to the moment of infusion (Time = 0).

✔ **The elimination half-life (λ):** The time it takes for half of the drug in the body to be eliminated.

Pharmacokinetic theory is pretty well developed, and it predicts that (under some reasonable assumptions), the drug concentration *(Conc)* in the blood following a bolus infusion should vary with time *(Time)* according to the equation:

$$Conc = C_0 e^{-k_e Time}$$

where k_e is the *elimination rate constant.* k_e is related to the elimination half-life (λ) according to the formula: $\lambda = 0.693/k_e$, where 0.693 is the natural logarithm of 2. So if you can fit the preceding equation to your *Conc*-versus-*Time* data in Table 21-3, you can get C_0, from which you can calculate V_d, and you can get k_e, from which you can calculate λ.

The preceding equation is nonlinear in the parameters (k_e appears in the exponent). In the old days, before nonlinear regression software became widely available, people would shoehorn this nonlinear regression problem into a straight-line regression program by working with the logarithms of the concentrations. But that approach has several problems, one of which is that it can't be generalized to handle more complicated equations that often arise.

Running a nonlinear regression

Nonlinear curve-fitting is supported by many modern statistics packages, like SPSS, SAS, GraphPad Prism, and R (see Chapter 4). You can also set up the calculations in Excel, although it's not particularly easy. Finally, the web page `http://StatPages.info/nonlin.html` can fit any function you can write, involving up to eight independent variables and up to eight parameters. Here I describe how to do nonlinear regression in R:

1. **Provide the concentration and time data.**

   R can read data files in various formats (Excel, Access, text files, and so on), or you can directly assign values to variables, using statements like the following (which come from Table 21-3):

   > Time = c(0.25, 0.5, 1, 1.5, 2, 3, 4, 6, 8, 12)

   > Conc = c(57.4, 54.0, 44.8, 52.7, 43.6, 40.1, 27.9, 20.6, 15.0, 10.0)

   In the two preceding equations, *c* is a built-in R function that creates an array (see Chapter 2) from a list of numbers.

2. **Specify the equation to be fitted to the data, using the algebraic syntax your software requires.**

   I write the equation this way (using R's algebraic syntax): Conc ~ C0 * exp(- ke * Time)

3. **Let the software know that C0 and ke are parameters to be fitted, and provide initial guesses for these values.**

   Nonlinear curve-fitting is a complicated task that works by iteration — you give it some rough guesses, and it refines them into closer estimates to the truth, repeating this process until it arrives at the best (least-squares) solution.

   Coming up with starting guesses can be tricky for some nonlinear regression problems; it's more of an art than a science. Sometimes, if the parameters have physiological meaning, you may be able to make a guess based on known physiology or past experience, but sometimes it just has to be trial and error. You can graph your observed data in Excel, and then superimpose a curve from values calculated from the function for various parameter guesses that you type in, and you can play around with the parameters until the curve is at least in the ballpark of the observed data.

   In this example, C0 is the concentration you expect at the moment of dosing (at t = 0). From Figure 21-6, it looks like the concentration starts out around 50, so you can use 50 as an initial guess for C0. The ke parameter affects how quickly the concentration decreases with time. Figure 21-6 indicates that the concentration seems to decrease by half about every few hours, so λ should be somewhere around 4 hours. Because $\lambda = 0.693/k_e$, a little algebra gives $k_e = 0.693/\lambda$, or 0.693/4, so you may try 0.2 as a starting guess for ke. You tell R the starting guesses by using the syntax: start=list(C0=50, ke=0.2).

The full R statement for doing the regression, using its built-in function nls (which stands for *nonlinear least-squares*) and summarizing the output is

> summary(nls(Conc ~ C0 * exp(-ke * Time), start = list(C0 = 50, ke = 0.2)))

Interpreting the output

As complicated as nonlinear curve-fitting may be, the output is quite simple — very much like the output from ordinary linear regression and not any more difficult to interpret. Figure 21-7 shows the relevant part of R's output for this example.

Figure 21-7:
Results of
nonlinear
regression
in R.

```
Formula: Conc ~ C0 * exp ( -ke * Time)

Parameters:
      Estimate Std. Error t value  Pr (>|t|)
C0    59.46203    2.29329  25.929  5.25e-09 ***
ke     0.16330    0.01644   9.931  8.94e-06 ***

Residual std. err. :  3.556 on 8 deg.of freedom
```

Illustration by Wiley, Composition Services Graphics

First is a restatement of the function you're fitting. Then comes the regression table, which has a row for every adjustable parameter that appears in the function. Like every other kind of regression table, it shows the fitted value for the parameter, its standard error, and the p value (the last column) indicating whether or not that parameter was significantly different from zero. C_0 is 59.5 ± 2.3 micrograms/deciliter ($\mu g/dL$); and k_e is 0.163 ± 0.0164 hr^1 (first-order rate constants have units of "per time"). From these values, you can calculate the PK parameters you want:

✔ **Volume of distribution:** V_d = Dose/C_0 = 10,000 $\mu g/59.5$ $\mu g/dL$ = 168 dL, or 16.8 liters. (This amount is several times larger than the blood volume of the average human, indicating that this drug is going into other parts of the body besides the blood.)

✔ **Elimination half-time:** $t_{\frac{1}{2}}$ = 0.693/k_e = 0.693/0.163 hr^1, or 4.25 hours. (After 4.25 hours, only 50 percent of the original dose is left in the body; after 8.5 hours, only 25 percent of the original dose remains; and so on.)

How precise are these PK parameters? (What is their SE?) Chapter 11 describes how SEs propagate through calculations, and gives you several ways to answer this question. Using the online calculator I describe in that chapter, you can calculate that the V_d = 16.8 ± 0.65 liters, and λ = 4.25 ± 0.43 hours.

R can also easily generate the predicted value for each data point, from which you can superimpose the fitted curve onto the observed data points, as in Figure 21-8.

R also provides the *residual standard error,* defined as the standard deviation of the vertical distances of the observed points from the fitted curve. The value of 3.556 means that the points scatter about 3.6 $\mu g/dL$ above and below the fitted curve. R can also provide Akaike's Information Criterion (AIC), which is useful in selecting which of several possible models best fits the data.

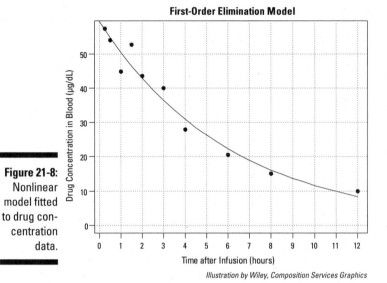

First-Order Elimination Model

Figure 21-8: Nonlinear model fitted to drug concentration data.

Using equivalent functions to fit the parameters you really want

It's inconvenient, annoying, and error-prone to have to perform calculations on the parameters you get from a nonlinear regression (like C_0 and the k_e rate constant) to get the parameters you really wanted (like V_d and $t_{1/2}$), and even more so to get their standard errors. Wouldn't it be nice if you could get V_d and λ and their SEs directly from the nonlinear regression program? Well, in many cases you can!

With nonlinear regression, there's usually more than one way to skin a cat. Very often you can express the formula in an equivalent form that directly involves the parameters you're interested in. Here's how it works for the PK example I use in the preceding sections.

Because $V_d = \text{Dose}/C_0$, that means (from high-school algebra) that $C_0 = \text{Dose}/V_d$, why not use Dose/V_d instead of C_0 in the formula you're fitting? If you do, it becomes $Conc = \left(\text{Dose} \middle/ V_d \right) e^{-k_e Time}$. And you can go even further than that. It turns out that a first-order exponential-decline formula can be written either as $e^{-k_e Time}$ or as the algebraically equivalent form $2^{-\left(Time / t_{1/2} \right)}$.

Applying both of these substitutions, you get the equivalent model:
$$C = \left(\text{Dose} \middle/ V_d \right) 2^{-Time/t_{1/2}}, \text{ which produces exactly the same fitted curve as the}$$

original model, but it has the tremendous advantage of giving you exactly the PK parameters you want (V_d and $t_{1/2}$), rather than other parameters (C_0 and k) that you have to do further calculations on.

You already know that *Dose* is 10,000 micrograms (from the original description of this example), so you can substitute this value for *Dose* in the formula to be fitted. You've already estimated $t_{1/2}$ as 4 hours and C_0 as about 50 μ g/dL from looking at Figure 21-6, as I describe earlier, so you can estimate V_d as 10,000/50, which is 200 deciliters. With these guesses, the final R statement is

summary(nls(Conc ~ (10000/Vd) * 2^(-Time/tHalf), start = list(Vd = 200, tHalf = 4)))

which produces the output shown in Figure 21-9.

Figure 21-9:
Nonlinear regression using the PK parameters you're interested in.

```
Formula: Conc ~ (10000/Vd) * 2^( -Time / tHalf)

Parameters:
        Estimate Std. Error t value Pr (>|t|)
Vd      168.1745   6.4860   25.929  5.25e-09 ***
tHalf     4.2446   0.4274    9.931  8.94e-06 ***

Residual std. err. :  3.556 on 8 deg.of freedom
```

Illustration by Wiley, Composition Services Graphics

Now you can directly see, with no further calculations required, that the volume of distribution is 168.2 ± 6.5 dL (or 16.8 ± 0.66 liters), and the elimination half-time is 4.24 ± 0.43 hours.

Smoothing Nonparametric Data with LOWESS

Sometimes you want to fit a smooth curve to a set of points that don't seem to conform to any curve (straight line, parabola, exponential, and so forth) that you're familiar with. You can't use the usual linear or nonlinear regression methods if you can't write an equation for the curve you want to fit. What you need is a kind of *nonparametric regression* — one that doesn't assume any particular model (formula) for the relationship, but rather just tries to draw a smooth line through the data points.

Several kinds of nonparametric data-smoothing methods have been developed. One popular one is called LOWESS, which stands for Locally Weighted Scatterplot Smoothing. Many statistical programs, like SAS and R, can do LOWESS regression. In the following sections, I explain how to run a LOWESS analysis and adjust the amount of smoothing (or "stiffness" of the curve).

Running LOWESS

Suppose you discover a new kind of hormone that is produced in the ovaries of women. The blood levels of this hormone should vary with age, being relatively low before puberty and after menopause, and high during child-bearing age. You want to characterize and quantify this age dependence as precisely as possible.

Now suppose you acquire 200 blood samples drawn from females of all ages (from 2 to 90 years) for another research project, and after addressing all human-subjects-protection issues, you analyze these specimens for your new hormone. A graph of hormone level versus age may look like Figure 21-10.

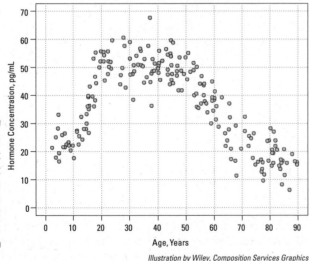

Figure 21-10: Data that doesn't seem to conform to any simple function.

Illustration by Wiley, Composition Services Graphics

You have quite a lot of scatter in these points, which makes it hard to see the more subtle aspects of the age dependency: At what age does the hormone level start to rise? When does it peak? Does it remain fairly constant throughout child-bearing years? When does it start to decline? Is the rate of post-menopause decline constant or does it change with advancing age?

It would be easier to answer those questions if you had a curve that represented the data without all the random fluctuations of the individual points. How would you go about fitting a curve to this data? LOWESS to the rescue!

Running LOWESS in R is quite simple; you need only to provide the program with the x and y variables, and it does the rest. If you have imported your data into R as two variables, x and y, the R instruction to run a LOWESS regression is very simple: lowess(x, y, f = 0.2). (I explain the f = 0.2 part in the following section.)

Unlike other forms of regression, LOWESS doesn't produce a coefficients table; the only output is a table of smoothed y values, one for each data point, from which (using another R instruction) you can plot the smoothed line superimposed on the scatter graph. Figure 21-11 shows the results of running the LOWESS routine provided with the R software.

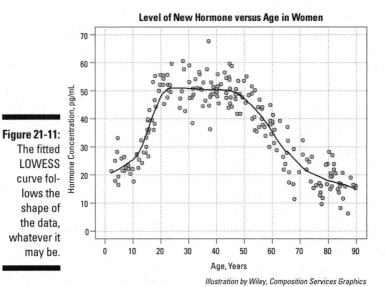

Figure 21-11: The fitted LOWESS curve follows the shape of the data, whatever it may be.

Illustration by Wiley, Composition Services Graphics

The smoothed curve seems to fit the data quite well, except possibly at the lowest ages. The individual data points don't show any noticeable upward trend until age 12 or so, but the smoothed curve starts climbing right from age 3. The curve completes its rise by age 20, and then remains flat until almost age 50, when it starts declining. The rate of decline seems to be greatest between ages 50 to 65, after which it declines less rapidly. These subtleties would be very difficult to spot just by looking at the individual data points without any smoothed curve.

Adjusting the amount of smoothing

R's LOWESS program allows you adjust the "stiffness" of the fitted curve by specifying a *smoothing fraction, f,* which is a number between 0 and 1. Figure 21-12 shows what the smoothed curve looks like for three different smoothing fractions.

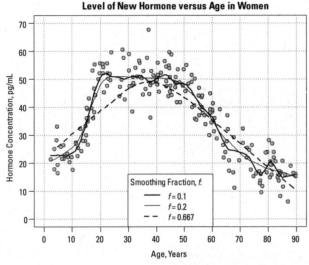

Illustration by Wiley, Composition Services Graphics

Figure 21-12:
You can adjust the smoothness of the fitted curve.

✔ Setting $f = 0.667$ (or ⅔, which is the value R uses if you leave the f parameter out of the LOWESS statement entirely) produces a rather "stiff" curve that rises steadily between ages 2 and 40, and then declines steadily after that. It misses important features of the data, like the low pre-puberty hormone levels, the flat plateau during child-bearing years, and the slowing down of the yearly decrease above age 65. You can say that this curve shows excessive *bias,* systematically departing from "the truth" in various places along its length.

✔ Setting $f = 0.1$, at the other extreme, produces a very jittery curve with a lot of up-and-down wiggles that can't possibly be real age dependencies, but reflect only random fluctuations in the data. You can say that this curve shows excessive *variance,* with too many random fluctuations along its length.

✔ Setting $f = 0.2$ produces a curve that's stiff enough not to have random wiggles, yet flexible enough to show that hormone levels are fairly low until age 10, reach their peak at age 20, stay fairly level until age 50, and then decline, with the rate of decline slowing down after age 70. This curve appears to strike a good balance, with low bias and low variance.

Whenever you do LOWESS regression, you have to explore different smoothing fractions to find the sweet spot that gives the best tradeoff between bias and variance — showing the real features while smoothing out the random noise. Used properly, LOWESS regression can be helpful in gleaning the most insight from noisy data.

Part V
Analyzing Survival Data

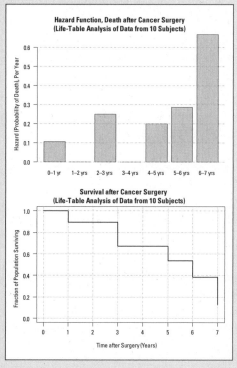

Illustration by Wiley, Composition Services Graphics

Estimate sample size in a variety of situations with the help of the Cheat Sheet at
www.dummies.com/extras/biostatistics.

In this part . . .

- ✔ Understand what survival data is and how to handle censoring (when you don't know whether the subject died).

- ✔ Prepare survival curves using the life-table and Kaplan-Meier methods.

- ✔ Estimate median survival times and survival rates at specified times.

- ✔ Compare survival curves between two or more groups, using the log-rank test.

- ✔ Analyze multiple predictors of survival using Cox proportional-hazards regression.

Chapter 22

Summarizing and Graphing Survival Data

*T*his chapter describes statistical techniques that deal with a special kind of numerical data — the interval from some starting point in time (such as a diagnosis date or procedure date) to the first (or only) occurrence of some particular kind of endpoint event. Because these techniques are so often applied to situations where the endpoint event is death, we usually call the use of these techniques *survival analysis,* even when the endpoint is something less drastic than death, like relapse, or even something desirable — for example, time to remission of cancer or time to recovery. Throughout this chapter, I use terms and examples that imply that the endpoint is death (like *survival time* instead of *time to event*), but everything I say also applies to other kinds of endpoints.

You may wonder why you need a special kind of analysis for survival data in the first place. Why not just treat survival times as ordinary numerical variables? Why not summarize them as means, medians, standard deviations, and so on, and graph them as histograms and box-and-whiskers charts? Why not compare survival times between groups with t tests and ANOVAs? Why not use ordinary least-squares regression to explore how various factors influence survival time?

In this chapter, I explain how survival data isn't like ordinary numerical data and why you need to use special techniques to analyze it properly. I describe two ways to construct survival curves: the life table and the Kaplan-Meier methods. I tell you what to watch out for when preparing and interpreting survival curves, and I show you how to glean useful information from these curves, such as median survival time and five-year survival rates.

Understanding the Basics of Survival Data

To understand survival analysis, you first have to understand survival data — that survival times are *intervals* between certain kinds of events, that these intervals are often affected by a peculiar kind of "partial missingness" called *censoring,* and that censored data must be analyzed in a special way to avoid biased estimates and incorrect conclusions.

Knowing that survival times are intervals

The techniques described in this chapter for summarizing, graphing, and comparing survival times deal with the time interval from a defined starting point to the first occurrence of an endpoint event. The event can be death; a relapse, like a recurrence of cancer; or the failure of a mechanical component, like a heart valve failure that requires an explant (surgical removal). For example, if a person had a heart valve implanted on January 10, but the body rejected the valve and it had to be removed on January 30, then the time interval from implant to explant is 30 – 10, or 20 days.

A person can die only once, but for other endpoints that can occur multiple times, such as stroke or seizure, the techniques I describe deal with only the first occurrence of the event. More advanced survival analysis methods, which can handle repeated occurrences, are beyond the scope of this book.

The starting point of the time interval is somewhat arbitrary, so it must be defined explicitly for every survival analysis. For example: If you're evaluating the natural history of some disease, like cancer or chronic obstructive pulmonary disease (COPD), the starting point can be the diagnosis date. If you're evaluating the efficacy of a treatment, the starting point is often defined as the date the treatment began.

Recognizing that survival times aren't normally distributed

Even though survival times are continuous or nearly continuous numerical quantities, they're almost never normally distributed. Because of this, it's generally *not* a good idea to use

✔ Means and standard deviations to describe survival times

✔ T tests and ANOVAs to compare survival times between groups

✔ Least-squares regression to investigate how survival time is influenced by other factors

If non-normality were the only problem with survival data, you'd be able to summarize survival times as medians and centiles instead of means and standard deviations, and you could compare survival between groups with nonparametric Mann-Whitney and Kruskal-Wallis tests instead of t tests and ANOVAs. But time-to-event data is susceptible to a special situation called *censoring,* which the usual parametric and non-parametric methods can't handle. So special methods have been developed to analyze censored data properly.

Considering censoring

What sets survival data apart from other kinds of numerical data is that, in many studies, you may not know the exact time of death (or other endpoint) for some subjects. This can happen in two general ways:

✔ **You may not (and usually don't) have the luxury of observing every subject until he dies.** Because of time constraints, at some point you have to end the study and analyze your data, while some of the subjects are still alive. You don't know how much longer these subjects will ultimately live; you know only that they were still alive up to the last time you or your colleagues saw them alive (such as at a clinic visit) or communicated with them in some way (such as a follow-up phone call). This is called the *date of last contact* or the *last-seen date.*

✔ **You may lose track of some subjects during the study.** Subjects can drop out of a study or leave town, never to be heard from again, becoming *lost to follow-up* (LFU). You don't know whether they're alive or dead now; you know only that they were alive at the date of last contact, before you lost track of them.

You can describe these two situations in a general way. You know that each subject either died on a certain date or was definitely alive up to some last-seen date (and you don't know how far beyond that date he may ultimately have lived). The latter situation is called a *censored* observation.

Figure 22-1 shows the results of a small study of survival in cancer patients after a surgical procedure to remove the tumor. Ten subjects were recruited and enrolled at the time of their surgery, during the period from Jan. 1, 2000, to the end of Dec. 31, 2001 (two years of enrollment). They were then followed until they died or until the conclusion of the study on Dec. 31, 2006 (five years of additional observation after the last enrollment). Each subject has a horizontal timeline that starts on the date of surgery and ends with either the death date or the censoring date.

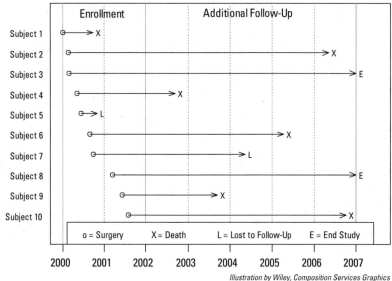

Typical Survival Data
Enroll for 2 years, then follow-up for 5 more years

Figure 22-1: Survival of ten subjects following surgery for cancer.

Six of the ten subjects (#1, 2, 4, 6, 9, and 10) died during the course of the follow-up study; two subjects (#5 and 7) were lost to follow-up at some point during the study, and two subjects (#3 and 8) were still alive at the end of the study. So this study has four subjects with censored survival times.

So how do you handle censored data like this? The following sections explain the right and wrong ways to proceed.

Dealing with censored data the right way

Statisticians have worked out the proper techniques to utilize the partial information contained in censored observations. I describe two of the most popular techniques later in this chapter — the life-table method and the Kaplan-Meier (K-M) method. To understand these methods, you need to understand two fundamental concepts — *hazard* and *survival*:

- **The hazard rate** is the probability of dying in the next small interval of time, assuming the subject is alive right now.

- **The survival rate** is the probability of living for a certain amount of time after some starting time point.

The first task when analyzing survival data is usually to describe how the hazard and survival rates vary with time. In this chapter, I show how to estimate the hazard and survival rates, and how to summarize them as tables and display them as graphs.

Most of the larger statistical packages (such as those in Chapter 4) provide the kinds of calculations I describe, so you may never have to work directly with a life table or perform a Kaplan-Meier calculation. But it's almost impossible to understand any aspect of survival analysis, from simple descriptive summaries to advanced analytical techniques, without first understanding how these two methods work.

Dealing with censored data the wrong way

Here are two ways *not* to handle censored survival data:

✔ You shouldn't exclude subjects with a censored survival time from any survival analysis.

✔ You shouldn't *impute* (replace) the censored (last-seen) date with some reasonable substitute value. One commonly used imputation scheme is to replace a missing value with the last observed value for that subject (called *last observation carried forward,* or LOCF imputation). So you may be tempted to set the death date to the last-seen date for a subject who didn't die during the observation period.

These techniques for dealing with missing data don't work for censored data. You can see why in Figure 22-2, in which the timelines for all the subjects have been slid to the left, as if they all had their surgery on the same date. The time scale now shows survival time (in years) after surgery instead of chronological time.

If you simply exclude all subjects with censored death dates from your analysis, you may be left with too few analyzable subjects (there are only six uncensored subjects in this example), which weakens (underpowers) your study. Worse, it will also bias your results in subtle and unpredictable ways.

Using the last-seen date in place of the death date for a censored observation may seem like a legitimate use of LOCF imputation, but it's not. It's equivalent to assuming that any subject who isn't known to have died must have died immediately after the last-contact date. But this assumption isn't reasonable — some subjects may live many years beyond the date you last saw them. Simply substituting last-seen dates for missing death dates will bias your results toward shorter survival times.

The problem is that a censored observation time isn't really missing; it's just not completely known. If you know that a person was last seen alive three years after treatment, you have partial information for that patient. You don't know exactly what the patient's true survival time is, but you do know that it's at least three years.

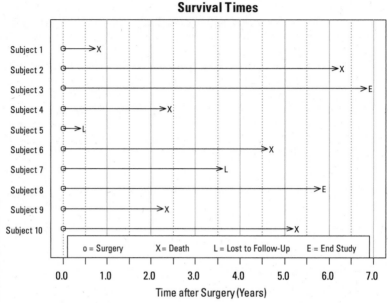

Figure 22-2: Survival times from the date of surgery.

Looking at the Life-Table Method

To estimate survival and hazard rates in a population from a set of observed survival times, some of which are censored, you must combine the information from censored and uncensored observations properly. How do you do that? First, forget about trying to get survival estimates simply by dividing the number of subjects alive at a certain time point by the total number of subjects in the study. That approach fails to account properly for the censored observations.

Instead, you have to think of the process in terms of a series of small slices of time, and think of the probability of making it through each time slice, assuming that the subject is alive at the start of that slice. The cumulative survival probability can then be obtained by successively multiplying all these individual time-slice survival probabilities together. For example, to survive three years, first the subject has to make it through Year 1, then she has to make it through Year 2, and then she has to make it through Year 3. The probability of making it through all three years is the product of the probabilities of making it through Year 1, Year 2, and Year 3.

These calculations can be laid out very systematically in a *life table,* sometimes called an *actuarial life table* because of its early use by insurance companies. The calculations involve only addition, subtraction, multiplication, and division and are simple enough to do by hand (which is how people did them before computers came along). They can also be set up very easily in a spreadsheet, and many life-table templates are freely available for Excel and other spreadsheet programs.

The following sections explain how to create, interpret, and graph information from a life table.

Making a life table

To create a life table from your survival-time data, first break the entire range of survival times into convenient slices (months, quarters, or years, depending on the time scale of the event you're studying). You should try to have at least five slices; otherwise, your survival and hazard estimates will be too coarse to show any useful features. Having very fine slices doesn't hurt the calculations, although the table will have more rows and may become unwieldy. For the survival times shown in Figure 22-2, a natural choice would be to use seven one-year time slices.

Next, count how many people died during each slice and how many were *censored* (that is, last seen alive during that slice, either because they became lost to follow-up or were still alive at the end of the study). From Figure 22-2, you see that

- During the first year after surgery, one subject died (#1), and one subject was censored (#5, who was lost to follow-up).
- During the second year, nothing happened (no deaths, no censoring).
- During the third year, two subjects died (#4 and 9), and none were censored.

Continue tabulating deaths and censored times for the fourth through seventh years, and enter these counts into the appropriate cells of a spreadsheet like the one shown in Figure 22-3:

- Put the description of the time interval that defines each slice into Column A.
- Enter the total number of subjects alive at the start into Column B, in the 0–1 yr row.
- Enter the counts of people who died within each time slice into Column C (Died).
- Enter the counts of people who were censored during each time slice into Column D (Last Seen Alive). Some statisticians prefer to split the censored subject counts into two separate columns — one for those lost to follow-up, and another for those still alive at the end of the study.

This practice makes the table a little more informative but isn't really necessary, because only the total number of censored subjects in each interval is used in the calculations. So it's a matter of personal preference; in this example, I use a single column for all censored counts.

	A	B	C	D	E	F	G	H
Formula:		B − C − D in Prev Row	(data)	(data)	B − D/2	C/E	1 − F	Running Product of G
	Time Slice	Alive at Start	Died	Last Seen Alive	At Risk	Probability of Dying	Probability of Surviving	Cumulative Survival
	0–1 yr	10	1	1				
	1–2 yr		0	0				
	2–3 yr		2	0				
	3–4 yr		0	1				
	4–5 yr		1	0				
	5–6 yr		1	1				
	6–7 yr		1	1				

Figure 22-3: A life table to analyze the survival times shown in Figure 22-2.

Illustration by Wiley, Composition Services Graphics

After you've entered all the counts, the spreadsheet will look like Figure 22-3. Then you perform the simple calculations shown in the "Formula" row at the top of the spreadsheet to generate the numbers in all the other cells of the table. In the following sections, I go through all the life-table calculations for this example, column by column.

TIP

I go through these calculations step by step to show you how they work, but you should never actually do these calculations yourself. Instead, put the formulas into the cells of a spreadsheet program so that it can do the calculations for you. Of course, if you use a preprogrammed life-table spreadsheet (which is even better), all the formulas will already be in place.

Columns B, C, and D

Column B shows the number of subjects known to be alive at the start of each year after surgery. This is equal to the number of subjects alive at the start of the preceding year minus the number of subjects who died (Column C) or were censored (Column D) during the preceding year. Here's the formula, written in terms of the column letters: B for any year = B − C − D from the preceding year.

Here's how this process plays out in Figure 22-3:

✔ Out of the ten subjects alive at the start, one died and one was last seen alive during the first year, so eight subjects (10 − 1 − 1) are known to still be alive at the start of the second year. The missing subject (#5, who was lost to follow-up during the first year) may or may not still be alive, so that censored subject isn't counted in any subsequent years.

✔ Nobody died or was last seen alive during the second year, so eight subjects are still known to be alive at the start of the third year.

✔ Calculations continue the same way for the remaining years.

Column E

Column E shows the number of subjects "at risk for dying" during each year. You may guess that this is the number of people alive at the start of the interval, but there's one minor correction. If any people were censored during that year, then they weren't really "available to die" (to use an awful expression) for the entire year. If you don't know exactly when, during that year, they became censored, then it's reasonable to "split the difference" and consider them at risk for only half the year. So the number at risk can be estimated as the number alive at the start of the year, minus one-half of the number who became censored during that year, as indicated by the formula for Column E: $E = B - D/2$.

Here's how this formula works in Figure 22-3:

✔ Ten people were alive at the start of Year 1, and one subject was censored during Year 1, so there were, in effect, only 9.5 people at risk of dying during Year 1 (1 divided by 2 is 0.5; subtract 0.5 from 10 to get 9.5).

✔ Eight people were alive at the start of Year 2, with none being censored during Year 2, so all eight people were at risk during Year 2.

✔ Calculations continue in the same way for the remaining years.

Column F

Column F shows the probability of dying during each interval, assuming the subject has survived up to the start of that interval. This is simply the number of people who died divided by the number of people at risk during each interval, as indicated by the formula for Column F: $F = C/E$.

Here's how this formula works in Figure 22-3:

✔ For Year 1, one death out of 9.5 people at risk gives a 1/9.5, or 0.105 probability of dying during Year 1.

✔ Nobody died in Year 2, so the probability of dying during Year 2 (assuming the subject has already survived Year 1) is 0.

✔ Calculations continue in the same way for the remaining years.

Column G

Column G shows the probability of surviving during each interval, assuming the subject has survived up to the start of that interval. Surviving means not dying, so the probability of surviving is simply 1 – the probability of dying, as indicated by the formula for Column G: $G = 1 - F$.

Here's how this formula works out in Figure 22-3:

✔ The probability of dying in Year 1 is 0.105, so the probability of surviving in Year 1 is 1 – 0.105, or 0.895.

✔ The probability of dying in Year 2 is 0.000, so the probability of surviving in Year 2 is 1 – 0.000, or 1.000.

✔ Calculations continue in the same way for the remaining years.

Column H

Column H shows the cumulative probability of surviving from the time of the operation all the way through the end of this time slice. To survive from the time of the operation through the end of any given year (year N), the subject must survive each of the years from Year 1 through Year N. Because surviving each year is an independent accomplishment, the probability of surviving all N of the years is the product of the individual years' probabilities. So Column H is a "running product" of Column G; that is, the value of Column H for Year N is the product of the first N values in Column G.

Here's what this looks like in Figure 22-3:

✔ For Year 1, H is the same as G: a 0.895 probability of surviving one year.

✔ For Year 2, H is the product of G for Year 1 times G for Year 2; that is, 0.895×1.000, or 0.895.

✔ For Year 3, H is the product of the Gs for Years 1, 2, and 3; that is, $0.895 \times 1.000 \times 0.750$, or 0.671.

✔ Calculations continue in the same way for the remaining years.

Putting everything together

Figure 22-4 shows the spreadsheet with the results of all the preceding calculations.

Figure 22-4: Life-table analysis of sample survival data.

	A	B	C	D	E	F	G	H
Formula:		B – C – D in Prev Row	(data)	(data)	B – D/2	C/E	1 – F	Running Product of G
	Time Slice	Alive at Start	Died	Last Seen Alive	At Risk	Probability of Dying	Probability of Surviving	Cumulative Survival
	0–1 yr	10	1	1	9.50	0.105	0.895	0.895
	1–2 yr	8	0	0	8.00	0.000	1.000	0.895
	2–3 yr	8	2	0	8.00	0.250	0.750	0.671
	3–4 yr	6	0	1	5.50	0.000	1.000	0.671
	4–5 yr	5	1	0	5.00	0.200	0.800	0.537
	5–6 yr	4	1	1	3.50	0.286	0.714	0.383
	6–7 yr	2	1	1	1.50	0.667	0.333	0.128

It's also possible to add another couple of columns to the life table to obtain standard errors and confidence intervals for the survival probabilities. The formulas aren't very complicated (they're based on the binomial distribution, described in Chapter 25), but I've omitted them from this simple example. The SEs are calculated for each year's survival probability and then combined according to the propagation-of-error rules (see Chapter 11) to get the SEs for the cumulative survival probabilities. Approximate CIs are then calculated as 1.96 SEs above and below the survival probability.

Interpreting a life table

Figure 22-4 contains the hazard rates (in Column F) and the cumulative survival probabilities (in Column H) for each year following surgery, based on your sample of ten subjects. Here are a few features of a life table that you should be aware of:

- ✔ The sample hazard and survival values obtained from a life table are only sample estimates (in this example, at 1-year time slices) of the true population hazard and survival functions.

- ✔ The slice widths are often the same for all the rows in a life table (as they are in this example), but they don't have to be. They can vary, perhaps being wider at greater survival times.

- ✔ The hazard rate obtained from a life table is equal to the probability of dying during each time slice (Column F) divided by the width of the slice, so the hazard rate for the first year would be expressed as 0.105 per year, or 10.5 percent per year.

- ✔ The cumulative survival probability, in Column H, is the probability of surviving from the operation date through to the end of the interval. It has no units, and it can be expressed as a fraction or as a percentage. The value for any time slice applies to the moment in time at the end of the interval.

- ✔ The cumulative survival probability is always 1.0 (100 percent) at time 0 (in this example, the time of surgery). This initial value isn't shown in the table.

- ✔ The cumulative survival function decreases only at the end of an interval that has at least one observed death. Censored observations don't cause a drop in the estimated survival, although they do influence the size of the drops when subsequent events occur (because censored events reduce the number of subjects at risk, which is used in the calculation of the death and survival probabilities).

- ✔ If an interval contains no events at all (no deaths and no censored subjects), like the second year (1–2 years) row in the table, it has no effect whatsoever on the calculations. All subsequent values for B and E through H remain the same as if that row had never been in the table.

Graphing hazard rates and survival probabilities from a life table

Graphs of hazard rates and survival probabilities can be prepared directly from the results of a life table calculation using almost any spreadsheet or program that can make graphs from numerical data. Figure 22-5 illustrates the way these results are typically presented.

- ✓ **Figure 22-5a is a graph of hazard rates.** Hazard rates are often graphed as bar charts, because the hazard rates are calculated for (and pertain to) each time slice in a life table.

- ✓ **Figure 22-5b is a graph of survival probabilities.** Survival values are usually graphed as *stepped line charts,* where the survival value calculated in each row of a life table "takes effect" at the end of that row's time slice. You might think it makes more sense to "connect the dots" with straight-line segments that descend gradually during each year rather than drop suddenly at the end of each year. (I certainly thought so in my early days!) But statisticians have good reasons for graphing survival "curves" as step charts, and that's how they're always shown.

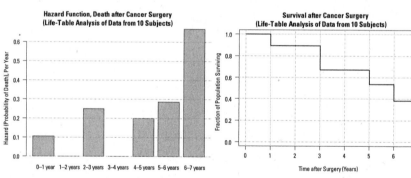

Figure 22-5: Hazard function (a) and survival function (b) results from life-table calculations.

Illustration by Wiley, Composition Services Graphics

Digging Deeper with the Kaplan-Meier Method

Using very narrow time slices doesn't hurt life-table calculations. In fact, you can define slices so narrow that each subject's survival time falls within its own private little slice. With N subjects, N rows would have one subject each; All the rest of the rows would be empty. And because empty rows don't affect the life-table calculations, you can delete them entirely, leaving a table with only *N* rows, one for each subject. (If you happen to have two or more subjects with exactly the same survival or censoring time, it's okay to put each of the subjects in a separate row.)

The life-table calculations work fine with only one subject per row and produce what's called *Kaplan-Meier (K-M) survival estimates.* You can think of the K-M method as a very fine-grained life table or a life table as a grouped K-M calculation.

A K-M worksheet for the survival times shown in Figure 22-2, based on the one-subject-per-row idea, looks like Figure 22-6. It's laid out much like the usual life-table worksheet in Figure 22-5 but with a few differences in the raw data cells and minor differences in the calculations:

- ✔ Instead of a column identifying the time slices, there are two columns (A and B) identifying the subject and the survival or censoring time, in order from the shortest time to the longest.

- ✔ Instead of two columns containing the number of subjects who died and the number of subjects who were censored in each interval, you need only one column (C) indicating whether or not the subject in that row died. You use 1 if the subject died and 0 if the subject was censored (alive at the end of the study or lost to follow-up).

- ✔ The Alive at Start column (D) now decreases by 1 for each subject.

- ✔ The At Risk column in Figure 22-5 isn't needed; the probability can be calculated from the Alive at Start column. That's because if the subject is censored, the probability of dying is calculated as 0, regardless of the value of the denominator.

- ✔ The probability of dying (Column E) is calculated as E = C/D; that is, by dividing the "Died" indicator (1 or 0) by the number of subjects alive at that time.

- ✔ The probability of surviving and the cumulative survival (Columns F and G) are calculated exactly as in the life-table method.

Figure 22-7 shows graphs of the K-M hazard and survival estimates from Figure 22-6. These charts were created using the R statistical software, but most statistics software that performs survival analysis can create graphs similar to this. The K-M survival curve in Figure 22-7b is now more fine-grained (has smaller steps) than the life-table survival curve in Figure 22-5b, because the step curve now has a drop at every time point at which a subject died (0.74 years for Subject 1, 2.27 years for Subject 9, 2.34 years for Subject 4, and so on).

A	B	C	D	E	F	G
Formula:	(data)	(data)	B − D/2	C/E	1 − E	Running Product of F
Subject	Death/Cens Time After Surgery (years)	Died	Alive at Start	Probability of Dying	Probability of Surviving	Cumulative Survival
5	0.40	0	10	0.000	1.000	1.000
1	0.74	1	9	0.111	0.889	0.889
9	2.27	1	8	0.125	0.875	0.778
4	2.34	1	7	0.143	0.857	0.667
7	3.61	0	6	0.000	1.000	0.667
6	4.62	1	5	0.200	0.800	0.533
10	5.18	1	4	0.250	0.750	0.400
8	5.80	0	3	0.000	1.000	0.400
2	6.21	1	2	0.500	0.500	0.200
3	6.85	0	1	0.000	1.000	0.200

Figure 22-6: Kaplan-Meier calculations.

Illustration by Wiley, Composition Services Graphics

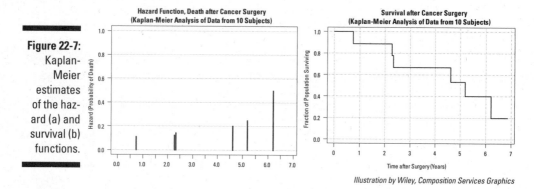

Figure 22-7: Kaplan-Meier estimates of the hazard (a) and survival (b) functions.

Illustration by Wiley, Composition Services Graphics

While the K-M survival curve tends to be smoother than the life-table survival curve, just the opposite is true for the hazard curve. In Figure 22-7a, each subject has his own very thin bar, and the resulting chart isn't easy to interpret.

Heeding a Few Guidelines for Life Tables and the Kaplan-Meier Method

Most of the larger statistical packages (SPSS, SAS, OpenStat, R, and so on; see Chapter 4) can perform life-table and Kaplan-Meier calculations for you and directly generate survival curves. The process is usually quite simple; you just have to provide the program with two variables: the survival time for each subject, and an indicator of whether that survival time represents the actual time to death or is a censored time. But you still have several golden opportunities to mess things up royally if you're not careful. Here are some pointers for setting up your data and interpreting the results properly.

Recording survival times the right way

When dealing with intervals between time points, you should enter the actual dates and times of time points and let the computer calculate the intervals between those time points. And when recording the raw data that will ultimately be used in a survival analysis, it's best to enter all the relevant dates and times — diagnosis, start of therapy, end of therapy, start of improvement or remission, relapse, event (each event if it's a recurring one), death, last seen date, and so on. Then you'll be able to calculate intervals between any starting point (diagnosis or treatment, for example) and any event (such as remission, relapse, death, and so forth).

Dates (and times) should be recorded to suitable precision. If you're dealing with things that happen over the course of months or years (like cancer), you may get by recording dates to the nearest month. But if you're interested in intervals that span only a few days (such as studying treatments for postoperative ileus), you should record dates and times to the nearest hour. When studying duration of labor, you should record time to the nearest minute. You can even envision laboratory studies of intracellular events where time would have to be recorded with millisecond — or even microsecond — precision!

Most modern spreadsheet, database, and statistical software lets you enter dates and times into a single variable (or a single cell of the spreadsheet). This is much better than having two different variables (or using two columns in a spreadsheet) — one for date and one for time of day. Having a single date/time variable lets the computer perform *calendar arithmetic* — you can obtain intervals between any two events by simple subtraction of the starting and ending date/time variables.

Recording censoring information correctly

People usually get the survival time variable right, but they may miscode the censoring indicator. The software may want you to use 0 or 1, or any two different numerical or character codes to distinguish actual from censored observations. The most common way is to use 1 if the event actually occurred (the subject died), and 0 if the observation is censored. But you might think that a variable that's referred to as the "censored" indicator should be 1 if the observation is censored and 0 if it's not censored.

Bad news: If you code the censoring indicator one way and the software is expecting it another way, the program may mistakenly process all the censored observations as uncensored and vice versa. *Worse news:* You won't get any warning or error message from the program; you'll only get incorrect results. *Worst news:* Depending on how many censored and uncensored observations you have, the survival curve may not display any sign of trouble — it may look like a perfectly reasonable survival curve for your data, even though it's completely wrong.

You have to check the software manual very carefully to make sure you code the censoring indicator the right way. Also, check the program's output for the number of censored and uncensored observations and compare them to your own manual count of censored and uncensored subjects in your data file.

Interpreting those strange-looking survival curves

Survival curves (like those shown in Figures 22-5 and 22-7) look different from most other kinds of graphs you see in biological books and publications. Not only is their stepped appearance unusual, but they also contain several kinds of "artifacts" that can easily confuse people who aren't familiar with life-table and Kaplan-Meier calculations.

- ✔ **Drops and ticks:** The drops in a K-M survival curve occur at every time point where there's an observed death and *only* at those time points. The curves do *not* drop at the times of censored observations. Most statistical software places small, vertical tick marks along the survival curve at every censored time point, so that the graph visibly displays all the censored (ticks) and uncensored (drops) data points.

- ✔ **Indistinguishable curves:** When several survival curves are plotted on the same chart, they can be very difficult to tell apart, especially if they're close together or cross over each other. The individual curves must always be drawn using different colors, different line-widths, or different line-types (solid, dashed, dotted, and so on), or they'll be almost impossible to distinguish.

- ✔ **Drastic drops in survival:** Because the magnitude of each drop in survival depends on the number at risk (in the denominator), which decreases toward the bottom of the life-table or K-M calculation, the size of the drops becomes larger at the right side of the survival chart. An extreme "artifact" of this type occurs if the subject with the longest observed time to event happens to be uncensored (for example, the subject died), in which case the curve will drop to zero, which may be completely misleading.

- ✔ **Deceptive precision:** Survival curves are usually less precise than they appear to be, and this can lead to your misjudging whether the curves for two or more groups of subjects are significantly different from each other. I say more about that in Chapter 23, dealing with how to compare survival curves.

Doing Even More with Survival Data

Besides giving you an idea of what a true population survival function looks like (the fraction of subjects surviving over the course of time), life-table and Kaplan-Meier survival curves let you estimate several useful numbers that describe survival. Figure 22-8 shows the same K-M survival curve as Figure 22-7b, but with the *Y* axis labeled as percent (rather than fraction) surviving, and with annotations showing how to estimate

✔ **The median (or other centile) survival time:** The survival curve in Figure 22-8 declines to 50 percent survival at 5.18 years, so you can say that the median survival after surgery for this cancer is about 5.2 years. Similarly, the graph indicates that 80 percent of subjects are still alive after about 2.2 years.

✔ **The five-year (or other time value) survival rate:** You can estimate from Figure 22-8 that the five-year survival rate is 53 percent, and the 2-year survival rate is about 89 percent.

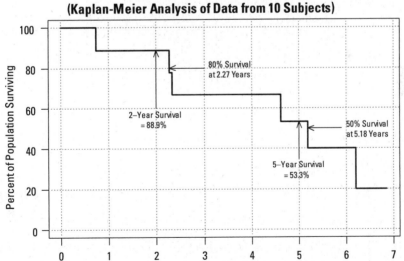

Figure 22-8:
Useful things you can get from a survival curve.

Illustration by Wiley, Composition Services Graphics

Besides preparing hazard and survival curves, you may want to do other things with your survival data:

- ✔ **Compare survival between two or more groups of subjects.** You may want to test whether subjects receiving a certain therapy survive longer than subjects receiving a placebo, whether males survive longer than females, or whether survival decreases with increasing stage or grade of disease. You can perform life-table or Kaplan-Meier calculations on each subgroup of subjects and then plot all the survival curves on the same graph. In Chapter 23, I describe how to test for significant differences in survival between two or more groups of subjects.

- ✔ **Determine whether survival is affected by other factors** (called *covariates*), such as stage of disease, subject age, prior medical history, and so on. And if so, you may want to quantify the size of that effect. You may also want to mathematically compensate for the effects of other variables when you're comparing survival between treatment groups. For other types of outcome data, this compensation is usually done by regression analysis, and you'll be happy to know that there's a special kind of regression designed just for survival outcomes. I describe it in Chapter 24.

- ✔ **Prepare a customized prognosis chart** — one that shows the expected survival curve for a particular person based on such factors as age, gender, stage of disease, and so forth. Survival regression can also generate these customized survival curves; I show you how in Chapter 24.

Chapter 23

Comparing Survival Times

In This Chapter

▶ Using the log-rank test to compare two groups

▶ Thinking about more complicated comparisons

▶ Calculating the necessary sample size

*T*he life table and Kaplan-Meier survival curves described in Chapter 22 are ideal for summarizing and describing the time to the first (or only) occurrence of some event, based on times observed in a sample of subjects. They correctly incorporate *censored* data (when a subject isn't observed long enough to experience the event). Animal studies or human studies involving endpoints that occur on a short time-scale (like duration of labor) might yield totally uncensored data, but most clinical studies will contain at least some censored observations.

In biological research (and especially in clinical trials), you often want to compare survival times between two or more groups of subjects. This chapter describes an important method — the *log-rank test* — for comparing survival between two groups and explains how to calculate the sample size you need to have sufficient statistical power (see Chapter 3) when performing this test. The log-rank test can be extended to handle three or more groups of subjects, but I don't describe that test in this book.

In this chapter, as in Chapters 22 and 24, I use the term *survival* and refer to the outcome event as death, but everything I say applies to any kind of outcome event.

A fair bit of ambiguity is associated with the name *log-rank test*. This procedure is also referred to as the Mantel-Cox test, a stratified Cochran-Mantel-Haenszel test, the Mantel-Haenszel test for survival data, the Generalized Savage's test, and the "Score Test" from the Cox Proportional Hazards model. (And I may have missed a few!) The log-rank test has also been extended in various ways; some of these variants have their own name (the Gehan-Breslow test, and Peto and Peto's modification of the Gehan test, among others). And different implementations of the log-rank test may calculate the test statistic differently, resulting in slightly different p values. In this chapter, I describe the most commonly used form of the log-rank test.

If you're lucky enough to have no censored observations in your data, you can skip most of this chapter. You simply have two (or more) groups of numbers (survival times) that you want to compare. One option is to use an unpaired Student t test to see whether one group has a significantly longer mean survival than the other (or an ANOVA if you have three or more groups), as described in Chapter 12. But because survival times are very likely to be non-normally distributed, it's safer to use a nonparametric test — you can use the Wilcoxon Sum of Ranks or Mann-Whitney U test to compare the median survival time between two groups, or the Kruskal-Wallis test for three or more groups.

Suppose you conduct a trial of a cancer drug with 90 subjects (randomized so that 60 receive the drug and 30 receive a placebo), following them for a total of five years and recording when each subject dies or is censored. You perform a life-table analysis on each group of subjects (drug and placebo) as described in Chapter 22 and graph the results, getting the survival curves shown in Figure 23-1. (The two life tables also provide the summary information you need for the log-rank test.)

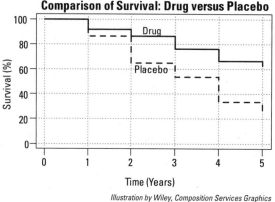

Figure 23-1: Survival curves for two groups of subjects.

Illustration by Wiley, Composition Services Graphics

The two survival curves look different — the drug group seems to be showing better survival than the placebo group. But is this apparent difference real, or could it be the result of random fluctuations only? The log-rank test answers this question.

Comparing Survival between Two Groups with the Log-Rank Test

The log rank test can be performed using individual-subject data or on data that has been summarized into a life-table format. I first describe how to run a log-rank test with statistical software; then I describe the log-rank test calculations in detail, as you might carry them out using a spreadsheet like Excel.

Understanding what the log-rank test is doing

Basically, the log-rank test asks whether deaths are split between the two groups in the same proportion as the number of at-risk subjects in the two groups. The difference between the observed and expected number of deaths in each time slice for one of the groups (it doesn't matter which one) is summed over all the time slices to get the total excess deaths for that group. The excess death sum is then *scaled down* — that is, divided by an estimate of its standard deviation. (I describe later in this chapter how that standard deviation estimate is calculated.) The scaled-down excess deaths sum is a number whose random sampling fluctuations should follow a normal distribution, from which a p value can be easily calculated.

Don't worry if the preceding paragraph makes your head spin; it's just meant to give you a general sense of the rationale for the log-rank test.

Running the log-rank test on software

Most commercial statistical software packages (like those in Chapter 4) can perform a log-rank test. You first organize your data into a file consisting of one record per subject, having the following three variables:

- ✔ A categorical variable that identifies which group each subject belongs to

- ✔ A numerical variable containing the subject's survival time (either the time to the event or the time to the end of observation)

- ✔ A variable that indicates the subject's status at the end of the survival time (usually 1 if the event was observed; 0 if the observation was censored)

You identify these three variables to the program, either by typing the variable names or by picking them from a list of variables in the data file.

The program should produce a p value for the log-rank test. If this p value is less than 0.05, you can conclude that the two groups have significantly different survival.

In addition to the p value, the program may produce the median survival time for each group as well as confidence intervals for the median times and the difference in median times between groups. It may also offer to produce analyses and graphs that assess whether your data is consistent with the hazard proportionality assumption that I describe later in this chapter. You should get these extra outputs if they're available. Consult the program's documentation for information about using the program's output to assess hazard proportionality.

Looking at the calculations

It's generally not a good idea to do log-rank tests by hand or with a home-written spreadsheet; things can go wrong in too many places. But, as with many tests that I describe in this book, you'll have a better appreciation of the strengths and limitations of the log-rank test if you understand how it works. So in this section, I describe how the log-rank calculations can be carried out in a spreadsheet environment.

The log-rank test utilizes some of the information from the life tables you prepared in order to graph the survival of the two groups in Figure 23-1. The test needs only the number of subjects at risk and the number of observed deaths for each group at each time slice. Figure 23-2 shows a portion of the life tables that produced the curves shown in Figure 23-1, with the data for the two treatment groups displayed side by side. The Drug group's results are in columns B through E, and the Placebo group's results are in columns F through I.

Figure 23-2:
Part of
life-table
calculations
for two
groups of
subjects.

A	B	C	D	E	F	G	H	I
Formula:	B – C – D in the Preceding Row	(data)	(data)	B – D/2	F – G – H in the Preceding Row	(data)	(data)	F – H/2
	Group 1: Drug				Group 2: Placebo			
Time Slice	Alive at Start	Died	Last Seen Alive	At Risk	Alive at Start	Died	Last Seen Alive	At Risk
0–1 yr	60	5	1	59.5	30	4	1	29.5
1–2 yrs	54	3	0	54.0	25	6	2	24.0
2–3 yrs	51	6	4	49.0	17	3	0	17.0
3–4 yrs	41	5	2	40.0	14	5	1	13.5
4–5 yrs	34	2	0	34.0	8	2	0	8.0

Illustration by Wiley, Composition Services Graphics

The calculations for the log-rank test are carried out in a second spreadsheet (as shown in Figure 23-3), with the following columns:

✔ Column A identifies the time slices, consistent with Figure 23-2.

✔ The log-rank test needs only the At Risk and Died columns for each group. Columns B and C of Figure 23-3 are taken from columns E and C, respectively, of Figure 23-2. Columns D and E of Figure 23-3 are taken from Columns I and G, respectively, of Figure 23-2.

✔ Columns F and G show the total number of subjects at risk and the total number of subjects who died; they're obtained by combining the corresponding columns for the two treatment groups.

✔ Column H shows Group 1's percentage of the total number of at-risk subjects.

✔ Column I shows the number of deaths you'd expect to see in Group 1 based on apportioning the total number of deaths (in both groups) by Group 1's percentage of total at-risk subjects. For the 0–1 year row, Group 1 had about 2/3 of the 89 subjects at risk, so you'd expect it to have about 2/3 of the nine deaths.

- ✔ Column J shows the excess number of actual deaths compared to the expected number for Group 1.

- ✔ Column K shows the variance (the square of the standard deviation) of the excess deaths. It's obtained from a rather complicated formula that's based on the properties of the binomial distribution (see Chapter 25):

$$V = D_T(N_1/N_T)(N_2/N_T)(N_T - D_T)/(N_T - 1)$$

For the first time slice (0–1 yr), this becomes: V = 9(59.5/89)(29.5/89) (89 – 9)/(89 – 1), which equals approximately 1.813.

N refers to the number of subjects at risk, D refers to deaths, the subscripts 1 and 2 refer to groups 1 and 2, and T refers to the total of both groups combined.

Figure 23-3:
Basic
log-rank
calcula-
tions (don't
try this
at home,
kids!).

	A	B	C	D	E	F	G	H	I	J	K
Formula:		Taken from Life Tables for Groups 1 & 2				B + D	C + E	B / F	H * G	C – I	Complicated (See Text)
		Group 1: Drug		Group 2: Placebo		Groups 1 & 2 Combined		Comparison of Observed and Expected in Group 1			
	Time Slice	At Risk	Died	At Risk	Died	At Risk	Died	% of At Risk	Expected Deaths	Excess Deaths	Variance
	0–1 yr	59.5	5	29.5	4	89.0	9	66.85%	6.02	–1.02	1.81
	1–2 yrs	54.0	3	24.0	6	78.0	9	69.23%	6.23	–3.23	1.72
	2–3 yrs	49.0	6	17.0	3	66.0	9	74.24%	6.68	–0.68	1.51
	3–4 yrs	40.0	5	13.5	1	53.5	6	74.77%	4.49	0.51	1.02
	4–5 yrs	34.0	2	8.0	2	42.0	4	80.95%	3.24	–1.24	0.57
									Sum:	–5.65	6.64

Illustration by Wiley, Composition Services Graphics

Next, you add up the excess deaths in all the time slices to get the total number of excess deaths for Group 1 compared to what you would have expected if the deaths had been distributed between the two groups in the same ratio as the number of at-risk subjects.

Then you add up all the variances, because the variance of the sum of a set of numbers is the sum of the variances of the individual numbers (from the error-propagation rules given in Chapter 11).

Then you divide the total excess deaths by the square root of the total variance to get a test statistic called Z:

$$Z = \sum ExcessDeaths \Big/ \sqrt{\sum Variances}$$

The Z value is approximately normally distributed, so you can obtain a p value from a table of the normal distribution or from an online calculator. For the data in Figure 23-3, $z = -5.65/\sqrt{6.64}$, which is 2.19, which corresponds to a p value of 0.028, so you can conclude that the two groups have significantly different survival.

Note: By the way, it doesn't matter which group (drug or placebo) you call Group 1 in these calculations; the final results are the same either way.

Assessing the assumptions

Like all statistical tests, the log-rank test assumes that you studied an unbiased sample from the population you're trying to draw conclusions about. It also assumes that any censoring that occurred was due to circumstances unrelated to the efficacy of the treatment (for example, subjects didn't drop out of the study because the drug made them sick).

One very important assumption is that the two groups have *proportional hazards.* I describe these hazards in more detail in Chapter 24, but for now the important thing to know is that the survival curves of the two groups must have generally similar shapes, as in Figure 23-4. (Flip to Chapter 22 for more about survival curves.)

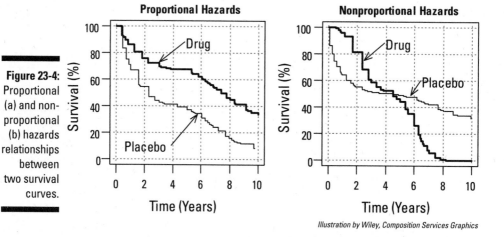

Figure 23-4: Proportional (a) and non-proportional (b) hazards relationships between two survival curves.

Illustration by Wiley, Composition Services Graphics

The log-rank test looks for differences in *overall* survival time; it's not good at detecting differences in shape between two survival curves with similar overall survival time, like the two curves shown in Figure 23-4b (which actually have the same median survival time). When two survival curves cross over each other, the excess deaths are positive for some time slices and negative for others, so they tend to cancel out when they're added up, producing a smaller test statistic (z value), and larger (less significant) p values.

Considering More Complicated Comparisons

The log-rank test is good for comparing survival between two or more groups of subjects. But it doesn't extend well to more complicated situations. What if you want to do one of the following?

- ✔ Test whether survival depends on age or some other continuous variable
- ✔ Test the simultaneous effect of several variables, or their interactions, on survival
- ✔ Correct for the presence of confounding variables or other covariates

In other areas of statistical testing, such situations are usually handled by regression techniques, so it's not surprising that statisticians have developed a special type of regression to deal with survival outcomes with censored observations. I describe this special kind of regression in Chapter 24.

Coming Up with the Sample Size Needed for Survival Comparisons

I introduce power and sample size in Chapter 3. Calculating the sample size for survival comparisons is complicated by several things:

- ✔ **The need to specify an alternative hypothesis:** This hypothesis can take the form of a hazard ratio, described in Chapter 24 (the null hypothesis is that the hazard ratio = 1), or the difference between two median survival times.

- ✔ **The effect of censoring:** This effect can depend on things like accrual rate, dropout rate, and the length of additional follow-up after the last subject has been enrolled into the study.

- ✔ **The shape of the survival curves:** This shape is often assumed, for the sake of the sample-size calculations, to be a simple exponential curve, but that may not be realistic.

I recommend using software like the free PS (Power and Sample Size Calculation; see Chapter 4) to do these calculations, because it can take a lot of these complications into account.

Suppose you're planning a study to compare a drug to a placebo. You'll have two equal-size groups, and you expect to enroll subjects for one year and then continue to follow the subjects' progress for another two years after enrollment is complete. You expect the median placebo time to be 20 months, and you think the drug should extend this to 30 months. If it truly does extend survival that much, you want to have an 80 percent chance of getting p ≤ 0.05 when you compare drug to placebo using the log-rank test.

You set up the PS program as shown in Figure 23-5. Note that time must always be entered in the same units (months, in this example) in the various fields: the median survival times for the two groups (*m1* and *m2*), the accrual interval (*A*), and the post-accrual follow-up period (*F*).

This tells you that you need to enroll 170 subjects in each group (a total of 340 subjects altogether).

Note that sample-size software often provides a brief paragraph describing the sample-size calculation, which you can copy and paste into your protocol (or proposal) document.

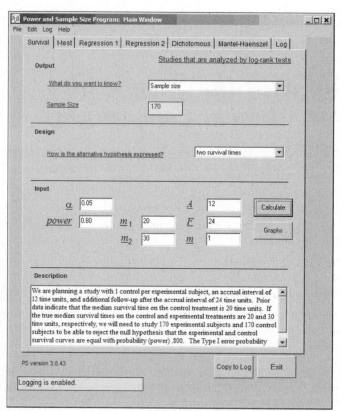

Figure 23-5: Sample-size calculation for comparing survival times using the PS program.

PS: Power and Sample Size Calculation by William D. Dupont

Chapter 24

Survival Regression

• •

In This Chapter

▶ Knowing when to use survival regression

▶ Describing the concepts behind survival regression

▶ Running and interpreting the outcome of survival regression

▶ Peeking at prognosis curves

▶ Estimating sample size for survival regression

• •

Survival regression is one of the most commonly used techniques in biostatistics. It overcomes the limitations of the log-rank test (see Chapter 23) and lets you analyze how survival time is influenced by one or more predictors (the X variables), which can be categorical or numerical (see Chapter 7). In this chapter, I introduce survival regression: when to use it, its basic concepts, running it and interpreting the output, building prognosis curves, and figuring out the sample size you need.

Note: Because time-to-event data is so often applied to survival, where the event is death, I use the terms *death* and *survival time* in this chapter, but everything I say applies also to analyzing times to the first occurrence of any event, like death, stroke, hospitalization, response to treatment, and recurrence of illness.

Knowing When to Use Survival Regression

In Chapter 22, I point out the special problems that come up when you can't follow a subject long enough to observe a death (called *censoring* of data). In that chapter, I explain how to summarize survival data with life tables and the Kaplan-Meier method, and how to graph time-to-event data as survival curves. In Chapter 23, I describe the log-rank test, which you can use to compare survival among a small number of groups — for example, drug versus placebo or four stages of cancer.

But the log-rank test has its limitations:

- ✔ **It doesn't handle numerical predictors well.** It compares survival among a small number of categories, but you may want to know how age (for example) affects survival. To use the log-rank test, you have to express the age as age-group categories (like 0–20, 21–40, 41–60, and so on) and compare survival among these categories. This test may be less efficient at detecting gradual trends across the whole age range.

- ✔ **It doesn't let you analyze the simultaneous effect of several predictors.** If you try to create subgroups of subjects for each distinct combination of categories for several predictors, you could have dozens or even hundreds of groups, most of which would have very few subjects. Suppose, for example, you have three predictors: stage of disease (four categories), age group (eight categories), and mode of treatment (five categories). There are a total of $4 \times 8 \times 5$, or 160, possible groups — one for each distinct combination of levels for the three predictors. If you have 250 subjects, most groups have only one or two subjects in them, and many groups are empty.

 Use survival regression when the outcome (the Y variable) is a time-to-event variable, like survival time; this regression lets you do any (or all) of the following:

- ✔ Determine whether there is a significant association between survival and one or more other variables

- ✔ Quantify the extent to which a variable influences survival, including testing whether survival is different between groups

- ✔ Adjust for the effects of confounding variables

- ✔ Generate a predicted survival curve (a *prognosis curve*) that is customized for any particular set of values of the predictor variables

Explaining the Concepts behind Survival Regression

Note: My explanation of survival regression has a little math in it, but nothing beyond high school algebra. For generality, I describe multiple survival regression (more than one predictor), but everything I say also applies when you have only one predictor variable.

Most kinds of regression require you to write a formula to fit to your data. The formula is easiest to understand and work with when the predictors appear in the function as a *linear combination* in which each predictor variable is multiplied by a coefficient, and these terms are all added together (perhaps with another coefficient, called an *intercept,* thrown in), like this: $y = c_0 + c_1 x_1 + c_2 x_2 + c_3 x_3$. This linear combination can also have terms with higher powers (like squares or cubes) of the predictor variables, and it can have *interaction terms* (products of two or more predictors).

Survival regression takes the linear combination and uses it to predict survival. But survival data presents some special challenges:

- ✔ **Censoring:** Censoring happens when the event doesn't occur during the time you follow the subject. You need special methods (such as life tables, the Kaplan-Meier method, and the log-rank test; see Chapters 22 and 23) to deal with this problem.

- ✔ **Survival curve shapes:** In some disciplines, such as industrial quality control, the times to certain kinds of events (like the failure of mechanical or electronic components) do tend to follow certain distribution functions, like the Weibull distribution (see Chapter 25), pretty well. These disciplines often use a *parametric* form of survival regression, which assumes that you can represent the survival curves by algebraic formulas. Early biological applications of survival regression also used parametric models. But biological data tends to produce *nonparametric* survival curves whose shapes can't be represented by any simple formulas.

Researchers wanted a hybrid, *semi-parametric* kind of survival regression: one that was partly *nonparametric* (didn't assume any mathematical formula for the shape of the overall survival curve) and partly *parametric* (assumed that the predictors influence the shape of that curve according to a mathematical relationship). Fortunately, in 1972, a statistician named David Cox came up with just such a method, called *proportional hazards (PH) regression.* His original paper is one of the most widely cited publications in the life sciences, and PH regression is often simply called *Cox regression.* In the following sections, I list the steps for Cox PH regression and explain hazard ratios.

The steps of Cox PH regression

You can understand Cox PH regression in terms of several conceptual steps, which statistical software (like the programs in Chapter 4) carry out in an integrated way during the regression:

1. **Figure out the overall shape of the survival curve by the Kaplan-Meier method.**

2. **Figure out how the predictor variables bend this curve upward or downward (how the predictors affect survival).**

3. **Determine the values of the regression coefficients that make the predicted survival times best fit your observed data.**

Figuring out the baseline

Your software may define *baseline survival function* in one of two ways:

- ✔ **The survival curve of an *average subject:*** One whose value of each predictor is equal to the group average value for that variable. The average-subject baseline is easy to understand — it's very much like the overall survival curve you get from a Kaplan-Meier calculation by using all the available subjects.

- ✔ **The survival curve of a hypothetical *zero subject:*** One whose value of each predictor is equal to 0. Some mathematicians prefer to use the *zero-subject* baseline because it makes some of their formulas simpler. But the zero-subject baseline corresponds to a hypothetical subject who can't possibly exist in the real world. Have you ever seen a person whose age is 0, weight is 0, or cholesterol level is 0? Neither have I. The survival curve for such an impossible person is so far away from reality that it usually doesn't even look like a survival curve.

Luckily, the way your software defines its baseline function doesn't affect regression coefficients, standard errors, hazard ratios, confidence intervals, p values, or goodness-of-fit measures, so you don't have to worry about it. But you should be aware of the two alternative definitions if you plan to generate prognosis curves, because the formulas to generate them are slightly different for the two different kinds of baseline function.

Bending the baseline

Now for the tricky part. How do you bend *(flex)* this baseline curve to express how survival may increase or decrease for different predictor values? Because survival curves always start at 1 (100 percent) at time 0, the bending process must leave this special point where it is. And the bending process must also leave a survival value of 0 unchanged. One very simple mathematical operation — raising a number to a power — can do the job: It leaves 1 at 1 and 0 at 0, but smoothly raises or lowers all the values between 0 and 1.

You can see how this plays out when you look at a simple baseline function: a straight line. (No actual biological survival curve would ever be exactly a straight line, but this line makes for a nice, simple example.) Look at Figure 24-1a, which is simply a graph of the equation $y = 1 - x$.

Look what happens when you raise this straight line to various powers, which I refer to as h and show in Figure 24-1b:

- ✔ Squaring ($h = 2$) the y value for every point on the line always makes the values smaller (for example, 0.8^2 is 0.64), because the y values are always less than 1.

✔ Taking the square root (h = 0.5) of the y value of every point on the line makes the y values larger (for example, the square root of 0.25 is 0.5).

✔ Both 1^2 and $1^{0.5}$ remain 1, and 0^2 and $0^{0.5}$ both remain 0, so those two ends of the line don't change.

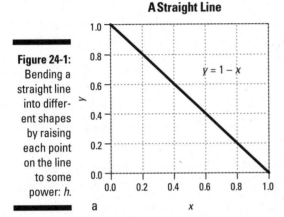

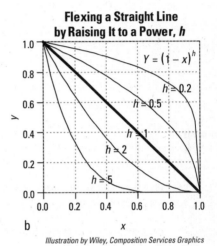

Figure 24-1: Bending a straight line into different shapes by raising each point on the line to some power: h.

Illustration by Wiley, Composition Services Graphics

Does the same trick work for a survival curve that doesn't follow any particular algebraic formula? Yes, it does; look at Figure 24-2.

✔ Figure 24-2a shows a typical survival curve. It's not defined by any algebraic formula; it exists simply as a table of values obtained by a life-table or Kaplan-Meier calculation.

✔ Figure 24-2b shows how the baseline survival curve is flexed by raising every baseline survival value to a power. You get the lower curve by squaring (h = 2) every baseline survival value; you get the upper curve by taking the square root (h = 0.5) of every baseline survival value. Notice that the two flexed curves keep all the distinctive zigs and zags of the baseline curve; every step occurs at the same time value as it occurs in the baseline curve.

• The lower curve represents a group of people who had a poorer survival outcome than those making up the baseline group. In other words, at any instant in time, they were somewhat more likely to die (had a greater hazard rate) than a baseline person at that same moment.

• The upper curve represents subjects who had better survival (had a lower hazard rate) than a baseline person at any given moment.

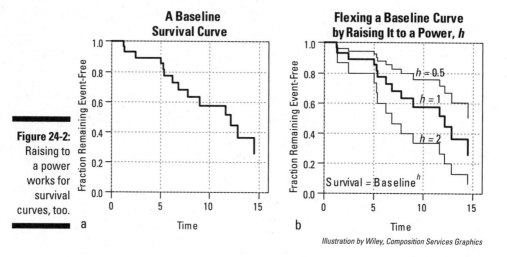

Illustration by Wiley, Composition Services Graphics

Figure 24-2: Raising to a power works for survival curves, too.

Because of the mathematical relationship between *hazard* (chance of dying at any instant in time) and *survival* (chance of surviving up to some point in time), it turns out that raising the survival curve to the *h* power is exactly equivalent to multiplying the hazard curve by the natural logarithm of *h*. Because every point in the hazard curve is being multiplied by the same amount — by *Log(h)* — raising a survival curve to a power is referred to as a *proportional hazards* transformation.

But what should the value of *h* be? The *h* value varies from one person to another. Keep in mind that the baseline curve describes the survival of a perfectly average person, but no individual is completely average. You can think of every subject as having her very own personalized survival curve, based on her very own *h* value, that provides the best estimate of that subject's chance of survival over time.

Seeing how predictor variables influence h

The final piece of the survival regression problem is to figure out how the predictor variables influence *h*, which influences survival. Any kind of regression finds the values of the coefficients that make the predicted values agree as much as possible with the observed values; likewise, Cox PH regression figures out the coefficients of the predictor variables that make the predicted survival curves agree as much as possible with the observed survival times of each subject.

How does Cox PH determine these regression coefficients? The short answer is, "Don't ask!" The longer answer is that, like all other kinds of regression, Cox PH is based on maximum likelihood estimation. You first build a big, complicated expression for the probability of one particular person dying at any point in time. This expression involves that person's predictor values and the regression coefficients. Then you construct a bigger expression giving the likelihood of getting exactly the survival times that you got for all the subjects in your data set. And as if this isn't already complicated enough, the expression has to deal with the complication of censored data. You then have to find the values of the regression coefficients that maximize this big likelihood expression. As with other kinds of regression, the calculations are far too difficult for any sane person to attempt by hand. Fortunately, computer software is available to do it for you.

Hazard ratios

Hazard ratios are among the most useful things you get from a Cox PH regression. Their role in survival regression is similar to the role of odds ratios in logistic regression (see Chapter 20), and they're even calculated the same way — by exponentiating the regression coefficients:

- **In logistic regression:** Odds ratio = $e^{\text{Regression Coefficient}}$
- **In Cox PH regression:** Hazard ratio = $e^{\text{Regression Coefficient}}$

Keep in mind that *hazard* is the chance of dying in any small period of time. Each predictor variable in a Cox PH regression has a *hazard ratio* that tells you how much the hazard increases in the relative sense (that is, by what amount it's multiplied) when you increase the variable by exactly 1.0 unit. Therefore, a hazard ratio's numerical value depends on the units in which the variable is expressed in your data. And for categorical predictors, the hazard ratio depends on how you code the categories.

For example, if a survival regression model in a study of emphysema subjects includes cigarettes smoked per day as a predictor of survival, and if the hazard ratio for this variable comes out equal to 1.05, then a person's chances of dying at any instant increase by a factor of 1.05 (5 percent) for every additional cigarette smoked per day. A 5 percent increase may not seem like much, but it's applied for every additional cigarette per day. A person who smokes one pack (20 cigarettes) per day has that 1.05 multiplication applied 20 times, which is like multiplying by 1.05^{20}, which equals 2.65. And a two-pack-per-day smoker's hazard increases by a factor of 2.65 over a one-pack-per-day smoker, which means a 2.65^2 (roughly sevenfold) increase in the chances of dying at any instant, compared to a nonsmoker.

If you change the units in which you record smoking levels from *cigarettes* per day to *packs* per day (using units that are 20 times larger), then the corresponding regression coefficient is 20 times larger, and the hazard ratio is raised to the 20th power (2.65 instead of 1.05 in this example).

Running a Survival Regression

As with all statistical methods dealing with time-to-event data, your dependent variable is actually a pair of variables:

- One variable is an event-occurrence indicator that's one of the following:

  - Equal to 1 if the event was known to occur *(uncensored)*

  - Equal to 0 if the event didn't occur during the observation period *(censored)*

- One variable is the time-to-event, which is the time from the start of observation to either the occurrence of the event (if it did occur) or to the end of the observation (if the event wasn't observed to occur). I describe time-to-event data in more detail in Chapter 22.

And as with all regression methods, you have one or more variables for the predictors. The rules for representing the predictor variables are the same as described in Chapter 19.

- For continuous numerical variables, choose units of a convenient magnitude.

- For categorical predictors, carefully consider how you record the data provided to the software and what the reference level is.

You may not be sure which variables in your data to include as predictors in the regression. I discuss this model-building problem in Chapter 19; the same principles apply to survival regression.

After you assemble and properly code the data, running the program is no more complicated than running it for ordinary least-squares or logistic regression. You need to specify the variables in the regression model:

1. **Specify the two components of the outcome event:**

   - Time to event

   - Censoring indicator

2. **Specify the predictor variables.**

   Specify the reference level (see Chapter 23) for categorical predictors if the software lets you do that.

Most software also lets you specify the kinds of output you want to see. You should always specify at least the following:

- Coefficients table, including hazard ratios and confidence intervals

- Tests of whether the hazard proportionality assumption is valid

You may also want to see some or all of the following:

✔ Summary descriptive statistics on the data, including number of censored and uncensored observations, median survival time, and mean and standard deviation for each predictor variable in the model

✔ One or more measures of goodness-of-fit for the model

✔ Baseline survival function (as a table of values and as a survival curve)

✔ Baseline hazard function values (as a table and graph)

After you specify all the input to the program, click the Start button, and let the computer do all the work.

Interpreting the Output of a Survival Regression

Suppose you have conducted a long-term survival study of 200 cancer patients who were enrolled at various stages of the disease (1 through 4) and were randomized to receive either chemotherapy or radiation therapy. Subjects were followed for up to ten years, after which the survival data was summarized by treatment (Figures 24-3a and 24-3b for the two treatments) and by stage of disease.

It would appear, from Figure 24-3, that chemotherapy and greater stage of disease are both associated with poorer survival, but are these apparent effects significant? Proportional-hazards regression can tell you that, and more.

Figure 24-3:
Kaplan-
Meier
survival
curves,
by treat-
ment and
by stage of
disease.

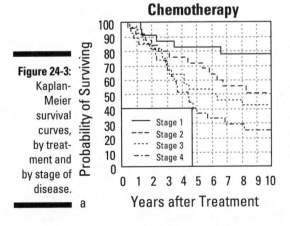

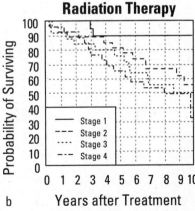

Illustration by Wiley, Composition Services Graphics

To run a proportional-hazards regression on the data from this example, you must provide the following data to the software:

✔ The time from treatment to death or censoring (a numerical variable *Time,* in years).

✔ The indicator of whether the subject died or was censored (a variable *Status,* set to 1 if the subject died or 0 if the subject was last seen alive).

✔ The treatment group (a categorical variable *Tx,* coded as Chemo or Radiation). In this example, I didn't say which treatment was the reference level (see the discussion of reference levels in Chapter 19), so R took Chemo (which came before Radiation alphabetically) as the reference level.

✔ The stage of disease at the time of treatment (a numerical variable *Stage,* equal to 1, 2, 3, or 4). Using a numerical variable as Stage implies the assumption that every successive increase in stage number by 1 is associated with a constant relative increase in hazard. If you don't want to make that assumption, you must code Stage as a categorical variable, with four levels (Stage 1 through Stage 4).

Using the R statistical software, the proportional hazards regression can be invoked with a single command:

```
coxph(formula = Surv(Time, Status) ~ Stage + Tx)
```

Figure 24-4 shows R's results, using the data that I graph in Figure 24-3. The output from other statistical programs won't look exactly like Figure 24-4, but you should be able to find the main components described in the following sections.

```
Call: coxph(formula = Surv(Time, Status) ~ Stage + Tx)

  n= 200, number of events= 92

                 coef exp(coef)  se(coef)     z Pr(>|z|)
Stage          0.4522    1.5717    0.1013 4.463 8.09e-06 ***
TxRadiation   -0.4323    0.6490    0.2116 -2.043  0.0411 *
---
Signif. codes:  0 '***' 0.001 '**' 0.01 '*' 0.05 '.' 0.1 ' ' 1

             exp(coef) exp(-coef) lower .95 upper .95
Stage            1.572     0.6362    1.2886    1.9170
TxRadiation      0.649     1.5407    0.4287    0.9826

Concordance= 0.642   (se = 0.031 )
Rsquare= 0.116    (max possible= 0.99 )
Likelihood ratio test= 24.64  on 2 df,    p=4.46e-06
Wald test            = 23.31  on 2 df,    p=8.67e-06
Score (logrank) test = 24.36  on 2 df,    p=5.124e-06
```

Figure 24-4:
Output of a Cox PH regression.

Illustration by Wiley, Composition Services Graphics

Testing the validity of the assumptions

When you're analyzing data by PH regression, you're assuming that your data is really consistent with the idea of flexing a baseline survival curve by raising all the points in the entire curve to the same power (shown as *h* in Figures 24-1b and 24-2b). You're not allowed to *twist* the curve so that it goes higher than the baseline curve ($h < 1$) for small time values and lower than baseline ($h > 1$) for large time values. That would be a non-PH flexing of the curve.

One quick check to see whether a predictor is affecting your data in a non-PH way is to take the following steps:

1. **Split your data into two groups, based on the predictor.**

2. **Plot the Kaplan-Meier survival curve for each group (see Chapter 22).**

If the two survival curves show the slanted figure-eight pattern shown in Figure 24-5, don't try to use Cox PH regression on that data. (At least don't include that predictor variable in the model.)

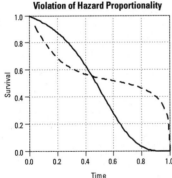

Figure 24-5: Don't try proportional-hazards regression on this kind of data.

Illustration by Wiley, Composition Services Graphics

Your statistical software may offer several options to test the hazard-proportionality assumption. Check your software's documentation to see what it offers (which may include the following) and how to interpret its output.

✔ Graphs of the hazard functions versus time, which let you see the extent to which the hazards are proportional.

✔ A statistical test for significant hazard non-proportionality. R provides a function called cox.zph for this purpose; other packages may offer a comparable option.

Checking out the table of regression coefficients

A regression coefficients table in a survival regression looks very much like the tables produced by almost all kinds of regression: ordinary least-squares, logistic, Poisson, and so on. The survival regression table has a row for every predictor variable, usually containing the following items:

- ✔ **The value of the *regression coefficient.*** Not too meaningful by itself, it tells how much the hazard ratio's logarithm increases when the predictor variable increases by exactly 1.0 unit. In Figure 24-4, the coefficient for Stage is 0.4522, indicating that every increase of 1 in the stage of the disease (going from 1 to 2, from 2 to 3, or from 3 to 4) increases the logarithm of the hazard by 0.4522 (more advanced stage of disease is associated with poorer survival). For a categorical predictor like treatment (Tx), there will be a row in the table for each non-reference level (in this case, a line for Radiation). The coefficient for Radiation is –0.4323; the negative sign indicates that Radiation has less hazard (better survival) than Chemo.

- ✔ **The coefficient's *standard error* (SE),** which is a measure of the precision of the regression coefficient. The SE of the Stage coefficient is 0.1013, so you would express the Stage coefficient as 0.45 ± 0.10.

- ✔ **The coefficient divided by its SE** (often designated as *t* or *Wald*).

- ✔ **The *p value.*** If less than 0.05, it indicates that the coefficient is significantly different from 0 (that is, the corresponding predictor variable is significantly associated with survival) after adjusting for the effects of all the other variables (if any) in the model. The p value for Stage is shown as 8.09e–06, which is scientific notation for 0.000008, indicating that Stage is very significantly associated with survival.

- ✔ **The *hazard ratio* and its confidence limits,** which I describe in the next section.

You may be surprised that no intercept (or constant) row is in the table. Cox PH regression doesn't include an intercept in the linear part of the model; the intercept is absorbed into the baseline survival function.

Homing in on hazard ratios and their confidence intervals

Hazard ratios from survival and other time-to-event data are used extensively as safety and efficacy outcomes of clinical trials, as well as in large-scale epidemiological studies. Depending on how the software formats its output, it may show the hazard ratio for each predictor in a separate column in the regression table, or it may create a separate table just for the hazard ratios and their confidence intervals.

If the software doesn't give hazard ratios or their confidence intervals, you can calculate them from the regression coefficients *(Coef)* and standard errors *(SE)* as follows:

- ✔ Hazard Ratio = e^{Coef}
- ✔ Low 95 percent CI = $e^{Coef - 1.96 \times SE}$
- ✔ High 95 percent CI = $e^{Coef + 1.96 \times SE}$

Hazard ratios are useful and meaningful measures of the extent to which a variable influences survival.

- ✔ A hazard ratio of 1 (which corresponds to a regression coefficient of 0) indicates that the variable has no effect on survival.

- ✔ The confidence interval around the hazard ratio estimated from your data sample indicates the range in which the true hazard ratio (of the population from which your sample was drawn) probably lies.

In Figure 24-4, the hazard ratio for Stage is $e^{0.4522}$ = 1.57, with a 95 percent confidence of 1.29 to 1.92 per unit of stage number, which means that every increase of 1 in the stage of the disease is associated with a 57 percent increase in hazard (multiplying by 1.57 is equivalent to a 57 percent increase). Similarly, the hazard ratio for Radiation relative to Chemo is 0.649, with a 95 percent confidence interval of 0.43 to 0.98.

Risk factors (such as smoking relative to nonsmoking) usually have hazard ratios greater than 1. *Protective factors* (such as drug relative to placebo) usually have hazard ratios less than 1.

Assessing goodness-of-fit and predictive ability of the model

There are several measures of how well a regression model fits the survival data. These measures can be useful when you're choosing among several different models:

- ✔ Should you include a possible predictor variable (like Age) in the model?

- ✔ Should you include the squares or cubes of predictor variables in the model (like Age^2 or Age^3 in addition to Age)?

- ✔ Should you include a term for the interaction between two predictors? (See Chapter 19 for details on interactions.)

Your software may offer one or more of the following goodness-of-fit measures:

- A measure of *concordance,* or agreement, between the observed and predicted outcomes — the extent to which subjects with higher predicted hazard values had shorter observed survival times (which is what you'd expect). Figure 24-4 shows a concordance of 0.642 for this regression.

- An R (or R^2) value that's interpreted like a correlation coefficient in ordinary regression — the larger the R^2 value, the better the model fits the data. In Figure 24-4, R-square is 0.116.

- A likelihood ratio number (and associated p value) that compares the full model (that includes all the parameters) to a model consisting of just the overall baseline function. In Figure 24-4, the likelihood ratio p value is shown as 4.46e–06, which is scientific notation for p = 0.00000446, indicating a model that includes the Tx and Stage variables can predict survival significantly better than just the overall (baseline) survival curve.

- *Akaike's Information Criterion* (AIC) or *Bayesian Information Criterion* (BIC), which are especially useful for comparing alternative models (see Chapter 19).

Focusing on baseline survival and hazard functions

The *baseline survival function* is represented as a table with two columns (time and predicted survival) and a row for each distinct time at which one or more events were observed.

The baseline survival function's table may have hundreds of rows for large data sets, so printing it isn't often useful. But if your software can save the table as a data file, you can use it to generate a customized prognosis curve for any specific set of values for the predictor variables. (I talk about prognosis curves in the following section.)

The software may also offer a graph of the baseline survival function. If your software is using an "average-subject" baseline, this graph is useful as an indicator of the entire group of subjects' overall survival. But if your software uses a "zero-subject" baseline, the curve is probably of no use.

The *baseline hazard function* may also be available as a table or as a graph, which provides insight into the course of the disease. Some diseases have a long *latency period* (time during which little seems to be happening) during which deaths are relatively infrequent, whereas other diseases are more aggressive, with many early deaths.

How Long Have I Got, Doc? Constructing Prognosis Curves

One of the (many) reasons for doing any kind of regression analysis is to predict outcomes from any particular set of predictor values, and survival regression is no exception: You can use the regression coefficients from a Cox PH regression, along with the baseline survival curve, to construct an *expected survival (prognosis)* curve for any set of predictor values.

Suppose you're an oncologist who's analyzing survival time (from diagnosis to death) for a group of cancer patients in which the predictors are age, tumor stage, and tumor grade at the time of diagnosis. You'd run a Cox PH regression on your data and have the program generate the baseline survival curve as a table of times and survival probabilities. Then, if you (or any other doctor) diagnose a patient with cancer, you can take that person's age, stage, and grade, and generate an expected survival curve tailored for that particular person. (I'm not sure I'd want to see that curve if I were the patient, but at least it could be done.)

You'll probably have to do these calculations outside of the software that you use for the survival regression, but the calculations aren't difficult, and can easily be done in a spreadsheet. The example in the following sections shows how it's done, using the rather trivial set of sample data that's preloaded into the online calculator for Cox PH regression at StatPages.info/prophaz.html. This particular example has only one predictor, but the basic idea extends to multiple predictors in a simple way, which I explain as I go.

Running the proportional-hazards regression

Figure 24-6 shows the output from the built-in example (omitting the Iteration History and Overall Model Fit sections). Pretend that this data represents survival, in years, as a function of Age (which, in this output, is referred to as Variable 1) for people just diagnosed with some particular disease.

First, consider the table in the Baseline Survivor Function section, which has two columns — time (years) and predicted survival (as a fraction) — and four rows — one for each time point in which one or more deaths was actually observed. The baseline survival curve for the dummy data starts (as survival curves always do) at 1.0 (100 percent survival) at time 0. (This row isn't shown in the output.) The survival curve remains flat at 100 percent until year two, when it suddenly drops down to 99.79 percent, where it stays until year seven, when it drops down to 98.20 percent, and so on.

```
Descriptive Stats...


Variable          Avg             SD
   1            51.1818        10.9778



Coefficients, Std Errs, Signif, and Conf Intervs...
   Var        Coeff.    StdErr       p       Lo95%      Hi95%
    1         0.3770    0.2542    0.1379    -0.1211    0.8752
```

Figure 24-6:

Output of Cox PH regression for generating prognostic curves.

```
Risk Ratios and Confidence Intervs...
   Var     Risk Ratio    Lo95%      Hi95%
    1         1.4580     0.8859     2.3993


Baseline Survivor Function (at predictor means)...
    2.0000     0.9979
    7.0000     0.9820
    9.0000     0.9525
   10.0000     0.8310
```

Illustration by Wiley, Composition Services Graphics

In the Descriptive Stats section near the start of the output, the average age of the 11 subjects in the test data set is 51.1818 years, so the baseline survival curve shows the predicted survival for a person who is exactly 51.1818 years old. But suppose you want to generate a survival curve that's customized for a person who is, say, 55 years old. According to the proportional-hazards model, you need to raise the entire baseline curve (in this case, each of the four tabulated points) to some power: h.

In general, h depends on two things:

✔ The particular value for that subject's predictor variables (in this example, an Age of 55)

✔ The values of the corresponding regression coefficients (in this example, 0.3770, from the regression table)

Finding h

To calculate the h value, do the following for each predictor:

1. **Subtract the average value from the patient's value.**

   In this example, you subtract the average age (51.18) from the patient's age (55), giving a difference of +3.82.

2. **Multiply the difference by the regression coefficient and call the product v.**

In this example, you multiply 3.82 from Step 1 by the regression coefficient for Age (0.377), giving a product of 1.44 for v.

3. **Calculate the v value for each predictor in the model.**

4. **Add all the v values; call the sum of the individual v values V.**

This example has only one predictor variable (Age), so V is just the v value you calculate for age in Step 2 (1.44).

5. **Calculate e^V.**

This is the value of h. In this example, $e^{1.44}$ gives the value 4.221, which is the h value for a 55-year-old person.

6. **Raise each of the baseline survival values to the power of h to get the survival values for the prognosis curve.**

In this example, you have the following prognosis:

- For year-zero survival $1.000^{4.221} = 1.000$, or 100 percent
- For two-year survival: $0.9979^{4.221} = 0.9912$, or 99.12 percent
- For seven-year survival $0.9820^{4.221} = 0.9262$, or 92.62 percent
- For nine-year survival $0.9525^{4.221} = 0.8143$, or 81.43 percent
- For ten-year survival $0.8310^{4.221} = 0.4578$, or 45.78 percent

You then graph these calculated survival values to give a customized survival curve for this particular person. And that's all there is to it!

Here's a short version of the procedure:

1. **V = sum of [(subject value – average value) * coefficient] summed over all the predictors**

2. **$h = e^V$**

3. **Customized survival = (baseline survival)^h**

Some points to keep in mind:

- ✔ If your software puts out a zero-based baseline survival function, then the only difference is that you don't subtract the average value from the subject's value; instead, calculate the v term as the simple product of the subject's predictor value multiplied by the regression coefficient.

- ✔ If a predictor is a categorical variable, you have to code the levels as numbers. If you have a dichotomous variable like gender, you could code male = 0 and female = 1. Then if, for example, 47.2 percent of the subjects are female, the "average gender" is 0.472, and the subtraction in Step 1 is (0 – 0.472), giving –0.472 if the patient is male, or (1 – 0.472), giving 0.528 if the subject is female. Then you carry out all the other steps exactly as described.

✔ It's even a little trickier for multivalued categories like race or district, because you have to code each of these variables as a set of dummy variables (see Chapter 19).

Estimating the Required Sample Size for a Survival Regression

Note: Elsewhere in this chapter, I use the word *power* in its algebraic sense (x^2 is x to the power of 2). But in this section, I use *power* in its statistical sense: the probability of getting a significant result when performing a statistical test.

Sample-size calculations for regression analysis tend to be difficult for all but the simplest straight-line regressions (see Chapter 18). You can find software for many types of regression, including survival, but it often asks you for things you can't readily provide.

Very often, sample-size estimates for studies that use regression methods to analyze the data are based on simpler analytical methods. I recommend that when you're planning a Cox PH regression, you base your sample-size estimate on the simpler log-rank test, which I describe in Chapter 23. The free PS-Power and Sample Size program handles these calculations very well.

You still have to specify the following:

✔ **Alpha level** (usually 0.05)

✔ **Desired power** (usually 80 percent)

✔ **Effect size of importance** (usually expressed as a hazard ratio or as the difference in median survival time between groups)

You also need some estimates of the following:

✔ **Anticipated enrollment rate:** How many subjects you hope to enroll per month or per year

✔ **Planned duration of follow-up:** How long, after the last subject has been enrolled, you plan to continue following all the subjects before ending the study and analyzing your data

I describe power calculations for survival comparisons in Chapter 23.

If this simpler approach isn't satisfactory, talk to a professional statistician, who will have access to more sophisticated software. Or, you can undertake a Monte-Carlo simulation of the proposed trial and regression analysis (see Chapter 3 for details on this simulation), but this task is seldom necessary.

Part VI
The Part of Tens

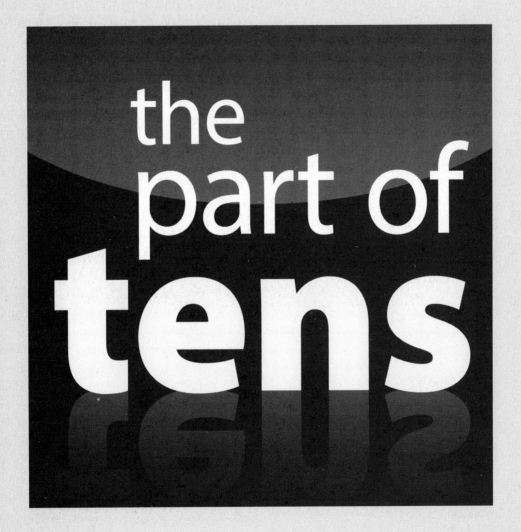

Check out an additional Part of Tens list all about names every biostatistician should know at www.dummies.com/extras/biostatistics.

In this part . . .

- ✔ Find common statistical distributions that describe how your data may fluctuate and common distribution functions that arise in statistical significance testing.

- ✔ Follow simple rules for getting quick estimates of the number of subjects you need for a properly designed study.

Chapter 25

Ten Distributions Worth Knowing

In This Chapter

▶ Delving into distributions that often describe your data

▶ Digging into distributions that arise during statistical significance testing

This chapter describes ten statistical distribution functions you'll probably encounter in biological research. For each one I provide a graph of what that distribution looks like as well as some useful or interesting facts and formulas.

You find two general types of distributions here:

✔ **Distributions that describe random fluctuations in observed data:** Your experimental data will often conform to one of the first seven common distributions. These distributions have one or two adjustable parameters that let them "fit" the fluctuations in your observed data.

✔ **Common test statistic distributions:** The last three distributions — the Student t, chi-square, and Fisher F distributions — don't describe your observed data; they describe how a test statistic (calculated as part of a statistical significance test) will fluctuate if the null hypothesis is true — that is, if the apparent effects in your data (differences between groups, associations between variables, and so on) are due only to random fluctuations. So, they're used to obtain p values, which indicate the statistical significance of the apparent effects. (See Chapter 3 for more information on significance testing and p values.)

This chapter provides a very short table of *critical values* for the t, chi-square, and F distributions — the value that your calculated test statistic must exceed in order for you to declare significance at the $p < 0.05$ level. For example, the critical value for the normal distribution is 1.96 for the 0.05 significance level.

The Uniform Distribution

The uniform distribution is one of the simplest distributions — a continuous number between 0 and 1 or (more generally) between a and b, with all values within that range equally likely (see Figure 25-1). The uniform distribution has a mean value of $(b + a)/2$ and a standard deviation of $(b - a)/\sqrt{12}$. The uniform distribution arises in the following contexts:

- ✔ Round-off errors are uniformly distributed. For example, a weight recorded as 85 kilograms can be thought of as a uniformly distributed random variable between 84.5 and 85.5 kilograms, with a standard error of 0.29 kilogram.

- ✔ The p value from any exact significance test is uniformly distributed between 0 and 1 if, and only if, the null hypothesis is true.

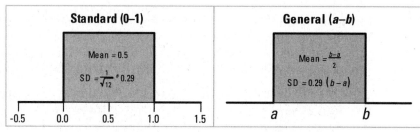

Figure 25-1:
The uniform distribution.

Illustration by Wiley, Composition Services Graphics

The Excel formula =RAND() generates a random number drawn from the standard uniform distribution.

The Normal Distribution

The normal distribution is the king of statistical distributions. It describes variables whose fluctuations are the combined result of many independent causes. Figure 25-2 shows the shape of the normal distribution for various values of the mean and standard deviation.

Many other distributions (binomial, Poisson, Student t, chi-square, Fisher F) become nearly normal-shaped for large samples.

The Excel statement =NORMSINV(RAND()) generates a normally distributed random number, with mean = 0 and SD = 1.

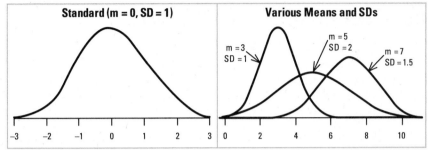

Figure 25-2: The normal distribution.

Illustration by Wiley, Composition Services Graphics

The Log-Normal Distribution

If a set of numbers (x) is log-normally distributed, then the logarithms of those numbers will be normally distributed (see the preceding section). Many enzyme and antibody concentrations are log-normally distributed. Hospital lengths of stay, charges, and costs are approximately log-normal.

You should suspect log-normality if the standard deviation of a set of numbers is comparable in magnitude to the mean of those numbers. Figure 25-3 shows the relationship between the normal and log-normal distributions.

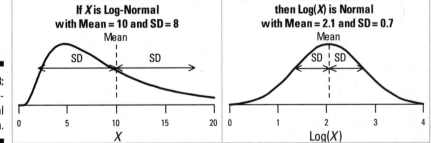

Figure 25-3: The log-normal distribution.

Illustration by Wiley, Composition Services Graphics

If a set of log-normal numbers has a mean A and standard deviation D, then the natural logarithms of those numbers will have a standard deviation $s = \text{Log}[1 + (D/A)^2]$, and a mean $m = \text{Log}(A) - s^2/2$.

The Binomial Distribution

The binomial distribution tells the probability of getting *x* successes out of *N* independent tries when the probability of success on one try is *p*. (See Chapter 3 for an introduction to probability.) The binomial distribution describes, for example, the probability of getting *x* heads out of *N* flips of a fair (*p* = 0.5) or lopsided (*p* ≠ 0.5) coin. Figure 25-4 shows the frequency distributions of three binomial distributions, all having *p* = 0.7 but having different *N* values.

Figure 25-4:
The binomial distribution.

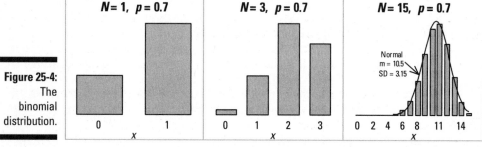

Illustration by Wiley, Composition Services Graphics

The formula for the probability of getting *x* successes in *N* tries when the probability of success on one try is *p* is $Pr(x, N, p) = p^x(1 - p)^{N-x}N!/[x!(N - x)!]$.

As *N* gets large, the binomial distribution's shape approaches that of a normal distribution with mean = *Np* and standard deviation = $\sqrt{Np(1-p)}$. (I talk about the normal distribution later in this chapter.)

The arc-sine of the square root of a set of proportions is approximately normally distributed, with a standard deviation of $1/\sqrt{4N}$. Using this "transformation," you can analyze data consisting of observed proportions (such as fraction of subjects responding to a treatment) with t tests, ANOVAs, regression models, and other methods designed for normally distributed data.

The Poisson Distribution

The Poisson distribution gives the probability of observing exactly *N* independent random events in some interval of time or region of space if the mean event rate is *m*. It describes, for example, fluctuations in the number of nuclear decay counts per minute and the number of pollen grains per square centimeter on a microscope slide. Figure 25-5 shows the Poisson distribution for three different values of the mean event rate.

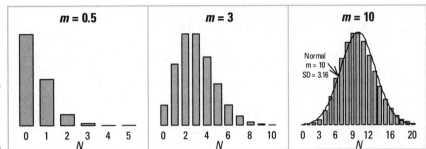

Figure 25-5:
The Poisson distribution.

Illustration by Wiley, Composition Services Graphics

The formula is $\Pr(N, m) = m^N e^{-m}/N!$

As *m* gets large, the Poisson distribution's shape approaches that of a normal distribution (see the next section), with mean = *m* and standard deviation = $\sqrt{m}$.

The square roots of a set of Poisson-distributed numbers are approximately normally distributed, with a standard deviation of 1/2.

The Exponential Distribution

If a set of events follows the Poisson distribution (which I discuss earlier in this chapter), the *time intervals* between consecutive events follow the exponential distribution and vice versa. Figure 25-6 shows the shape of two different exponential distributions.

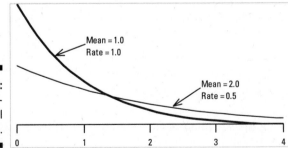

Figure 25-6:
The exponential distribution.

Illustration by Wiley, Composition Services Graphics

The Excel statement = –LN(RAND()) makes exponentially distributed random numbers with mean = 1.

The Weibull Distribution

This function describes failure times for people or devices (such as light bulbs), where the failure rate can be constant or can change over time depending on the *shape parameter, k*. The failure rate is proportional to time raised to the $k - 1$ power, as shown in Figure 25-7a.

- ✔ If $k < 1$, the failure rate declines over time (with lots of early failures).
- ✔ If $k = 1$, the failure rate is constant over time (corresponding to an exponential distribution).
- ✔ If $k > 1$, the failure rate increases over time (as items wear out).

Figure 25-7b shows the corresponding cumulative survival curves.

Figure 25-7:
The Weibull
distribution.

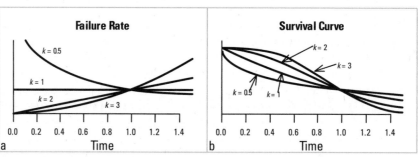

Illustration by Wiley, Composition Services Graphics

This distribution leads to survival curves of the form $Survival = 1 - e^{-Time^k}$, which are widely used in industrial statistics. But survival methods that don't assume any particular formula for the survival curve are more common in biostatistics.

The Student t Distribution

This family of distributions is most often used when comparing means between two groups or between two paired measurements. Figure 25-8 shows the shape of the Student t distribution for various degrees of freedom. (See Chapter 12 for more info about t tests and degrees of freedom.)

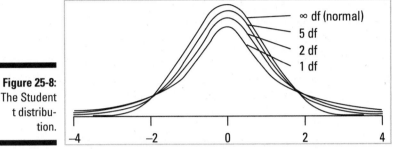

Figure 25-8:
The Student t distribution.

As the degrees of freedom increase, the shape of the Student t distribution approaches that of the normal distribution that I discuss earlier in this chapter.

Table 25-1 shows the "critical" t value for various degrees of freedom.

Random fluctuations cause t to exceed the critical t value (on either the positive or negative side) only 5 percent of the time. If the t value from your Student t test exceeds this value, the test is significant at $p < 0.05$.

Table 25-1	Critical Values of Student t for $p = 0.05$
Degrees of Freedom	t_{crit}
1	12.71
2	4.30
3	3.18
4	2.78
5	2.57
6	2.45
8	2.31
10	2.23
20	2.09
50	2.01
∞	1.96

For other p and df values, the Excel formula =TINV(p, df) gives the critical Student t value.

The Chi-Square Distribution

This family of distributions is used for testing goodness-of-fit between observed and expected event counts and for testing for association between categorical variables. Figure 25-9 shows the shape of the chi-square distribution for various degrees of freedom. (See Chapter 13 for more info about the chi-square test and degrees of freedom.)

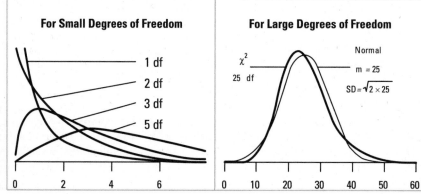

Figure 25-9: The chi-square distribution.

Illustration by Wiley, Composition Services Graphics

As the degrees of freedom increase, the shape of the chi-square distribution approaches that of the normal distribution that I discuss earlier in this chapter.

Table 25-2 shows the "critical" chi-square value for various degrees of freedom.

Random fluctuations cause chi-square to exceed the critical chi-square value only 5 percent of the time. If the chi-square value from your test exceeds the critical value, the test is significant at $p < 0.05$.

Table 25-2	Critical Values of Chi-Square for $p = 0.05$
Degrees of Freedom	$\chi^2 Crit$
1	3.84
2	5.99
3	7.81
4	9.49

Degrees of Freedom	χ^2Crit
5	11.07
6	12.59
7	14.07
8	15.51
9	16.92
10	18.31

For other p and df values, the Excel formula =CHIINV(p, df) gives the critical χ^2 value.

The Fisher F Distribution

This family of distributions is most frequently used to get p values from an analysis of variance (ANOVA). Figure 25-10 shows the shape of the Fisher F distribution for various degrees of freedom. (See Chapter 12 for more info about ANOVAs and degrees of freedom.)

Figure 25-10:
The Fisher F
distribution.

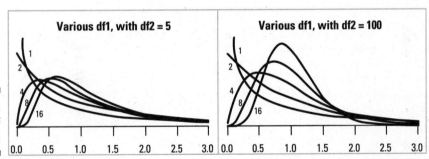

Illustration by Wiley, Composition Services Graphics

Figure 25-11 shows the "critical" Fisher F value for various degrees of freedom.

Random fluctuations cause F to exceed the critical F value only 5 percent of the time. If the F value from your ANOVA exceeds this value, the test is significant at $p < 0.05$.

	df₁							
	1	**2**	**3**	**4**	**5**	**6**	**7**	**8**
1	161.4	199.5	215.7	224.6	230.2	234.0	236.8	238.9
2	18.51	19.00	19.16	19.25	19.30	19.33	19.35	19.37
3	10.13	9.55	9.28	9.12	9.01	8.94	8.89	8.85
4	7.71	6.94	6.59	6.39	6.26	6.16	6.09	6.04
5	6.61	5.79	5.41	5.19	5.05	4.95	4.88	4.82
6	5.99	5.14	4.76	4.53	4.39	4.28	4.21	4.15
8	5.32	4.46	4.07	3.84	3.69	3.58	3.50	3.44
10	4.96	4.10	3.71	3.48	3.33	3.22	3.14	3.07
15	4.54	3.68	3.29	3.06	2.90	2.79	2.71	2.64
20	4.35	3.49	3.10	2.87	2.71	2.60	2.51	2.45
30	4.17	3.32	2.92	2.69	2.53	2.42	2.33	2.27
50	4.03	3.18	2.79	2.56	2.40	2.29	2.20	2.13
100	3.94	3.09	2.70	2.46	2.31	2.19	2.10	2.03
200	3.89	3.04	2.65	2.42	2.26	2.14	2.06	1.98
∞	3.84	3.00	2.60	2.37	2.21	2.10	2.01	1.94

(Left axis label: df_2)

Figure 25-11: Critical values of Fisher F for $p = 0.05$.

df_1 ("numerator" degrees of freedom) = # of Groups – 1.

df_2 ("denominator" degrees of freedom) = # of Cases – # of Groups.

Illustration by Wiley, Composition Services Graphics

For other values of p, df_1, and df_2, the Excel formula =FINV(p, df_1, df_2) will give the critical F value.

Chapter 26

Ten Easy Ways to Estimate How Many Subjects You Need

· ·

In This Chapter

▶ Quickly estimating sample size for several basic kinds of tests

▶ Adjusting for different levels of power and alpha

▶ Adjusting for unequal group sizes and for attrition during the study

· ·

Sample-size calculations tend to frighten researchers and send them running to the nearest statistician. But if you're brainstorming a possible research project and you need a ballpark idea of how many subjects to enroll, you can use the ten quick and (fairly) easy rules of thumb in this chapter.

Before you begin, look at Chapter 3, especially the sections on hypothesis testing and the power of a test, so that you have the basic idea of what power and sample-size calculations are all about. Think about the *effect size of importance* (such as the difference in some variable between two groups, or the degree of correlation between two variables) that you want to be able to detect. Then find the rule for the statistical test that's appropriate for the primary objective of your study.

The first six sections tell you how many analyzable subjects you need to analyze in order to have an 80 percent chance of getting a p value that's less than 0.05 when you run the test. Those parameters (80 percent power at 0.05 alpha) are widely used in biological research. The remaining four sections tell you how to modify this figure for other power or alpha values and how to adjust for unequal group size and dropouts from the study.

Comparing Means between Two Groups

- ✔ **Applies to:** Unpaired Student t test, Mann-Whitney U test, or Wilcoxon Sum-of-Ranks test (see Chapter 12).

- ✔ **Effect size (E):** The difference between the means of two groups divided by the standard deviation (SD) of the values within a group. (See Chapter 8 for details on means and SD.)

- ✔ **Rule:** You need $16/E^2$ subjects in each group, or $32/E^2$ subjects altogether.

For example, if you're comparing a blood pressure (BP) drug to a placebo, an improvement of 10 millimeters of mercury (mmHg) is important, and the SD of the BP changes is known to be 20 mmHg, then $E = 10/20$, or 0.5, and you need $16/(0.5)^2$, or 64 subjects in each group (128 subjects altogether).

Comparing Means among Three, Four, or Five Groups

- ✔ **Applies to:** One-way Analysis of Variance (ANOVA) or Kruskal-Wallis test (see Chapter 12).

- ✔ **Effect size (E):** The difference between the largest and smallest means among the groups divided by the within-group SD.

- ✔ **Rule:** You need $20/E^2$ subjects in each group.

Continuing the example from the preceding section, if you're comparing two BP drugs and a placebo (for a total of three groups), and if any difference of 10 mmHg between any pair of drugs is important, then E is still $10/20$, or 0.5, but you now need $20/(0.5)^2$, or 80 subjects in each group (240 subjects altogether).

Comparing Paired Values

- ✔ **Applies to:** Paired Student t test or Wilcoxon Signed-Ranks test.

- ✔ **Effect size (E):** The average of the paired differences divided by the SD of the paired differences.

- ✔ **Rule:** You need $8/E^2$ subjects (pairs of values).

So, if you're studying test scores before and after tutoring, a six-point improvement is important, and the SD of the changes is ten points, then $E = 6/10$, or 0.6, and you need $8/(0.6)^2$, or about 22 students, each of whom provides a "before" score and an "after" score.

Comparing Proportions between Two Groups

- ✔ **Applies to:** Chi-square test of association or Fisher Exact test (see Chapter 13).
- ✔ **Effect size (*D*):** The difference between the two proportions, P_1 and P_2, that you're comparing. You also have to calculate the average of the two proportions: $P = (P_1 + P_2)/2$.
- ✔ **Rule:** You need $16 \times P \times (1 - P)/D^2$ subjects in each group.

For example, if a disease has a 60 percent mortality rate but you think your drug can cut this rate in half (to 30 percent), then $P = (0.6 + 0.3)/2$, or 0.45, and $D = 0.6 - 0.3$, or 0.3. You need $16 \times 0.45 \times (1 - 0.45)/(0.3)^2$, or 44 subjects in each group (88 subjects altogether).

Testing for a Significant Correlation

- ✔ **Applies to:** Pearson correlation test (see Chapter 17) and is also a good approximation for the nonparametric Spearman correlation test.
- ✔ **Effect size:** The correlation coefficient (*r*) you want to be able to detect.
- ✔ **Rule:** You need $8/r^2$ subjects (pairs of values).

So, if you're studying the association between weight and blood pressure, and you want the correlation test to come out significant if these two variables have a true correlation coefficient of at least 0.2, then you need to study $8/(0.2)^2$, or 200 subjects.

Comparing Survival between Two Groups

- ✔ **Applies to:** Log-rank test or Cox proportional-hazard regression (see Chapter 23).
- ✔ **Effect size:** The hazard ratio (*HR*) you want to be able to detect.
- ✔ **Rule:** The required *total* number of observed deaths (or events) = $32/(\text{natural log of } HR)^2$.

Here's how the formula works out for several values of *HR:*

Hazard Ratio	Total Number of Events
1.1	3,523
1.2	963
1.3	465
1.4	283
1.5	195
1.75	102
2.0	67
2.5	38
3.0	27

Your enrollment must be large enough, and your follow-up must be long enough, to ensure that you get the required number of events. The required enrollment may be difficult to estimate beforehand, because it involves recruitment rates, censoring rates, the shape of the survival curve, and other things that are difficult to foresee and difficult to handle mathematically. So some protocols provide only a tentative estimate of the expected enrollment (for planning and budgeting purposes), and state that enrollment and/or follow-up will continue until the required number of events has been observed.

Scaling from 80 Percent to Some Other Power

Here's how you take a sample-size estimate that provides 80 percent power (from one of the preceding rules) and scale it up or down to provide some other power:

- ✔ **For 50 percent power:** Use only half as many subjects (multiply by 0.5).

- ✔ **For 90 percent power:** Increase the sample size by 33 percent (multiply by 1.33).

- ✔ **For 95 percent power:** Increase the sample size by 66 percent (multiply by 1.66).

For example, if you know (from some power calculation) that a study with 70 subjects provides 80 percent power to test its primary objective, then a study that has 1.33×70, or 93 subjects, will have about 90 percent power to test that objective.

Scaling from 0.05 to Some Other Alpha Level

Here's how you take a sample-size estimate that was based on testing at the 0.05 alpha level and scale it up or down to correspond to testing at some other alpha level:

- **For 0.10 alpha:** Decrease the sample size by 20 percent (multiply by 0.8).
- **For 0.025 alpha:** Increase the sample size by 20 percent (multiply by 1.2).
- **For 0.01 alpha:** Increase the sample size by 50 percent (multiply by 1.5).

For example, if you've calculated a sample size of 100 subjects based on using $p < 0.05$ as your criterion for significance, and then your boss says you have to apply a two-fold Bonferroni correction (see Chapter 5) and use $p < 0.025$ as your criterion instead, you need to increase your sample size to 100×1.2, or 120 subjects, to have the same power at the new alpha level.

Making Adjustments for Unequal Group Sizes

When comparing means or proportions between two groups, it's usually most efficient (that is, you get the best power for a given total sample size) if both groups are the same size. If you want to have unbalanced groups, you need more subjects overall in order to preserve the statistical power of the study. Here's how to adjust the size of the two groups to keep the same statistical power:

- **If you want one group twice as large as the other:** Increase one group by 50 percent and reduce the other group by 25 percent. This increases the total sample size by about 13 percent.

- **If you want one group three times as large as the other:** Reduce one group by a third and double the other group. This increases the total sample size by about 33 percent.

- **If you want one group four times as large as the other:** Reduce one group by 38 percent and increase the other group by a factor of 2.5. This increases the total sample size by about 56 percent.

Suppose, for example, you're comparing two equal-size groups (drug and placebo), and you've calculated that you need 64 subjects (two groups of 32). But then you decide you want to randomize drug and placebo subjects in a 2:1 ratio. To keep the same power, you'll need 32×1.5, or 48 drug subjects, (an increase of 50 percent) and 32×0.75, or 24 placebo subjects (a decrease of 25 percent), for a total of 72 subjects altogether.

Allowing for Attrition

Most sample-size calculations (including the quick formulas shown in this chapter) tell you how many *analyzable* subjects you need. But you have to enroll more than that number because some subjects will drop out of the study or be unanalyzable for other reasons. Here's how to scale up the number of analyzable subjects (from a power calculation) to get the number of subjects you need to *enroll:*

$$\text{Enrollment} = \text{Number Analyzable} \times 100/(100 - \%\text{Attrition})$$

Here are the enrollment scale-ups for several attrition rates:

Expected Attrition	Increase the Enrollment by
5%	5%
10%	11%
15%	18%
20%	25%
25%	33%
33%	50%
50%	100%

So, if a power calculation indicates that you need a total of 60 analyzable subjects and you expect a 25 percent attrition rate, you need to enroll 60×1.33, or 80 subjects. That way, you'll still have 60 subjects left after a quarter of the original 80 subjects have dropped out.

Index

good doses, defined, 84
goodness-of-fit indicators, 247–248, 351–352
G*Power software, 57
GraphPad InStat software, 54
GraphPad Prism software, 53–54
graphs and charts. *See also* scatter plots;
   tables
  bar charts, 105, 118–119
  box-and-whiskers charts, 119–120
  of categorical data, 105
  hazard rates and survival probabilities, 324
  histograms, 35, 116–118
  logistic regression data, 269–270
  nomograms (alignment charts), 59–60,
     170–171, 208
  of numerical data, 115–120
  pie charts, 105
  of probability distributions, 37
  Receiver Operator Characteristics,
     283–285
  of relationships between numerical
     variables, 120
  residuals versus fitted, 242–243, 249
  S-shaped function for logistic regression,
     270–273
  3D charts, avoiding, 105

• H •

H_0 (null hypothesis), 41, 43–45
$H_{1 \text{ or }} H_{Alt}$ (alternate hypothesis), 41
hazard rate
  defined, 316
  estimating censored data, 318–328
  graphing from a life table, 324
  interpreting life-table output, 323
hazard ratios, 345, 350–351
hierarchical testing strategy, 75
hierarchy rules for formulas, 25–26
histograms, 35, 116–118
historical control, comparing results to, 156
Hood, Greg (ecologist), 56
Hosmer-Lemeshow (H-L) test, 277
human error, 124
hypotheses, identifying, 62
hypothesis testing, 41–43

• I •

icons in this book, explained, 5–6
identification (ID) numbers, recording,
     95–96
imprecision. *See* precision
imputing values, 74, 317
in silico studies, 79
in vitro studies, 79
in vivo studies, 79
inaccuracy. *See* accuracy
incidence, 204
incidence rate (R), 204–207
inclusion criteria, 64, 126, 128
index of an array, 27
Informed Consent Form (ICF), 71–72
inner mean, 109
Institutional Review Boards (IRBs), 71, 72, 76
intent-to-treat (ITT) population, 67
inter- and intra-rater reliability, 201–202
intercept, 231, 244
interim analyses, 76
inter-quartile range (IQR), 112
interval data, 94, 100–101, 314
interval of uncertainty (IOU), 145

• K •

Kaplan-Meier (K-M) method, 324–328
kappa (κ)
  for Cohen's Kappa, 202
  for Pearson kurtosis index, 114
Kendall test, 185–187
Krukal-Wallis test, 158
kurtosis, 113–114

• L •

Last Observation Carried Forward
     (LOCF), 74
LazStats software, 55
least-squares regression, 291–292. *See also*
     nonlinear regression
leptokurtic distribution, 114
lethal doses on logistic curve, 280